WQ 175 SYM

THE S

WITHDRAWN

Maternal-Fetal Nutrition during Pregnancy and Lactation

Maternal-Fetal Nutrition during Pregnancy and Lactation

Editors

Michael E. Symonds and Margaret M. Ramsay
University of Nottingham and Nottingham University Hospitals, Nottingham, UK

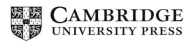

CAMBRIDGE UNIVERSITY PRESS
Cambridge, New York, Melbourne, Madrid, Cape Town,
Singapore, São Paulo, Delhi

Cambridge University Press
The Edinburgh Building, Cambridge CB2 8RU, UK

Published in the United States of America by
Cambridge University Press, New York

www.cambridge.org
Information on this title: www.cambridge.org/9780521887090

First published 2010

Printed in the United Kingdom at the University Press, Cambridge

*A catalog record for this publication is available from the
British Library*

Library of Congress Cataloging in Publication data
Maternal-fetal nutrition during pregnancy and lactation / editors, Michael
E. Symonds and Margaret M. Ramsay.
    p.   ;   cm.
Includes bibliographical references and index.
ISBN 978-0-521-88709-0 (hardback)
1. Pregnancy – Nutritional aspects.   I. Symonds, Michael E., 1960–
II. Ramsay, M. M., M.D.   III. Title.
[DNLM: 1. Maternal Nutritional Physiological Phenomena.   2. Child
Development.   3. Fetal Development.   4. Infant Nutritional Physiological
Phenomena.   5. Infant.   6. Nutritional Requirements.   7. Pregnancy.
WQ 175 M4225 2010]
RG559.M365   2010
618.2′42 – dc22   2009043217

ISBN 978-0-521-88709-0 hardback

Additional resources for this publication at
www.cambridge.org/9780521887090

Contents

Contributors

Annie S. Anderson BSc PhD
Centre for Public Health Nutrition Research, Department of Medicine, University of Dundee, Ninewells Hospital and Medical School, Dundee, UK

James Barry MD
Perinatal Research Center, Department of Pediatrics, University of Colorado Denver, Aurora, Colorado, USA

Eve Blair PhD
Centre for Child Health Research, University of Western Australia, West Perth, WA, Australia

Laura Brown MD
Perinatal Research Center, Department of Pediatrics, University of Colorado Denver, Aurora, Colorado, USA

Sirinuch Chomtho MD PhD
Childhood Nutrition Research Centre, University College London Institute of Child Health, London, UK

Rana Conway PhD BSc RPHNutr
Freelance Public Health Nutritionist, London, UK

Adrienne Cullum BSc PhD RPHNutr
Centre for Public Health Excellence, National Institute for Health and Clinical Excellence, London, UK

Alan T. Davis PhD
Department of Surgery, Michigan State University, and GRMERC Department of Research, Grand Rapids, Michigan, USA

Mary Fewtrell MD MA FRCPCH
Childhood Nutrition Research Centre, University College London Institute of Child Health, London, UK

Lorraine Gambling BSc PhD
Rowett Institute of Nutrition and Health, University of Aberdeen, Aberdeen, UK

Y. Ingrid Goh HBSc PhD
Division of Clinical Pharmacology and Toxicology, The Hospital for Sick Children, Toronto, Ontario, Canada

William W. Hay Jr. MD
Perinatal Research Center, Department of Pediatrics, University of Colorado Denver, Aurora, Colorado, USA

William C. Heird MD
Children's Nutrition Research Center, Baylor College of Medicine, Houston, Texas, USA

Louise Kenny PhD MRCOG
Anu Research Centre, Department of Obstetrics and Gynaecology, Cork University Maternity Hospital, University College Cork, Wilton, Cork, Ireland

Christopher H. Knight PhD
University of Copenhagen Faculty of Life Sciences, Frederiksberg, Denmark

Wing Yee Kwong
School of Biosciences, University of Nottingham, Sutton Bonington, Leicestershire, UK

Barbara Luke ScD MPH
Department of Obstetrics, Gynecology, and Reproductive Biology, and Department of Epidemiology, Michigan State University, East Lansing, Michigan, USA

Harry J. McArdle BSc PhD
Rowett Institute of Nutrition and Health, University of Aberdeen, Aberdeen, UK

Fergus McCarthy MRCPI
Anu Research Centre, Department of Obstetrics and Gynaecology, Cork University Maternity Hospital, University College Cork, Wilton, Cork, Ireland

Karin B. Michels ScD PhD
Obstetrics and Gynecology Epidemiology Center, Department of Obstetrics, Gynecology and Reproductive Biology, Brigham and Women's Hospital, Harvard Medical School; and Department of Epidemiology, Harvard School of Public Health; Boston, MA, USA

Ian M. Morison MBChB PhD FRCPA
Department of Pathology, Dunedin School of Medicine, University of Otago, Dunedin, New Zealand

Leslie Myatt PhD
University of Texas Health Science Center, San Antonio, Texas, USA

James D. Paauw MD PhD
Spectrum Health Metabolic Nutrition Support Service and Department of Surgery, Michigan State University, Grand Rapids, Michigan, USA

Theresa Powell PhD
Department of Obstetrics and Gynecology, University of Cincinnati College of Medicine, Cincinnati, Ohio, USA

Shobha Rao, PhD
Biometry and Nutrition Unit, Agharkar Research Institute, Pune, India

Tim Regnault PhD
Departments of Physiology and Pharmacology and Obstetrics and Gynaecology, University of Western Ontario, London, Ontario, Canada

Wolf Reik MD FMedSci
Babraham Institute, Babraham, Cambridge; Professor of Epigenetics, Centre for Trophoblast Research, Department of Physiology, Development & Neuroscience, University of Cambridge, Cambridge, UK

Jacques Rigo MD PhD
Pediatrics and Neonatal Department, University of Liège, CHR Citadelle, Liège, Belgium

Paul Rozance MD
Perinatal Research Center, Department of Pediatrics, University of Colorado Denver, Aurora, Colorado, USA

Thibault Senterre MD
Pediatrics and Neonatal Department, University of Liège, CHR Citadelle, Liège, Belgium

Kevin D. Sinclair PhD
School of Biosciences, University of Nottingham, Sutton Bonington, Leicestershire, UK

Alison C. Tse SM
Department of Epidemiology, Harvard School of Public Health, Boston, MA, USA

Wendy L. Wrieden PhD
Public Health Nutrition Research Group, Section of Population Health, Institute of Applied Health Science, University of Aberdeen, Aberdeen, UK

Chittaranjan Yajnik MD FRCP
Diabetes Unit, King Edward Memorial Hospital Research Center, King Edward Memorial Hospital, Pune, India

Maternal adaptations to pregnancy and the role of the placenta

Leslie Myatt and Theresa Powell

Delivery of an optimally grown, viable infant defines a successful pregnancy. Optimal growth is achieved by the interaction of maternal, placental, and fetal systems to deliver maternal nutrients to the placenta, transfer them to the fetus, and maximize their utilization for fetal growth. Pregnancy is characterized by profound changes in the maternal immune, metabolic, cardiovascular, and renal systems to ensure a successful pregnancy and adequate fetal growth. The fetal-placental unit secretes many hormonal signals, the roles of which include redirecting maternal physiology and metabolism to direct substrate toward the fetus and support normal fetal growth. The physiological adaptations of pregnancy begin shortly after conception, indeed before the establishment of a fetal-placental unit, and thus in their early phases must be directed by maternal signals, including those from the corpus luteum. Subsequently feto-placental signals play a major role in regulation of maternal metabolism. This chapter describes the maternal adaptation to pregnancy and the role of the placenta in nutrient transfer to the fetus.

Adaptive changes in maternal physiology

Cardiovascular system

The changes in the cardiovascular system seen in pregnancy are by far the largest physiological challenge this system will face throughout the life cycle and include anatomical changes, increased blood volume and cardiac output, and a decrease in systemic vascular resistance. Ventricular wall muscle mass increases in the first trimester [1], followed by an increase in end-diastolic volume in the second and early third trimesters to increase cardiac compliance. Collagen softening is seen, resulting in increased compliance of capacitive and conductive vessels; this change occurs

within 5 weeks of conception [2]. Blood volume increases from 6 to 8 weeks gestation onward by 45% to reach approximately 5 l at 32 weeks gestation [3]. This increase is greater with multifetal gestation and correlates with fetal weight. The mechanism is unknown but occurs in the absence of a fetus and may be related to the renin-angiotensin system or relaxin. Red blood cell mass also increases by 20% to 30% in pregnancy, reflecting increased production of red blood cells, but the net result is physiological hemodilution, potentially a protective effect because it reduces blood viscosity to counter the predisposition for thromboembolic events in pregnancy [4] and may also be beneficial for placental perfusion.

Cardiac output (heart rate × stroke volume) increases by 30% to 50% in pregnancy [5] because of increases in both stroke volume and heart rate. The early increase is due to the rise in stroke volume [5], reflecting the increase in ventricular mass and end-diastolic volume. Stroke volume declines toward term, but heart rate increases from 5 to 32 weeks gestation by 15 to 20 beats per min and is maintained thereafter to maintain cardiac output. Blood flow to the uterus increases 10-fold (from 2% to 17% of cardiac output) in gestation, reaching 500 to 800 ml/min at term. Arterial blood pressure and systemic vascular resistance decrease from as early as 5 weeks gestation and reach a nadir in the second trimester, after which blood pressure increases again. This is thought to be hormonally regulated, perhaps by progesterone, the endothelial-derived vasodilator nitric oxide, or prostaglandins, but also potentially by the introduction of the low-resistance uteroplacental circulation [6]. The decrease in systemic vascular resistance may be the stimulus to increase heart rate, stroke volume, and cardiac output in early gestation. Maternal tidal volume increases by 40% in pregnancy, resulting in hyperventilation and a decrease in partial pressure of carbon dioxide in blood.

Renal system

Renal size, weight, and volume increase in gestation because of increases in renal vascular and interstitial volume [7] together with a marked increase in dilation of the collecting system. Renal blood flow increases 60% to 80% by mid-gestation and is 50% greater at term [8]. Glomerular filtration rate increases up to 50% at the end of the first trimester, with a modest increase in creatinine clearance. These changes are initiated in the luteal phase of the menstrual cycle [9]. In the rat, there is strong evidence that the ovarian hormone relaxin is responsible for renal hemodynamic and osmoregulatory changes in pregnancy [10]. Similarly, in humans, relaxin appears to play a role in establishing the renal response [11]. However in the absence of relaxin, as in patients with ovum donation and no corpus luteum, a renal response, although subdued, is still seen, suggesting that some other mechanism may also operate. In the luteal phase of the cycle, luteinizing hormone stimulates relaxin secretion from the corpus luteum, and this response is augmented and maintained by human chorionic gonadotropin (hCG) after conception.

The endocrinology of pregnancy

The concept of the feto-placental unit originated in the 1950s but it is now recognized that the placenta and in particular the syncytiotrophoblast is a powerful endocrine organ that synthesizes many steroid and peptide hormones whose role is to ensure fetal survival and growth by directing maternal metabolism and fetal growth and development. Human chorionic gonadotropin (hCG) is the earliest biochemical marker of pregnancy produced by the embryo (7–8 days after fertilization) and with a doubling time of 31 hours after implantation [12]. The major biological role of hCG in early pregnancy is to rescue the corpus luteum from demise and maintain progesterone (and presumably relaxin) production until the luteal-placental shift in progesterone production at 9 weeks gestation. Following this time, the placenta is the major source of progesterone synthesis from maternal cholesterol, reaching 250 mg/day at term from 25 mg/day in the luteal phase. The major roles of progesterone in pregnancy may be in dampening immune responses and maintaining smooth muscle quiescence. Indeed, in animal species, high circulating progesterone is associated with myometrial quiescence and delayed onset of labor [13]. Similarly progesterone

may have major nongenomic relaxatory effects on the vasculature [14].

The placenta is also the major site for estrogen synthesis. The predominant estrogen in pregnancy is estriol, formed as a result of interaction of fetal and placental tissues through which fetal adrenal dehydroepiandrosterone sulfate (DHEAS) is converted to estrogens by placental sulfatase and aromatase. Placental estrogen production increases throughout gestation. Estrogen has been shown to have a powerful effect in increasing uterine blood flow and may therefore facilitate fetal nutrition by increasing placental oxygenation and nutrient delivery. It also prepares the breast for lactation, affects the renin-angiotensin system, and stimulates production of hormone-binding globulins in the liver.

Maternal metabolic changes in gestation

During pregnancy, an adaptation of maternal metabolism functions to ensure normal fetal growth throughout gestation and neonatal growth during lactation. Thus, there is a period of adipose tissue accretion in early gestation followed by insulin resistance to increase glucose availability for the fetus and lipolysis to increase fatty acid availability. The maternal metabolic reprogramming is believed to be directed by placental hormones. Insulin secretion increases during early pregnancy and more than doubles, resulting in a 30% higher mean insulin level by the third trimester. Skeletal muscle, which is the major site of glucose disposal, and adipose tissue both become highly insulin resistant during the second half of pregnancy. There is a 50% reduction in insulin-mediated glucose disposal, requiring an increase in insulin secretion to maintain euglycemia [16]. Failure of the mother to increase insulin will lead to maternal hyperglycemia and thus fetal hyperglycemia with consequent fetal hyperinsulinemia, macrosomia, and fetal hypoxia. Insulin also loses its ability to suppress whole-body lipolysis, leading to increased postprandial free fatty acid levels and a decline in maternal adipose tissue [17]. Total plasma lipids, triglycerides, free fatty acids, and cholesterol increase after 24 weeks gestation [18] with increases in pre-B lipoprotein, high-density lipoprotein (HDL) cholesterol in early pregnancy, and low-density lipoprotein (LDL) cholesterol in late pregnancy. The action of insulin is mediated through insulin receptors that are regulated by phosphorylation. The degree of glucose uptake and insulin resistance is also regulated by the level of insulin receptor substrate-1 (IRS-1) protein and levels of the p85α subunit of phosphoinositide 3-kinase, which docks to IRS-1 (reviewed by Barbour et al. [19]).

Early pregnancy as a determinant of placental and fetal growth

Maternal nutrition around the time of conception may have important effects on gestational length, fetal growth trajectory, and postnatal growth and health (for review, see Cross and Mickelson [20]. Specific nutrients and general nutritional status of the mother may play key roles in altering the development of the placenta, effects that have direct consequences on the fetus [21]. Blastocyst development and subsequent implantation potential are reduced in diabetic mothers and when culturing embryos in high D-glucose [22]. Both essential and nonessential amino acids affect mouse blastocyst development during in vitro culture by enhancing postimplantation development and increasing implantation potential [23]. The mammalian target of rapamycin (mTOR) signaling pathway mediates the effects of amino acids in stimulating blastocyst growth and invasion. Adequacy of amino acids is detected by the mTOR system, and invasive capacity is upregulated if nutrients are available. Insufficient nutrients result in a lack of invasiveness, and the implantation window may be lost [24]. Ghrelin, a hormone known to stimulate appetite, may also affect early development. Treatment with ghrelin reduces the number of inner cell mass and trophectoderm cells in blastocysts, similar to the effect of a low protein diet [25].

Once implantation is successful and the pregnancy is established, there is little variation in the size of the human fetus up to 16 weeks gestation, and the early conceptus has low absolute energetic and anabolic needs. Excluding chromosomal and genetic disorders, the dominant determinant of variation in fetal size is supply of nutrients and oxygen. Early fetal nutrition may be provided by endometrial glands that remain functional until at least 10 weeks gestation. These glands have intact pathways to the intervillous space and secrete carbohydrates and lipids as well as growth factors, which provide a source of histotrophic nutrients and direct the differentiation of the developing villous tissue (for review, see Burton et al. [26]).

The effect of maternal nutrient availability

In light of the low total nutrient requirements in early pregnancy, data are rapidly accumulating implicating early gestation as a pivotal period for determining placental and fetal growth trajectories. Maternal nutrient availability and metabolic status may not be fully equivalent as determinants of fetal growth, as is apparent in the analysis of exposure to food shortage during different periods of gestation for individuals born around the time of the Dutch famine. In pregnancies affected by famine primarily during early gestation, offspring were of normal size at birth and showed increased risk for cardiovascular disease later in life [27]. The early pregnancy effect may be related to insufficient fat deposition in the mother during this critical period of pregnancy [28]. Likewise, hyperemesis in the first half of pregnancy, which could be considered a form of maternal undernutrition in early pregnancy, generally results in only small reductions in birth weight [29]. In pregnancies in which the Dutch famine was experienced later in pregnancy, growth restriction as well as increased risk for metabolic diseases in adulthood resulted [30].

In animal models in which nutrient restriction can be manipulated to distinct periods of gestation, differential long-term effects on the offspring have been documented. In pregnant sheep, early maternal nutrient restriction appears to have effects primarily on the brain (smaller brain and impaired cognitive function), whereas maternal nutrient restriction later in pregnancy results in small fetuses that have an increased risk of developing glucose intolerance, insulin resistance, and increased fat mass (for review, see Symonds et al. [31]). These data suggest that nutrient availability alone is not the primary factor regulating fetal and placental growth rates or birth weight. In fact, several observational studies suggest that only in quite severe maternal malnutrition is birth size affected. The balance of macronutrients in the diet of pregnant women has been suggested to play a role in determining birth weight, with dietary protein in early pregnancy likely to be an important factor [32]. The metabolic status of the mother – that is, insulin sensitivity, glycemic control, and inflammatory status during the early pregnancy window – may have profound effects on the fetus in utero and later in life. The relationship between maternal nutritional availability and the mother's ability to maintain a healthy metabolic environment for her fetus may depend on her nutritional status before pregnancy [33] or her ability to mobilize stores during pregnancy. The interaction between maternal nutrition and metabolic status in pregnancy requires additional study.

Mechanisms linking maternal nutrition and fetal growth

The genetic contribution to fetal size at birth is primarily of maternal origin and may relate to maternal size – in particular, maternal height. Although overall genetic contributions to birth weight are low, the non-genetic maternal environmental and phenotypic influences are more important. Generally speaking, maternal nutrition may contribute to fetal growth regulation through several mechanisms.

Insulin-like growth factor 1 (IGF-1) is the primary fetal growth–stimulating factor in response to altered nutrient supply during late gestation and is under the control of fetal insulin [34]. Maternal undernutrition is associated with reduced fetal IGF-1 levels and reduced fetal growth [35].

Repeat exposure to maternal glucocorticoid leads to growth restriction. The fetus is normally protected by the action of the placental enzyme 11-βHSD. This enzyme is downregulated in periods of maternal undernutrition, which exposes the fetus to maternal glucocorticoids [36].

Maternal glycemic control in early pregnancy has been shown in both animal models and humans to be a major factor in predicting fetal growth. In humans, first-trimester maternal glycosylated hemoglobin ($Hb1_{AC}$) is the best predictor of macrosomia in pregnancies complicated by Type I diabetes [37], suggesting that growth trajectories are established early in pregnancy and are responsive to maternal metabolic signaling. Similarly, in pregnant rats, episodic hyperglycemia in early but not late pregnancy resulted in placental and fetal overgrowth [38].

Insulin and leptin are maternal metabolic indicators that may be involved in fetal intrauterine growth adaptation and long-term health. Decreases in leptin and insulin during periods of maternal nutrient restriction or high levels of these hormones in pregnant obese women may provide a signaling pathway for altering fetal growth in utero [39]. Both of these hormones have been shown to regulate placental nutrient transport functions, providing a direct link between maternal nutritional status and nutrient delivery to the fetus.

Nutritionally mediated alterations in epigenetic regulation during gestation may lead to alterations in placental function. Changes in maternal nutrition can affect the degree of DNA methylation – for example, through altered availability of methyl donors (folate) in the diet. This provides an inheritable alteration in gene expression without a change in the DNA sequence and may be important in modifying fetal and placental growth in utero and in developmental origins of adult disease [40].

Maternal nutrition also affects both placental and fetal vascular development. In pregnant rats, global undernutrition of the dam leads to intrauterine growth restriction (IUGR) and whereas the placental villous surface area increases to compensate for insufficient nutrient delivery from the mother, the extent of fetal vasculature does not [41]. In experimental iron restriction in rodents, the villous surface area is also increased, but fetal vasculature is not [42]. In sheep models of nutrition in pregnancy, both increased and decreased overall caloric intake leads to IUGR and fewer, smaller, less vascularized cotyledons [43]. The developmental signaling systems that lead to changes in placental vascular and fetal growth are not yet clearly defined and are likely to be different for early and late gestation. The interaction between developmental signaling systems and nutrient availability is an area that requires investigative attention to define more accurately the exact nature of maternal nutrient requirements in early pregnancy.

The role of the placenta in regulation of maternal metabolism and fetal growth

Secretion of human chorionic somatomammotropin and growth hormone

Human chorionic somatomammotropin (hCS; also called human placental lactogen, hPL) has structural and biological similarities to human growth hormone (hGH) and prolactin. hCS is produced only by syncytiotrophoblast, but production increases 30-fold in gestation, reaching 1 to 4 g/day at term. However the role of hCS is still not fully elucidated. It is suggested to control maternal metabolism, resulting in reductions

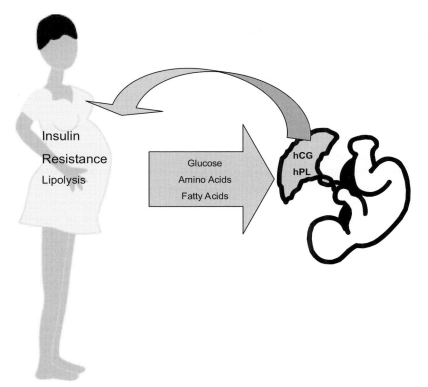

Figure 1.1 Schematic representation of maternal adaptation to pregnancy.

in fasting maternal glucose, increased maternal plasma free fatty acids, increased insulin secretion from the pancreas, but insulin resistance and reduced maternal glucose uptake to facilitate transfer to the fetus. Despite its structural similarity, hCS has little growth-promoting and lactogenic activity in humans, and normal pregnancies occur in the near absence of hCS, suggesting that hCS is not essential for pregnancy but serves a redundant function for hGH and prolactin.

Placental GH occurs in nonglycosylated and glycosylated forms and increases six- to eightfold in maternal plasma in the second trimester, replacing normal pituitary GH in the maternal circulation. In transgenic mice, overexpression of hPGH causes severe peripheral insulin resistance [44]. Placental GH may also stimulate IGF-1 production in maternal liver. Insulin resistance in pregnancy is associated with maternal islet cell hyperplasia and may be affected by hCS and placenta GH, which reduce insulin receptor number and glucose transport in insulin-sensitive tissues. In Figure 1.1, the interaction among placental hormone release, maternal metabolic state, and placental function is illustrated.

Role of adipokines

The term *adipokines* includes leptin, adiponectin, tumor necrosis factor–alpha (TNFα), interleukin-6 (IL-6), resistin, and other mediators. These are produced by many cell types including the placenta, making difficult the dissection of the roles of maternal versus placental synthesis and paracrine versus endocrine action.

TNFα, in addition to monocytes, macrophages, and adipocytes, is produced by the placenta. In obese individuals, there is a positive correlation between TNFα levels, hyperinsulinemia, and body mass index (BMI) [45]. TNFα increases insulin resistance when added to human skeletal muscle cells in culture [46]. This may be due to increased phosphorylation of IRS-1 [45] and reduced insulin receptor tyrosine kinase activity [47].

Adiponectin is synthesized only in adipocytes and possibly placenta. Adiponectin expression and secretion from white adipose tissue decrease with advancing gestation [48] and correlate with whole-body insulin sensitivity. Adiponectin acts as an endogenous insulin-sensitizing hormone through receptors on skeletal muscle, where it stimulates glucose uptake, and liver, where it reduces uptake via adenosine monophosphate-activated protein kinase alpha (AMPK α).

Leptin, the product of the *LEP* gene, was originally described in the adipocyte and thought to modulate satiety and energy homeostasis. It is now known to be synthesized in other tissues including the placenta and to assume other roles. Serum leptin concentrations increase throughout human gestation, beginning to rise in the first trimester and correlating with hCG levels. Therefore, leptin alterations are seen before changes in body weight, suggesting another mechanism of regulation [49]. However, serum leptin levels correlate to maternal adiposity rather than placenta mass. Both leptin and leptin receptors are found in syncytiotrophoblast and will stimulate hCG secretion [50].

Placental growth factors

The placenta is also a major source of growth factors and their binding proteins that affect placental and fetal growth and development. Of these IGF-1 and -2 are the most important mediators of fetal growth. The *Igf1* and *Igf2* genes are expressed in many fetal and placental tissues where the proteins have metabolic, mitogenic, and differentiative actions and may act as local growth regulators [51]. In addition, the IGFs appear to have a role in trophoblast invasion [52]. Umbilical levels of IGFs are correlated to birth weight in many species, including humans [53], with IGF-2 concentrations being up to 10-fold higher than IGF-1. Placental IGF-2 mRNA was also positively correlated with placental weight in a group of normal and diabetic pregnancies [54]. *Igf2* is an imprinted gene expressed from the paternal allele in the placenta [55] and is expressed in syncytiotrophoblast and invasive trophoblast [56]. Deletion of either *Igf1* or *Igf2* genes results in fetal growth restriction, but deletion of the IGF type 1 receptor gene results in a more severe growth restriction, suggesting that both IGFs act through the type 1 receptor. Conversely, fetal growth is enhanced by overexpression of IGF-2 or deletion of the IGF type 2 clearance receptor [57]. In the mouse, manipulation of the *Igf2* gene reduces placental growth by 30% to 40%, involving all cell types in *Igf2*-null mice [58] or just the labyrinthine trophoblast in a placenta-specific knockdown of the *Igf2* gene [59],

whereas overexpression of IGF-2 increases placental growth. In cultured human trophoblast, both IGF-1 and -2 alter glucose and amino acid transport, and in sheep, IGF-1 administration alters feto-placental protein and carbohydrate transfer and metabolism [60]. Placental System A transporter activity is increased in the placental-specific *Igf2* mutant mouse, perhaps as a compensatory mechanism, and passive diffusion is reduced [59]. Thus, the promotional effect of IGF-2 on fetal growth may be an indirect one mediated through the placenta through the IGF type 1 receptor.

The level of nutrients appears to regulate IGF concentrations in the fetus because reducing both nutrients and oxygen lowers IGF-1, although to a greater extent than IGF-2 [61]. Conversely infusion of insulin or glucose increases IGF-1 in the fetus of fasted sheep [34]. Nutritionally sensitive hormones including insulin, thyroxine, and glucocorticoids affect IGF concentrations in the fetus [62], again with deficiency affecting IGF-1 more than IGF-2. Insulin and IGF-1 levels are positively correlated in the fetus and appear to act synergistically to enhance accumulation of glucose and amino acids in the fetus [62]. Glucocorticoids affect both *Igf1* and *Igf2* gene expression in a tissue-specific manner in the fetus [63]. Hence, placental glucocorticoid metabolism may affect fetal growth in a gestational specific manner.

IGF bioavailability is regulated by expression of the IGF binding proteins (IGFBP), of which there are at least six functionally redundant isoforms, with IGFBP-1 through -4 being found in humans. Changes in IGFBP expression modulate IGF levels and thus fetal growth and are sensitive to nutritional and endocrine regulation [61]. The placenta also expresses all the IGFBPs, with IGFBP-1 being predominant. They show differential localization, with IGFBP-3 being found on the microvillous and basal trophoblast membranes and IGFBP-1 predominantly found on the fetal-facing basal surface [64].

Nutrient partitioning across the placenta

Although it is well accepted that maternal nutritional status, diet, and body size are closely correlated with birth weight, fetal nutrition is clearly not equivalent to maternal nutrition because the intervening placental syncytiotrophoblast (ST) constitutes a distinct barrier between the two circulations. The ST is a syncytial, polarized, epithelial cell layer separating the maternal blood in the intervillous space from the fetal capillary. The ST forms by fusion of underlying cytotrophoblast cells and is composed of an apical plasma membrane or microvillous membrane (MVM) facing the maternal blood and a basal plasma membrane (BM) toward the fetal capillary. The syncytial cell layer thins in the terminal villous region, and the total transporting distance at term is 10 microns. This short transport distance between the two blood supplies allows for rapid transfer of small hydrophobic molecules and blood gases. Larger hydrophilic molecules require specialized transporting systems in the epithelial membranes to provide adequate support for fetal growth.

Fetal blood sampling and the use of stable isotopes in human pregnancy have allowed for description of maternal and fetal nutrient concentrations [65]. These recent advances have established that glucose concentrations are lower in fetuses and change in parallel to maternal levels. Amino acids are significantly higher in fetal plasma than their mothers' plasma, with glutamate being the only exception. Fatty acids on the whole are much lower in fetal than in maternal circulation. A preferential transfer of essential long-chain polyunsaturated fatty acids (LCPUFA) such as docosahexaenoic acid (DHA) and arachidonic acid across the placenta to the fetus [66] ensures adequate supply for brain and retinal development.

The cellular mechanisms for transport of key nutrients across the human placental ST have been described in detail and recently reviewed [67, 68]. The key features can be summarized as follows.

Glucose is transported across the placenta by facilitated diffusion. Abundant expression of the glucose transport protein isoform 1 (GLUT1) on the MVM allows for rapid uptake into the ST from the maternal circulation. A concentration gradient toward the fetus allows for continuous transport to the fetal circulation and maintains fetal glucose levels that mirror but never exceed those in the maternal compartment.

Active transport allows for fetal accumulation of amino acids in concentrations considerably higher than those found in maternal blood in both mid- and late gestation. The use of the sodium gradient to drive amino acid transport into the ST on the MVM, followed by passive diffusion out of the cell toward the fetus, constitutes one important mechanism for amino acid accumulation in the fetal compartment.

Circulating maternal triglycerides (TG) in very low-density lipoproteins (VLDL), as well as both chylomicrons and TG bound to albumin, are hydrolyzed by lipase enzymes in the MVM of the placental epithelium. This liberates free fatty acids for uptake by the epithelial cell. Preferential binding of LCPUFA by a placental-specific fatty acid binding protein (FABP-pm) allows for specificity of transfer of these crucial cellular components.

Vectorial transport of calcium to the fetus is accomplished by influx of calcium through a variety of channels on the MVM, cytoplasmic binding to calbindin9K and sequestration in the endoplasmic reticulum, and, finally, active transport to the fetus by calcium pumps localized exclusively to the basal plasma membrane of the ST.

Placental nutrient transport capacity and fetal growth

The placental transport capacity for a number of important nutrients has been shown to be correlated to birth weight (for review, see Sibley et al. [69]). Transport capacity for essential amino acids by System L for leucine, System y+L for lysine, and System tau for taurine and nonessential neutral amino acid transport by System A have been shown to be reduced in cases of small for gestational age (SGA) and IUGR. Increased amino acid transport capacity in the placenta of large-for-gestational-age (LGA) babies of diabetic mothers has likewise been reported. In contrast to amino acids, glucose transport capacity appears to be unchanged in the placenta of small babies. There are, however, indications that glucose transport capacity is increased in the placenta of LGA babies of diabetic mothers. Maternal circulating triglycerides are hydrolyzed by lipase enzymes at the microvillous surface of the ST, and several reports indicate alterations in hydrolase enzyme activity and expression in growth-restricted fetuses and LGA fetuses of diabetic mothers. With respect to ion transport, placental calcium pump activity has been shown to be upregulated in both SGA/IUGR and LGA babies. Taken together, these data suggest that specific regulation of placental nutrient transporter activity occurs in association with altered fetal growth, as shown in Table 1.1 (for review, see Jansson and Powell [70]).

Recently, investigations using a nutrient-restricted pregnant rodent model suggested that reductions in placental amino acid transport precede deviations in fetal growth [71]. These data have led to the hypothesis that the human placenta may act as a nutrient sensor to coordinate fetal growth with the ability of the

Table 1.1 Directional changes seen in placental transport capacity in pregnancies complicated by altered fetal growth.

Transporter	IUGR MVM	IUGR BM	Diabetes + LGA MVM	Diabetes + LGA BM
System A	↓	↔	↔	↔
Leucine	↔	↓	↔	↔
Glucose	↔	↔	↔	
Ca 2± ATPase	—		—	
Na±/H± exchanger	↓	—	↔	—
Na± K± ATPase	↓	↔	↔	↔
Lipoprotein lipase	↓	—	↑	—

mother to provide nutrients in individual pregnancies [70]. This would allow for generation of a smaller fetus when nutrient availability was low and takes advantage of periods of nutrient abundance by producing a larger, potentially more viable fetus. Pathologies in fetal growth occur when the maternal supply of nutrients is severely disrupted, as in cases of shallow placental invasion or long-term famine, or when nutrient supply is chronically in excess, as in maternal diabetes and obesity.

Regulation of placental nutrient transport

If the ability of the placenta to transport nutrients is regulated in response to the ability of the mother to supply those nutrients, then it is logical that maternal nutritional signals would be involved in this regulation. IGF-1, insulin, and leptin have been shown to upregulate placental System A amino acid uptake in a variety of experimental systems, suggesting that maternal markers of adequate nutrition stimulate transport of nutrients to the fetus (for review, see Jones et al. [68]). Interestingly, the nature of the regulation of nutrient transport differs in early pregnancy compared with term. The placenta in early pregnancy responds to insulin by increasing glucose uptake, but the term placenta responds to insulin stimulation by increasing amino acid uptake. Other factors that indicate an inability of the maternal blood supply to deliver sufficient nutrients could include oxygen levels, cytokines, and substrates. Although the exact nature of the nutrient-sensing function of the human placenta has not been fully delineated, one intracellular signaling system may in part account for this type of regulation. The mTOR controls cell growth by initiating or inhibiting protein translation in response to amino acid availability – in particular, leucine – through its actions as a phosphatidylinositol kinase–related kinase. mTOR has been localized to the ST, and phosphorylation of downstream mediators of mTOR activity is correlated with fetal size. Inhibition of the mTOR system in placental explant cultures by rapamycin resulted in a reduction in leucine uptake, suggesting a direct link between mTOR and nutrient transport to the fetus [72].

Maternal nutrition and metabolic status in the periconceptual period are critical for successful establishment of pregnancy. The early-gestation placenta secretes a number of critical hormones that alter maternal metabolism and cardiovascular and renal physiology to allow for maintenance of the pregnancy. The developing placenta appears to respond to maternal metabolic status, nutrient levels, and/or placental blood flow to regulate nutrient delivery to the fetus. These events lead to a careful coordination between maternal mobilization of nutrient stores, delivery of those nutrients to the placenta by altering maternal blood flow dynamics, and transport across the placental epithelial barrier to the fetus. The successful integration of these three diverse systems through maternal/placental/fetal endocrine signaling networks defines the ultimate pregnancy outcome – a normally grown, healthy fetus with low risk for adult disease.

References

1. Thompson JA, Hays PM, Sagar KB, and Cruikshank DP, Echocardiographic left ventricular mass to differentiate chronic hypertension from preeclampsia during pregnancy. *Am J Obstet Gynecol* (1986), **155**:994–9.

2. Spaanderman ME, Willekes C, Hoeks AP, Ekhart TH, and Peeters LL, The effect of pregnancy on the compliance of large arteries and veins in healthy parous control subjects and women with a history of preeclampsia. *Am J Obstet Gynecol* (2000), **183**:1278–86.

3. Pritchard JA, Changes in the blood volume during pregnancy and delivery. *Anesthesiology* (1965), **26**:393–9.

4. Koller O, The clinical significance of hemodilution during pregnancy. *Obstet Gynecol Surv* (1982), **37**:649–52.

5. Robson SC, Hunter S, Boys RJ, and Dunlop W, Serial study of factors influencing changes in cardiac output during human pregnancy. *Am J Physiol* (1989), **256**:H1060–5.

6. Greiss FC Jr. and Anderson SG, Effect of ovarian hormones on the uterine vascular bed. *Am J Obstet Gynecol* (1970), **107**:829–36.

7. Christensen T, Klebe JG, Bertelsen V, and Hansen HE, Changes in renal volume during normal pregnancy. *Acta Obstet Gynecol Scand* (1989), **68**:541–3.

8. Dunlop W, Serial changes in renal haemodynamics during normal human pregnancy. *Br J Obstet Gynaecol* (1981), **88**:1–9.

9. Davison JM and Noble MC, Serial changes in 24 hour creatinine clearance during normal menstrual cycles and the first trimester of pregnancy. *Br J Obstet Gynaecol* (1981), **88**:10–17.

10. Danielson LA, Sherwood OD, and Conrad KP, Relaxin is a potent renal vasodilator in conscious rats. *J Clin Invest* (1999), **103**:525–33.

11. Smith MC, Murdoch AP, Danielson LA, Conrad KP, and Davison JM, Relaxin has a role in establishing a renal response in pregnancy. *Fertil Steril* (2006), **86**:253–5.

12. Lenton EA and Woodward AJ, The endocrinology of conception cycles and implantation in women. *J Reprod Fertil Suppl* (1988), **36**:1–15.

13. Zakar T and Hertelendy F, Progesterone withdrawal: key to parturition. *Am J Obstet Gynecol* (2007), **196**:289–96.

14. Van Buren GA, Yang DS, and Clark KE, Estrogen-induced uterine vasodilatation is antagonized by L-nitroarginine methyl ester, an inhibitor of nitric oxide synthesis. *Am J Obstet Gynecol* (1992), **167**:828–33.

15. Hagedorn KA, Cooke CL, Falck JR, Mitchell BF, and Davidge ST, Regulation of vascular tone during pregnancy: a novel role for the pregnane X receptor. *Hypertension* (2007), **49**:328–33.

16. Catalano PM, Tyzbir ED, Wolfe RR, Calles J, Roman NM, Amini SB, and Sims EA, Carbohydrate metabolism during pregnancy in control subjects and women with gestational diabetes. *Am J Physiol* (1993), **264**:E60–7.

17. Homko CJ, Sivan E, Reece EA, and Boden G, Fuel metabolism during pregnancy. *Semin Reprod Endocrinol* (1999), **17**:119–25.

18. Freinkel N, Herrera E, Knopp RH, and Ruder HJ, Metabolic realignments in late pregnancy: a clue to diabetogenesis. *Adv Metab Disord* (1970), **1**(Suppl 1):205+.

19. Barbour LA, McCurdy CE, Hernandez TL, Kirwan JP, Catalano PM, and Friedman JE, Cellular mechanisms for insulin resistance in normal pregnancy and gestational diabetes. *Diabetes Care* (2007), **30**(Suppl 2):S112–9.

20. Cross JC and Mickelson L, Nutritional influences on implantation and placental development. *Nutr Rev* (2006), **64**:S12–8; discussion S72–91.

21. Oliver MH, Jaquiery AL, Bloomfield FH, and Harding JE, The effects of maternal nutrition around the time of conception on the health of the offspring. *Soc Reprod Fertil Suppl* (2007), **64**:397–410.

22. Leunda-Casi A, Genicot G, Donnay I, Pampfer S, and De Hertogh R, Increased cell death in mouse blastocysts exposed to high D-glucose in vitro: implications of an oxidative stress and alterations in glucose metabolism. *Diabetologia* (2002), **45**:571–9.

23. Lane M and Gardner DK, Increase in postimplantation development of cultured mouse embryos by amino acids and induction of fetal retardation and exencephaly by ammonium ions. *J Reprod Fertil* (1994), **102**:305–12.

24. Martin PM and Sutherland AE, Exogenous amino acids regulate trophectoderm differentiation in the mouse blastocyst through an mTOR-dependent pathway. *Dev Biol* (2001), **240**:182–93.

25. Kawamura K, Sato N, Fukuda J, Kodama H, Kumagai J, Tanikawa H, et al., Ghrelin inhibits the development of mouse preimplantation embryos in vitro. *Endocrinology* (2003), **144**:2623–33.

26. Burton GJ, Jauniaux E, and Charnock-Jones DS, Human early placental development: potential roles of the endometrial glands. *Placenta* (2007), **28**(Suppl A):S64–9.

27. Roseboom T, de Rooij S, and Painter R, The Dutch famine and its long-term consequences for adult health. *Early Hum Dev* (2006), **82**:485–91.

28. Herrera E, Lopez-Soldado I, Limones M, Amusquivar E, and

Ramos MP, Lipid metabolism during the perinatal phase, and its implications on postnatal development. *Int J Vitam Nutr Res* (2006), **76**:216–24.

29. Bailit JL, Hyperemesis gravidarium: epidemiologic findings from a large cohort. *Am J Obstet Gynecol* (2005), **193**:811–14.

30. Lumey LH, Stein AD, and Ravelli AC, Timing of prenatal starvation in women and offspring birth weight: an update. *Eur J Obstet Gynecol Reprod Biol* (1995), **63**:197.

31. Symonds ME, Stephenson T, Gardner DS, and Budge H, Long-term effects of nutritional programming of the embryo and fetus: mechanisms and critical windows. *Reprod Fertil Dev* (2007), **19**:53–63.

32. Moore VM, Davies MJ, Willson KJ, Worsley A, and Robinson JS, Dietary composition of pregnant women is related to size of the baby at birth. *J Nutr* (2004), **134**:1820–6.

33. Oliver MH, Hawkins P, and Harding JE, Periconceptional undernutrition alters growth trajectory and metabolic and endocrine responses to fasting in late-gestation fetal sheep. *Pediatr Res* (2005), **57**:591–8.

34. Oliver MH, Harding JE, Breier BH, and Gluckman PD, Fetal insulin-like growth factor (IGF)-I and IGF-II are regulated differently by glucose or insulin in the sheep fetus. *Reprod Fertil Dev* (1996), **8**:167–72.

35. Gallaher BW, Breier BH, Harding JE, and Gluckman PD, Periconceptual undernutrition resets plasma IGFBP levels and alters the response of IGFBP-1, IGFBP-3 and IGF-1 to subsequent maternal undernutrition in fetal sheep. *Prog Growth Factor Res* (1995), **6**:189–95.

36. Stocker CJ, Arch JR, and Cawthorne MA, Fetal origins of insulin resistance and obesity. *Proc Nutr Soc* (2005), **64**:143–51.

37. Rey E, Attie C, and Bonin A, The effects of first-trimester diabetes control on the incidence of macrosomia. *Am J Obstet Gynecol* (1999), **181**:202–6.

38. Ericsson A, Saljo K, Sjostrand E, Jansson N, Prasad PD, Powell TL, and Jansson T, Brief hyperglycaemia in the early pregnant rat increases fetal weight at term by stimulating placental growth and affecting placental nutrient transport. *J Physiol* (2007), **581**:1323–32.

39. Jansson N, Nilsfelt A, Gellerstedt M, Wennergren M, Rossander-Hulthén L, Powell TL, and Jansson T, Maternal hormones linking maternal body mass index and dietary intake to birth weight. *Am J Clin Nutr* (2008), **87**:1743–9.

40. Gluckman PD, Lillycrop KA, Vickers MH, Pleasants AB, Phillips ES, Beedle AS, et al., Metabolic plasticity during mammalian development is directionally dependent on early nutritional status. *Proc Natl Acad Sci U S A* (2007), **104**:12796–800.

41. Doherty CB, Lewis RM, Sharkey A, and Burton GJ, Placental composition and surface area but not vascularization are altered by maternal protein restriction in the rat. *Placenta* (2003), **24**:34–8.

42. Lewis RM, Doherty CB, James LA, Burton GJ, and Hales CN, Effects of maternal iron restriction on placental vascularization in the rat. *Placenta* (2001), **22**:534–9.

43. Reynolds LP, Borowicz PP, Vonnahme KA, Johnson ML, Grazul-Bilska AA, Redmer DA, and Caton JS, Placental angiogenesis in sheep models of compromised pregnancy. *J Physiol* (2005), **565**:43–58.

44. Barbour LA, Shao J, Qiao L, Pulawa LK, Jensen DR, Bartke A, et al., Human placental growth hormone causes severe insulin resistance in transgenic mice. *Am J Obstet Gynecol* (2002), **186**:512–17.

45. Hotamisligil GS and Spiegelman BM, Tumor necrosis factor alpha: a key component of the obesity-diabetes link. *Diabetes* (1994), **43**:1271–8.

46. Frost RA and Lang CH, Skeletal muscle cytokines: regulation by pathogen-associated molecules and catabolic hormones. *Curr Opin Clin Nutr Metab Care* (2005), **8**:255–63.

47. Peraldi P and Spiegelman B, TNF-alpha and insulin resistance: summary and future prospects. *Mol Cell Biochem* (1998), **182**:169–75.

48. Catalano PM, Hoegh M, Minium J, Huston-Presley L, Bernard S, Kalhan S, and Hauguel-De Mouzon S, Adiponectin in human pregnancy: implications for regulation of glucose and lipid metabolism. *Diabetologia* (2006), **49**:1677–85.

49. Sagawa N, Yura S, Itoh H, Mise H, Kakui K, Korita D, et al., Role of leptin in pregnancy – a review. *Placenta* (2002), **23**(Suppl A):S80–6.

50. Islami D, Bischof P, and Chardonnens D, Possible interactions between leptin, gonadotrophin-releasing hormone (GnRH-I and II) and human chorionic gonadotrophin (hCG). *Eur J Obstet Gynecol Reprod Biol* (2003), **110**:169–75.

51. Fant M, Munro H, and Moses AC, An autocrine/paracrine role for insulin-like growth factors in the regulation of human placental growth. *J Clin Endocrinol Metab* (1986), **63**:499–505.

52. Hamilton GS, Lysiak JJ, Han VK, and Lala PK, Autocrine-paracrine regulation of human trophoblast invasiveness by insulin-like growth factor (IGF)-II and IGF-binding protein (IGFBP)-1. *Exp Cell Res* (1998), **244**: 147–56.

53. Ong K, Kratzsch J, Kiess W, Costello M, Scott C, and Dunger D, Size at birth and cord blood levels of insulin, insulin-like growth factor I (IGF-I), IGF-II, IGF-binding protein-1 (IGFBP-1), IGFBP-3, and the soluble IGF-II/mannose-6-phosphate receptor in term human infants. The ALSPAC Study Team. Avon Longitudinal Study of Pregnancy and Childhood. *J Clin Endocrinol Metab* **85** (2000):4266–9.

54. Liu YJ, Tsushima T, Onoda N, Minei S, Sanaka M, Nagashima T, et al., Expression of messenger RNA of insulin-like growth factors (IGFs) and IGF binding proteins (IGFBP1–6) in placenta of normal and diabetic pregnancy. *Endocr J* (1996), **43**(Suppl):S89–91.

55. Ferguson-Smith AC, Cattanach BM, Barton SC, Beechey CV, and Surani MA, Embryological and molecular investigations of parental imprinting on mouse chromosome 7. *Nature* (1991), **351**:667–70.

56. Han VK and Carter AM, Spatial and temporal patterns of expression of messenger RNA for insulin-like growth factors and their binding proteins in the placenta of man and laboratory animals. *Placenta* (2000), **21**:289–305.

57. Lau MM, Stewart CE, Liu Z, Bhatt H, Rotwein P, and Stewart CL, Loss of the imprinted IGF2/cation-independent mannose 6-phosphate receptor results in fetal overgrowth and perinatal lethality. *Genes Dev* (1994), **8**:2953–63.

58. DeChiara TM, Efstratiadis A, and Robertson EJ, A growth-deficiency phenotype in heterozygous mice carrying an insulin-like growth factor II gene disrupted by targeting. *Nature* (1990), **345**:78–80.

59. Constancia M, Hemberger M, Hughes J, Dean W, Ferguson-Smith A, Fundele R, et al., Placental-specific IGF-II is a major modulator of placental and fetal growth. *Nature* (2002), **417**:945–8.

60. Harding JE, Liu L, Evans PC, and Gluckman PD, Insulin-like growth factor 1 alters feto-placental protein and carbohydrate metabolism in fetal sheep. *Endocrinology* (1994), **134**:1509–14.

61. Iwamoto HS, Murray MA, and Chernausek SD, Effects of acute hypoxemia on insulin-like growth factors and their binding proteins in fetal sheep. *Am J Physiol* (1992), **263**:E1151–6.

62. Fowden AL, Endocrine regulation of fetal growth. *Reprod Fertil Dev* (1995), **7**:351–63.

63. Fowden AL, Li J, and Forhead AJ, Glucocorticoids and the preparation for life after birth: are there long-term consequences of the life insurance? *Proc Nutr Soc* (1998), **57**:113–22.

64. Fang J, Furesz TC, Smith CH, and Fant ME, IGF binding protein-1 (IGFBP-1) is preferentially associated with the fetal-facing basal surface of the syncytiotrophoblast in the human placenta. *Growth Horm IGF Res* (1999), **9**:438–44.

65. Pardi G and Cetin I, Human fetal growth and organ development: 50 years of discoveries. *Am J Obstet Gynecol* (2006), **194**:1088–99.

66. Larque E, Demmelmair H, Berger B, Hasbargen U, and Koletzko B, In vivo investigation of the placental transfer of (13)C-labeled fatty acids in humans. *J Lipid Res* (2003), **44**:49–55.

67. Jansson T and Powell TL, Role of the placenta in fetal programming: underlying mechanisms and potential interventional approaches. *Clin Sci (Lond)* (2007), **113**:1–13.

68. Jones HN, Powell TL, and Jansson T, Regulation of placental nutrient transport – a review. *Placenta* (2007), **28**:763–74.

69. Sibley CP, Turner MA, Cetin I, Ayuk P, Boyd CA, D'Souza SW, et al., Placental phenotypes of intrauterine growth. *Pediatr Res* (2005), **58**:827–32.

70. Jansson T and Powell TL, IFPA 2005 Award in Placentology Lecture. Human placental transport in altered fetal growth: does the placenta function as a nutrient sensor? – a review. *Placenta* (2006), **27**(Suppl A):S91–7.

71. Jansson N, Pettersson J, Haafiz A, Ericsson A, Palmberg I, Tranberg M, et al., Down-regulation of placental transport of amino acids precedes the development of intrauterine growth restriction in rats fed a low protein diet. *J Physiol* (2006), **576**:935–46.

72. Roos S, Jansson N, Palmberg I, Saljo K, Powell TL, and Jansson T, Mammalian target of rapamycin in the human placenta regulates leucine transport and is down-regulated in restricted fetal growth. *J Physiol* (2007), **582**:449–59.

Nutritional regulation and requirements for pregnancy and fetal growth

2 Pregnancy and feto-placental growth: macronutrients

Laura Brown, Tim Regnault, Paul Rozance, James Barry, and William W. Hay Jr.

Introduction

Nutrient substrates for placental and fetal metabolism

The principal metabolic nutrients in the fetus are glucose and amino acids. Glucose is the principal energy substrate for basal metabolism and protein synthesis and contributes to energy storage in glycogen and fat. Amino acids provide the building blocks for protein synthesis and growth; they are also oxidative substrates for energy production, especially when glucose is deficient. Fatty acids are also taken up by the fetus; they are primarily used for structural components of membranes and for fat production in adipose tissue. The principal anabolic hormones, insulin and the insulin-like growth factors (IGFs), are important regulators of the synthesis of amino acids into protein, cell growth, and cell turnover, but their contributions to fetal metabolism and growth are secondary to the supply of nutrient substrates [1–3].

Growth of the placenta and its transport capacity

Placental nutrient transfer capacity increases over gestation by increased placental growth, primarily of membrane surface area, allowing for the increase in nutrient supply required for the growing fetus. Placental size, morphology, and membrane transporter abundance are regulated by imprinted paternally derived genes, such as the placental-specific *Igf2-H19* gene complex [4]. A larger paternal versus maternal *Igf2* gene allele supply leads to a larger placenta and the potential for a larger fetus. Activity of the imprinted genes can also be affected by epigenetic modification, which allows for considerable environmental influence over gene expression. Thus, DNA methylation can limit placental-specific *Igf2* gene activity, leading to intrauterine growth restriction (IUGR) of the placenta and, in turn, the fetus.

Glucose

Placental glucose transport and metabolism

Glucose is the primary energy substrate for the mammalian fetus and placenta. Normally, the fetus does not produce glucose [5]. Therefore, fetal glucose concentration is dependent on the placental supply from the maternal circulation according to placental facilitated transport mediated by sodium-independent transport proteins. Glucose entry into the fetal circulation depends on three steps: (1) uptake from the maternal circulation by transporters in the maternal-facing microvillous membrane of the trophoblast, (2) transport across the cytoplasm of the trophoblast, and (3) transporter-dependent transport across the fetal-facing basal membrane of the trophoblast into the fetal circulation. Glucose transport to the fetus is increased by placental glucose transporter density, trophoblast membrane surface area, the maternal-fetal glucose concentration gradient, and uterine and umbilical blood flows; it is decreased by the thickness of cellular and interstitial layers between the maternal and fetal vasculature.

At present, only glucose transport proteins 1 (GLUT1) and 3 (GLUT3) have been found in placental tissue locations that would allow for maternal-to-fetal glucose transport [6]. GLUT1 has been localized on both maternal- and fetal-facing membranes of the synciotrophoblast, whereas GLUT3 has been found on maternal facing microvillous membranes of the trophoblast. In the trophoblast, GLUT1 protein concentrations are threefold higher in the maternal-facing membranes than in the fetal-facing membranes. In vitro dual cotyledon perfusion studies have demonstrated a twofold greater uptake of glucose from the maternal than the fetal vasculature [7]. These functional data are supported by placental studies showing a sixfold greater maternal-facing trophoblast membrane surface area and a threefold higher GLUT1 concentration compared with the fetal-facing basal membrane [8, 9]. This unique arrangement of transporters allows for the high rate of glucose transport from maternal to fetal plasma, which is directly related to the maternal plasma glucose concentration and the maternal-to-fetal plasma glucose concentration gradient [10]. In contrast, uteroplacental glucose consumption is regulated by fetal glucose concentrations [11]. Thus, when fetal plasma glucose concentrations are relatively higher, glucose is shunted toward placental consumption. Conversely, if fetal plasma glucose concentrations are relatively lower, glucose transport into the fetal circulation increases, but placental glucose consumption diminishes. This unique reciprocal relationship regulates fetal and placental glucose utilization in relation to maternal glucose concentration.

From mid-gestation to term, fetal glucose demand increases 14-fold [1]. To meet this higher fetal glucose demand, placental-to-fetal glucose transfer increases through two discrete developmental changes. First, the maternal-to-fetal glucose concentration gradient increases as the fetal glucose concentration decreases in relation to maternal plasma glucose concentrations [12]. The decrease in fetal glucose concentration is the result of increased glucose utilization in the placenta and the fetus. Near term, in vivo and in vitro studies have shown that as much as 60% to 80% of glucose taken up by the placenta is not transferred to the fetus but is instead consumed by the placenta [11, 12], thereby lowering the concentration of glucose in the uterine and umbilical veins. Increased fetal glucose utilization occurs in response to increased fetal insulin production and growth of fetal insulin-sensitive tissues (primarily skeletal muscle). Quantitatively more important, placental glucose transport capacity also increases significantly as a function of the increase in placental trophoblast surface area and its directly related increase in glucose transporter abundance [8, 13].

Physiological and clinical points for placental glucose and metabolism

1. Glucose is the primary energy substrate for the mammalian fetus and placenta.

2. The placenta is a highly metabolically active organ. Its significant nutrient requirements are necessary to increase its growth, metabolism, and transport capacity to support the increasing metabolic needs of the growing fetus as gestation advances.

3. Glucose transport to the fetus is increased by trophoblast membrane surface area, the maternal-fetal glucose concentration gradient, and uterine and umbilical blood flows but is decreased by the thickness of cellular and interstitial layers between the maternal and fetal vasculature.

4. When fetal plasma glucose concentrations are relatively higher, glucose is shunted toward placental consumption. Conversely, if fetal plasma glucose concentrations are relatively lower, glucose transport into the fetal circulation increases, and placental glucose consumption diminishes.

5. From mid-gestation to term, fetal glucose demand increases 14-fold.

Fetal glucose utilization

The fetus metabolizes glucose in several ways, including oxidation for energy requirements (55% of total glucose utilization) and as a carbon source for production of various macromolecules, such as glycogen, glycolytic products (e.g. lactate, riboses, and glycerol), proteins, and fatty acids. The fraction of fetal oxygen consumption provided by glucose oxidation is approximately 30%, with most of the remainder provided by lactate and, to a lesser extent, amino acids [10, 14]. In humans the estimated fetal glucose utilization rate in late gestation is 5 to 6 mg/kg/min [15]. This is similar to the rate determined in large animal models near term [1, 2] and corresponds to glucose utilization rates in human newborn infants. Fetal glucose utilization rates normalized to fetal weight decrease from mid- to late gestation as a result of the growth of organs, such as muscle, bone, and adipose tissue, which have lower rates of glucose utilization.

Acutely, the rate of fetal glucose utilization is regulated by maternal plasma glucose concentration and placental glucose transport to the fetus. This regulation is partly due to fetal insulin secretion. Increased placental transport of glucose to the fetus increases glucose concentrations, which stimulate fetal insulin secretion. Insulin then acts to increase fetal glucose utilization and lower glucose concentrations [10].

In addition, glucose and insulin clamp experiments in fetal sheep, in which glucose is infused to produce desired concentrations and increases in insulin concentration are blocked by simultaneous infusions of somatostatin, have demonstrated that fetal glucose concentrations regulate glucose utilization independently of fetal insulin concentrations. Despite the changes in overall glucose utilization, the fraction of glucose oxidized in these short-term studies is unchanged (approximately 55% in fetal sheep) [14]. Therefore, in the acute setting, fetal glucose utilization is regulated by acute changes in fetal insulin and glucose concentrations.

Physiological and clinical points for fetal glucose utilization

1. Fetal glucose concentration is dependent on the placental supply through facilitated transport mediated by sodium-independent transport proteins.
2. From mid-gestation to term, fetal glucose utilization increases 14-fold, which is met by an increase in the maternal-to-fetal glucose concentration gradient and in the placental trophoblast surface area and glucose transporter abundance. However, fetal glucose utilization rates normalized to fetal weight decrease from mid- to late gestation.
3. Late in gestation the estimated fetal glucose utilization rate in late gestation is 5 to 6 mg/kg/min.
4. Fetal glucose utilization is regulated by acute changes in fetal insulin and glucose concentrations.

Fetal insulin secretion

Insulin is secreted by the β-cell, located in the islets of Langerhans within the pancreas, which develops during the first trimester. Data from fetal sheep indicate that baseline insulin concentrations and the capacity for insulin secretion increase from mid-gestation toward term, although this secretory capacity is significantly less than in neonatal animals [14]. In humans glucose-stimulated insulin secretion has been demonstrated in the mid third trimester, although functioning islets are present, as in the sheep, by mid second trimester [16].

Fetal glucose production

Although fetal glucose production has not been demonstrated in humans [5], glucose production from glycogenolysis and gluconeogenesis has been demonstrated under certain conditions in laboratory animals. Glycogen is normally produced in the fetal liver from glucose, although lactate and certain amino acids also can act as precursors. Hepatic glycogen content normally increases during the later part of gestation. Following experimental manipulation, the fetal liver can acutely produce glucose from glycogen, a process that is rapidly activated by pharmacologic concentrations of catecholamines and glucagon, as well as by hypoxia (which probably acts by increasing catecholamine secretion). Sustained glucose production by the fetal liver occurs under experimental conditions through gluconeogenesis – for example, in certain models of IUGR or sustained fetal hypoglycemia [17, 18] – and sustained glucose production, though of modest degree, does develop naturally in late-gestation fetal sheep. Functional activities of the hepatic gluconeogenic pathway are usually present late in fetal life, following stimulation by the late-gestation increase in fetal cortisol secretion.

Intrauterine growth restriction

IUGR is characterized by fetal hypoglycemia and hypoinsulinemia and serves as an example of how the placenta and fetus adapt to such chronic changes to maintain normal glucose metabolic rates. On an absolute basis, placental glucose transport is reduced by 65% at near term in IUGR gestations, but on a relative weight basis, it is similar to control transport rates [19]. Many studies have confirmed, in fact, that the severity of the fetal growth restriction and placental insufficiency may affect the degree and causal mechanisms of fetal hypoglycemia.

Several animal models of IUGR or experimental fetal hypoglycemia have shown that weight-specific fetal glucose utilization rates are not severely decreased from control rates [14, 19]. Recent data from these models have shown maintained or increased insulin sensitivity as a mechanism that maintains the glucose utilization rates. This is consistent with data in human IUGR infants obtained within the first 48 hours of life showing increased insulin sensitivity [20]. Increased insulin sensitivity for glucose utilization is required to maintain normal glucose utilization rates because another adaptation of the severely IUGR fetus is decreased baseline and glucose stimulated insulin concentrations, probably due to decreased numbers of pancreatic β-cells [16, 21]. Again, a wide variety of many animal models of IUGR and selective fetal hypoglycemia also show decreased insulin concentrations, decreased glucose stimulated insulin secretion, and decreased abundance of pancreatic β-cells in the resulting smaller islets [14, 22].

If fetal adaptations to IUGR, such as increased insulin sensitivity despite decreased insulin secretion and β-cell mass, persist into postnatal life and into late childhood and adulthood, they could underlie the increased risk that IUGR infants have of developing obesity and Type II diabetes mellitus as adults. Increased insulin sensitivity might predispose the formerly IUGR infant to have abnormally increased rates of fatty acid deposition, leading to obesity and eventually insulin resistance. If a β-cell defect persists that limits the insulin response to peripheral insulin resistance, then Type II diabetes mellitus would follow. This problem raises two important areas for future research. One area is in the prenatal treatment of IUGR. Previous human studies using nutritional interventions have demonstrated variable results with potential fetal toxicity. However, mechanisms of fetal toxicity are unknown, and large animal models are particularly useful for determining these mechanisms and investigating safe interventions for established IUGR. In addition, future research is needed to determine whether postnatal feeding practices should be modified in the previously IUGR infant during the period of increased insulin sensitivity with the goal of preventing future insulin resistance and obesity without sacrificing long-term neurodevelopmental outcomes.

Physiological and clinical points for intrauterine growth restriction

1. IUGR is characterized by fetal hypoglycemia as well as by hypoinsulinemia and adaptations that maintain normal glucose metabolic rates.
2. On an absolute basis, placental glucose transport is reduced by 65% near term in IUGR gestations, but on a relative weight basis, it is similar to control transport rates.
3. Recent data from animal models have shown maintained or increased insulin sensitivity as a mechanism that maintains the glucose utilization rates in IUGR.

Amino acids

Protein (nitrogen) requirements during pregnancy

Current dietary recommendations for increased protein intake during pregnancy are based on estimates of overall accumulation of nitrogen in the conceptus. Total nitrogen concentration measurements have been used to estimate the rate of protein accretion in tissues, because most of the total nitrogen is represented by amino acid nitrogen uptake [3]. Several methods have been used to estimate total nitrogen accretion during pregnancy. Measurements of total body potassium, which estimate lean body mass, predict an additional nitrogen accretion of 90 g (550 g protein, $N \times 6.25$) during pregnancy from increased protein deposition in the placenta, fetus, uterus, red blood cells, plasma, and other maternal tissues. Nitrogen balance studies in pregnant women consistently show an increase in nitrogen retention as pregnancy progresses and estimate nitrogen deposition to be approximately 1.2 to 1.8 g of nitrogen/day by the third trimester of pregnancy [23]. Because the fetus contributes most to nitrogen requirements, both anthropometric measurements and postmortem chemical composition studies of infants born at different gestational ages have predicted fetal protein accretion to be 64 g nitrogen (400 g protein) at term [24]. Nonfat dry weight and nitrogen content are linearly related to fetal weight; the rate of fetal growth, therefore, determines the macronutrient requirements for fetal protein accretion gain. On the basis of such information, 6 to 10 g of protein per day is generally recommended for pregnant women.

Fetal and placental amino acid requirements for net protein accretion, however, do not appear to depend only or directly on maternal diet. A positive correlation between fetal weight and maternal protein intake has not been demonstrated. It also has been shown that when pregnant women receive high protein supplementation, there is a significantly increased risk of small-for-gestational-age birth [25]. Furthermore, stable isotope studies performed during pregnancy indicate that lower rates of urea synthesis (reflecting decreased amino acid oxidation) and lower rates of branch chain amino acid transamination function to conserve nitrogen accretion for both maternal and fetal requirements [26]. Therefore, changes in maternal protein metabolism independent of protein intake contribute significantly to protein delivery to the fetus. Increased maternal lean body mass also may positively affect protein turnover and fetal growth [26]. With contributions from diet, maternal body composition, and maternal protein turnover, protein delivery to the growing fetus ultimately depends on umbilical amino acid uptake from the placenta and the ability to transport amino acids from the maternal to the fetal circulation.

Placental transport of amino acids from mother to fetus

The net uptake of amino acids by umbilical circulation through the placenta represents the dietary supply of amino acids for fetal growth and protein metabolism. In fetal sheep at term, total fetal umbilical nitrogen uptake is 0.91 g nitrogen/kg/day, similar to the calculated total fetal nitrogen requirement of approximately 1 g nitrogen/kg/day based on nitrogen accretion data and estimated fetal urea production rates [27]. The net uptake of most amino acids exceeds their net accretion by considerable amounts, indicating that the fetus must oxidize the balance not used for net protein accretion. As in postnatal life, several amino acids (primarily the branch chain amino acids leucine, isoleucine, and valine, as well as lysine) cannot be synthesized in the fetus. Thus, limitation of supply of these essential or indispensable amino acids is likely to lead to reduced fetal protein accretion and growth. For the nonessential amino acids, fetal requirements can be met by production within fetal tissues. The placenta also contributes to fetal amino acid and nitrogen balance through placental-fetal amino acid cycling. In other words, certain amino acids (e.g. glutamine and glycine and their metabolic products glutamate and serine) are produced in the placenta, metabolized in the placenta, or taken up from the fetal pool to optimize metabolic processes such as signaling of protein synthesis and oxidation for energy production [28].

Amino acids are transported across the placental trophoblast by energy-dependent amino acid transporter systems. Because the concentration of most amino acids is higher in the fetal than the maternal plasma, transport usually occurs actively against a concentration gradient. Amino acid transport systems are present on both the maternal-facing (apical) and fetal-facing (basal) surfaces of the trophoblast in the human placenta. Each system transports a collection of pre-ferred amino acids (reviewed in Regnault et al. [28]). Not only amino acids are transported from the maternal circulation to the fetus, they are also transported from the fetus to the placenta, so the net uptake a fetus receives is the sum of these movements. Amino acids supplied to the placenta from the maternal and fetal circulations are metabolized for energy production and amino acid synthesis.

As pregnancy advances, placental amino acid transport capacity must increase to meet the nutrient demands of the developing fetus. Factors that change with advancing gestation to affect the total placental transport of amino acids include uteroplacental blood flow, trophoblast villous surface area, competition among amino acids for the same transporter, placental metabolism of amino acids, and transport system location and activity. Therefore, these changes associated with advancing gestational age, in conjunction with maternal diet and metabolic condition, alter amino acid transport and fetal growth potential. The nutritional requirements for amino acids are highest during mid-gestation because of high fractional protein synthetic and growth rates during this time [29]. It is important to note that placental transport rates of amino acids are not significantly affected by moderate fluctuations in uterine or placental blood flow, because they are actively transported and thus clearance is diffusion limited. However, during the second half of gestation, increasing placental surface area falls short of the increase in fetal size [8]. Therefore, increasing amino acid transporter abundance and activity, in combination with villous surface area, appear necessary to support fetal growth, and both have been shown to increase over gestation [30].

Fetal amino acid metabolism

Accretion of amino acids is an essential component of fetal protein synthesis and growth. In the growing fetus, net protein synthesis exceeds net protein degradation, yielding net protein accretion, although both processes continue simultaneously. Direct measurements of fetal protein synthesis, breakdown, and oxidation have been made with carbon-labeled isotopic tracers of selected amino acids. A net uptake of amino acids by the fetus in excess of accretion requirements for growth implies that this excess portion of amino acid uptake is used for oxidation, and several tracer studies have documented $^{14}CO_2$ production from amino acid oxidation [3].

Insulin and insulin-like growth factor 1 (IGF-1) are important growth hormones for the fetus and promote the utilization of substrates such as amino acids in fetal life. In vivo studies in the ovine fetus have demonstrated that both hormones increase cellular amino acid uptake, promoting their direct synthesis both into protein and into oxidative metabolism and energy production [31, 32]. Insulin and IGF-1 regulate translation initiation and protein synthesis through well-recognized intermediates in their signal transduction pathways, including mitogen activated pathway (MAP) kinase and mammalian target of rapamycin (mTOR) [33, 34]. In mammals, mTOR functions as a sensor for growth factors, nutrients, energy, and stress and coordinates these signals to regulate cell growth and proliferation. Amino acids also have been documented to function as direct-acting nutrient signals that activate mRNA translation initiation via mTOR. Leucine has been documented as the major regulator of this pathway, as well as an important regulator of gene expression during cellular stress [35].

Abnormal delivery of amino acids to the fetus with IUGR

Amino acid and protein insufficiency produces growth failure of the whole fetus and preterm infant. Placental amino acid transport studies in both humans and sheep have consistently found reduced placental transport of amino acids, and in particular leucine, across the IUGR placenta [3, 36]. Furthermore, in vitro studies on isolated human syncytiotrophoblast plasma membranes have demonstrated reduced expression, activity, or both in several specific amino acid transport systems on both the maternal- and fetal-facing plasma membranes of the trophoblast from IUGR pregnancies [37]. Although reduced placental transport of selected or all amino acids might be expected from such IUGR placentas and thus contribute to lower fetal plasma amino acid concentrations during mid-gestation and term, other IUGR studies have reported maintenance of circulating fetal concentrations [37]. Many factors contribute to fetal plasma amino acid concentrations in utero, such as amino acid supply and the balance of rates of fetal protein synthesis, breakdown, and catabolism (Fig. 2.1). Thus, reliance on fetal plasma concentration data alone in assessing the transport capacity of a placenta may not be entirely accurate. Reduced placental

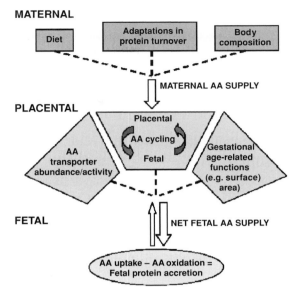

Figure 2.1 Schematic diagram showing maternal, placental, and fetal influences on fetal protein accretion and growth.

surface area has been reported for the IUGR placenta, indicating that morphometric changes also contribute to overall reduction in placental amino acid transport capacity in cases of IUGR [38]. Further investigation into mechanisms involved in the development of IUGR in relation to amino acid uptake and utilization in fetal life is critical because of the short- and long-term consequences for neonates born with this condition, including increased morbidity and mortality in the neonatal period as well as the predisposition to abnormal muscle development, peripheral insulin resistance, obesity, diabetes, and cardiovascular disease later in life [39].

Physiological and clinical points for placental and fetal amino acid metabolism

1. Placental and fetal requirements for protein accretion during pregnancy are met by adaptations in maternal protein turnover and, to a lesser degree, maternal protein intake.

2. Amino acids are transported from mother to fetus across the placental trophoblast against a concentration gradient by energy-dependent amino acid transporter systems.

3. Amino acid transporter abundance and activity and villous surface area increase during the second half of gestation to support fetal growth.

4. Placental insufficiency will result in intrauterine fetal growth restriction, in part as a result of

reduced placental surface area, reduced expression and/or activity of amino acid transporters, as well as decreased flux of amino acids across the placenta.

Lipids

Placental lipid metabolism and fetal lipid supply

The transport of fatty acids and other lipid substances across the placenta and the deposition of lipids in fetal adipose tissue are primarily late-gestation phenomena. Essential fatty acid transport, however, begins early in gestation, allowing membrane lipids, particularly those of neurons and glial cells, to develop throughout gestation.

Fetal uptake and plasma concentrations of all fatty acids and structural lipids correlate directly with the fatty acid/lipid composition of the maternal plasma and, therefore, indirectly with maternal diet, metabolic conditions (fed vs. fasting), and disease states (e.g. diabetes). Experimentally, diabetic animal models and those fed oil-rich diets produce fetuses and newborns at term gestation that have increased whole-body adipose tissue and fat stores as well as organ (particularly liver) lipid contents [40]. Quantitatively in pregnant women, the net flux of free fatty acids (FFAs) into the fetus from the maternal circulation can account for 50% to 100% of the fetal requirement of fatty acids during the end of pregnancy, although lipid synthesis in the fetus from glucose and FFAs does contribute significant amounts of fat in late gestation. Overall, there is a general relationship between the permeability of the placenta to lipids, especially fatty acids, and the adiposity of the fetus at term. Among mammals, human fetuses develop the most fat, 15% to 18% of body weight at term, compared with other mammals in which fetal fat content at term is 3% or less of body weight [2].

Direct placental FFA uptake and transfer to the fetus increases over gestation by increased placental lipoprotein lipase activity, which appears to be increased by glucose and insulin and expression and activity of the fatty acid transporter binding protein L-FAB [41]. These processes contribute to the greater lipid transport to the fetus and fetal macroscomia (obesity) common in gestational diabetics. Maternal lipid metabolism changes to a catabolic state in late gestation, with increased adipose tissue lipolysis and reduced uptake of circulating triglycerides as adipose tissue lipoprotein lipase activity decreases. The maternal liver also overproduces triglycerides under these conditions, and the maternal intestine increases its absorption of dietary lipids, particularly in late gestation. These changes in maternal lipid metabolism produce increasing concentrations of nearly all types of circulating plasma lipids, including free fatty acids, glycerol, and triglyceride-rich very low-density lipoproteins (VLDLs) and chylomicron particles. Maternal plasma concentrations of keto acids (β-hydroxybutyrate and acetoacetate) increase rapidly during fasting and can contribute significantly to the supply of lipid substrates to the placenta and fetus [2].

Placental uptake, synthesis, and metabolism of fatty acids

After entering the placenta, fatty acids can be used for triglyceride synthesis, cholesterol esterification, membrane biosynthesis, direct transfer to the fetus, or oxidation [42]. Placental tissue from different species expresses lipoprotein lipase activity as well as phospholipase A$_2$ [43]. Maternal plasma triglycerides are hydrolyzed by these enzymes, and the fatty acids that are released are then taken up by the placenta. In the trophoblast cells, the fatty acids are then re-esterified and further hydrolyzed, facilitating their diffusion into fetal circulation. Most of these processes increase in late gestation and recent gene expression patterns show upregulation of the genes responsible for placental lipid metabolism and transport early during this period. Normally, increased maternal lipolysis during pregnancy provides substrate for maternal energy metabolism, which spares glucose for the fetus and also increases maternal plasma FFA concentrations. Furthermore, placental triglyceride content increases in women who are fasting, who deliver preterm infants, or who have diabetes mellitus – all conditions in which maternal plasma free fatty acid concentrations are increased. In contrast, lipolysis is lower in pregnancies complicated by IUGR, in which both placenta and fetus have reduced lipid concentrations and fat mass [44].

Fatty acid transport into the fetal circulation is primarily determined by the transplacental gradient of FFAs and the fetal plasma concentrations and binding site availabilities of fatty acid binding proteins in the fetal circulation; normal conditions generally favor maternal-to-fetal transport. All fatty acids cross lipid bilayers, such as those in the syncytiotrophoblast, by rapid simple diffusion. In addition, fatty acid transport across membranes is facilitated by fatty acid binding proteins (FABPs), which aid in intracellular channeling of fatty acids [45].

Another major effect of maternal fatty acids taken up by the placenta involves their role as signals for additional metabolism in the placenta and fetus [46]. For example, the nuclear receptor peroxisome proliferator-activated receptor gamma (PPAR gamma) is expressed in placental trophoblast cells and is essential for placental development, trophoblast invasion, differentiation of cytotrophoblasts into syncytium, and regulation of fat accumulation in trophoblasts, and even produce fetal membrane signals that lead to parturition. Low-density lipoprotein cholesterol is also taken up by endocytosis into trophoblast cells; it is the major precursor for placental production of progesterone and estrogen. Some of this cholesterol is transferred directly to the fetus, although most of fetal cholesterol is synthesized in the fetal liver.

Essential fatty acid metabolism and transfer by the placenta

The supply of essential, long-chain polyunsaturated fatty acids (LCPUFAs: linoleic acid or 18:2 omega-6, and α-linolenic acid or 18:3 omega-3) is critical to the synthesis of structural lipids. All of the omega-6 and omega-3 fatty acid structures acquired by the fetus must come from the mother via the placenta, either in the form of these two essential fatty acids or their principal LCPUFA derivatives, arachidonic acid (AA, 20:4 omega-6) and docosahexaenoic acid (DHA, 22:6 omega-3) [47].

Essential fatty acids are not synthesized in the placenta, even though concentrations of the EFAs are higher in the fetus than in the mother [48]. Although these results indicate that fetal AA acid and DHA are transferred directly from the mother to a higher binding capacity in the fetal plasma, they do not exclude the possibility that some might be synthesized from linoleic and linolenic acids in the fetal liver.

Maternal diet and essential fatty acid supply

In general, there is a direct correlation between maternal essential fatty acid nutrition and neonatal growth and head circumference in humans; this correlation parallels those for maternal and fetal (or neonatal) concentrations of LCPUFAs and other essential fatty acids such as DHA in healthy women eating normal, unsupplemented diets and after fish oil supplementation during pregnancy [49]. In fact, because the developing fetus depends primarily on the maternal supply of essential fatty acids and AA status in preterm infants has also been correlated with birth weight, maternal dietary supplementation with LCPUFA-rich oils during the last trimester of pregnancy to increase levels in fetus has been advised. However, foods containing lipid peroxides are potentially toxic, and the higher the content of LCPUFAs in the diet, the more likely that peroxidation will occur, because excess intake of PUFAs could reduce antioxidant capacity and enhance susceptibility to oxidative damage. Furthermore, experimental animal studies have shown improvements in fetal and neonatal growth rates and neurodevelopmental indices with maternal λ-linolenic acid supplementation, in agreement with previous observations in humans fed diets rich in AA in which the proportion of linolenic acid in plasma phospholipids was decreased, likely as a consequence of replacing linolenic acid with AA in tissues [50]. Furthermore, although n-3 LCPUFA supplementation during human pregnancy does enhance pregnancy duration and fetal head circumference at term gestation, the mean effect size is small, making it difficult to determine the implications for later growth and development. Therefore, because the benefits and risks of modifying maternal fat intake in pregnancy and lactation are not yet completely established and the safety of high intakes of LCPUFAs during pregnancy is still unclear, further studies are required before definitive recommendations to markedly increase LCPUFA intake in pregnancy can be made.

This point, however, must be considered in light of data showing that pregnant women in some countries, particularly the United States, have remarkably lower LCPUFA concentrations, and their key metabolic derivatives than found in other populations, such as in Scandinavia, where natural dietary fish oil intake is relatively higher. More recent studies are now showing potentially important and statistically significant benefit to the offspring of pregnant mothers supplemented with dietary oils that increase DHA and related essential fatty acids in the fetus. For example, children who were born to mothers who had taken cod liver oil, rich in DHA, AA, and eicosapentaenoic acid, during pregnancy and lactation scored higher on mental processing tests at age 4 years compared with children whose mothers had taken corn oil [51]. Thus, maternal intake of very long-chain n-3 PUFAs during pregnancy and lactation may be favorable for later mental development of children.

Fetal accumulation of essential fatty acids

Production of AA acid and DHA from essential fatty acid precursors occurs in term and preterm infants, but it is not clear whether the fetus is capable of fatty acid desaturation and elongation [52]. Both AA and DHA are readily incorporated into the structural lipids of the developing brain, where, besides their role in maintaining membrane fluidity, permeability, and conformation, they play an important functional role. For example, once released from phospholipids by the action of phospholipase A_2, AA is the main precursor for eicosanoids, prostaglandins, and leukotrienes and is essential for fetal and neonatal growth [53]. DHA has a key role in the development of visual function. Depletion of DHA from the retina and brain results in reduced visual function and learning deficits, emphasizing the critical roles of DHA in membrane-dependent signaling pathways and neurotransmitter metabolism. Increasing evidence from human studies of maternal n-3 fatty acid supplementation during pregnancy does indicates beneficial effects on visual function of the offspring, but primarily in infants born preterm; similar results relate to maternal n-3 intake during pregnancy and infant neurodevelopmental outcome [54]. Specificity of most of the beneficial effects, however, is confounded by improved postnatal n-3 dietary intake of the preterm infants.

Fetal lipid metabolism

The fetus also develops its own mechanisms that enhance lipid uptake, including insulin secretion that increases fatty acid utilization (largely to develop adipose tissue) [1]. Such increased fetal lipid metabolism also lowers fetal plasma fatty acid concentrations relative to those in the maternal plasma and thereby increases the maternal-to-fetal fatty acid concentration gradient and the diffusion of fatty acids into the fetal plasma. Increased fetal albumin synthesis and plasma concentrations directly increase the transfer of fatty acids across the placenta by providing increased esterification capacity in the fetal plasma.

Fatty acid oxidation in the fetus

There is little evidence for much fatty acid oxidation in the fetus. RNA expression and activity of long-chain fatty acid oxidation enzymes are low in fetal tissues, although they subsequently increase rapidly after birth, even in preterm infants. The abundant glucose supply to the fetus also limits fatty acid oxidation by producing high concentrations of malonyl-CoA, which inhibits carnitine palmitoyl transferase 1 (CPT1) activity, the rate-limiting enzyme for long-chain fatty acid entry into mitochondria that already is low in fetal tissues.

Physiological and clinical points for placental and fetal lipid metabolism

1. Human fetuses are unique among land mammals in the large amount of "white" fat that they accumulate over the last trimester of pregnancy – 12% to 18% of body weight.
2. Placental and fetal lipid uptake and fetal plasma lipid concentrations are directly related to maternal plasma lipid concentrations and thus to maternal diet.
3. Placental lipid transfer occurs directly for FFAs and indirectly by active metabolism for many other lipid products.
4. Essential fatty acids are transported by specific transporters over the bulk of gestation.
5. Fetal and neonatal neurological development is positively affected by EFA supply.
6. Most of fetal lipid uptake and production is used for fat production in adipose tissue and not for oxidation.

Acknowledgments

Preparation of this manuscript was supported in part by research grants HD42815, HD28794, and DK52138 (WW Hay, PI) and by NIH-GCRC grant M01 RR00069 (W. Hay, Associate Director) from the National Institutes of Health (NIH). Dr. Brown was supported by The Children's Hospital of Denver Research Institute Research Scholar Award and the Colorado Clinical Nutrition Research Unit, which is funded by NIH P30 DK048520. Dr. Regnault was supported by NIH grant HD41505. Dr. Barry and Dr. Rozance were supported by The Children's Hospital of Denver Research Institute Research Scholar Award.

References

1. Hay WW Jr., Energy and substrate requirements of the placenta and fetus. *Proc Nutr Soc* (1991), **50**:321–36.

2. Hay WW Jr., Metabolic interrelationships of placenta and fetus. *Placenta* (1995), **16**:19–30.

3. Hay WW Jr., Brown LD, and Regnault TRH, Fetal requirements and placental transfer of nitrogenous compounds. In Polin RA, Fox WW, Abman SH, eds., Fetal and Neonatal Physiology, 4th edn (Philadelphia: Elsevier/W. B. Saunders Co., in press, 2008).

4. Fowden AL, Sibley C, Reik W, and Constancia M, Imprinted genes, placental development and fetal growth. *Horm Res* (2006), 65 Suppl **3**:50–8.

5. Marconi AM, Cetin I, Davoli E, Baggiani AM, Fanelli R, Fennessey PV, et al., An evaluation of fetal glucogenesis in intrauterine growth-retarded pregnancies. *Metab Clin Exp* (1993), **42**:860–4.

6. Wooding FB, Fowden AL, Bell AW, Ehrhardt RA, Limesand SW, and Hay WW, Localisation of glucose transport in the ruminant placenta: implications for sequential use of transporter isoforms. *Placenta* (2005), 626–405.

7. Schneider H, Reiber W, Sager R, and Malek A, Asymmetrical transport of glucose across the in vitro perfused human placenta. *Placenta* (2003), **24**:27–33.

8. Teasdale F and Jean-Jacques G, Intrauterine growth retardation: morphometry of the microvillous membrane of the human placenta. *Placenta* (1998), **9**:47–55.

9. Quraishi AN and Illsley NP, Transport of sugars across human placental membranes measured by light scattering. *Placenta* (1999), **20**:167–74.

10. Hay WW Jr. and Meznarich HK, Effect of maternal glucose concentration on uteroplacental glucose consumption and transfer in pregnant sheep. *Proc Soc Exp Biol Med* (1988), **190**:63–9.

11. Hay WW Jr., Molina RA, DiGiacomo JE, and Meschia G. Model of placental glucose consumption and glucose transfer. *Am J Physiol* (1990), **258**:R569–77.

12. Molina RD, Meschia G, Battaglia FC, and Hay WW Jr., Gestational maturation of placental glucose transfer capacity in sheep. *Am J Physiol* (1991), **261**:R697–704.

13. Ehrhardt RA and Bell AW, Developmental increases in glucose transporter concentration in the sheep placenta. *Am J Physiol* (1997), **273**:R1132–41.

14. Hay WW Jr., Recent observations on the regulation of fetal metabolism by glucose. *J Phys* (2006), **572**:17–24.

15. Marconi AM, Davoli E, Cetin I, Lanfranchi A, Zerbe G, Fanelli R, et al., Impact of conceptus mass on glucose disposal rate in pregnant women. *Am J Physiol* (1993), **264**:E514–E518.

16. Nicolini U, Hubinont C, Santolaya J, Fisk NM, and Rodeck CH, Effects of fetal intravenous glucose challenge in normal and growth retarded fetuses. *Horm Metab Res* (1990), **22**:426–30.

17. DiGiacomo JE and Hay WW Jr., Fetal glucose metabolism and oxygen consumption during sustained hypoglycemia. *Metabolism* (1990), **39**:193–202.

18. Limesand SW, Rozance PJ, Smith D, and Hay WW Jr., Increased insulin sensitivity and maintenance of glucose utilization rates in fetal sheep with placental insufficiency and intrauterine growth restriction. *Am J Physiol Endocrinol Metab* (2007), **293**:E1716–1725.

19. Thureen PJ, Trembler KA, Meschia G, Makowski EL, and Wilkening RB, Placental glucose transport in heat-induced fetal growth retardation. *Am J Physiol* (1992), **263**:R578–R585.

20. Bazaes RA, Salazar TE, Pittaluga E, Pena V, Alegria A, Iniguez G, et al., Glucose and lipid metabolism in small for gestational age infants at 48 hours of age. *Pediatrics* (2003), **111**:804–9.

21. Van Assche FA, De Prins F, Aerts L, and Verjans M, The endocrine pancreas in small-for-dates infants. *Br J Obstet Gynaecol* (1977), **84**:751–3.

22. Limesand SW, Jensen J, Hutton JC, and Hay WW Jr., Diminished beta-cell replication contributes to reduced beta-cell mass in fetal sheep with intrauterine growth restriction. *Am J Physiol Regul Integr Comp Physiol* (2005), **288**:R1297–R1305.

23. Mojtahedi M, de Groot LC, Boekholt HA, and van Raaij JM, Nitrogen balance of healthy Dutch women before and during pregnancy. *Am J Clin Nutr* (2002), **75**:1078–83.

24. Widdowson EM, Chemical composition and nutritional needs of the fetus at different stages of gestation. In: Maternal Nutrition during Pregnancy and Lactation, eds. Aebi H, Whitehead R. (Bern: Hans Huber, 1980), pp. 39–48.

25. Kramer MS and Kakuma R, Energy and protein intake in pregnancy. Cochrane Database Syst Rev (2003), CD000032.

26. Kalhan SC, Protein metabolism in pregnancy. *Am J Clin Nutr* (2000), **71**:1249S–55S.

27. Marconi AM, Battaglia FC, Meschia G, and Sparks JW, A comparison of amino acid arteriovenous differences across the liver and placenta of the fetal lamb. *Am J Physiol* (1989), **257**:E909-E915.

28. Regnault TR, de Vrijer B, and Battaglia FC, Transport and metabolism of amino acids in

placenta. *Endocrine* (2002), **19**:23–41.

29. Kennaugh JM, Bell AW, Teng C, Meschia G, and Battaglia FC, Ontogenetic changes in the rates of protein synthesis and leucine oxidation during fetal life. *Pediatr Res* (1987), **22**:688–92.

30. Ayuk PT, Sibley CP, Donnai P, D'Souza S, and Glazier JD, Development and polarization of cationic amino acid transporters and regulators in the human placenta. *Am J Physiol Cell Physiol* (2000), **278**:C1162–C1171.

31. Brown LD, and Hay WW Jr., Effect of hyperinsulinemia on amino acid utilization and oxidation independent of glucose metabolism in the ovine fetus. *Am J Physiol Endocrinol Metab* (2006), **291**:E1333–E1340.

32. Shen W, Wisniowski P, Ahmed L, Boyle DW, Denne SC, and Liechty EA, Protein anabolic effects of insulin and IGF-I in the ovine fetus. *Am J Physiol Endocrinol Metab* (2003), **284**:E748–E756.

33. Shen W, Mallon D, Boyle DW, and Liechty EA, IGF-I and insulin regulate eIF4F formation by different mechanisms in muscle and liver in the ovine fetus. *Am J Physiol Endocrinol Metab* (2002), **283**:E593–E603.

34. Stephens E, Thureen PJ, Goalstone ML, Anderson MS, Leitner JW, Hay WW Jr., et al., Fetal hyperinsulinemia increases farnesylation of p21 Ras in fetal tissues. *Am J Physiol Endocrinol Metab* (2001), **281**:E217–E223.

35. Kimball SR and Jefferson LS, Molecular mechanisms through which amino acids mediate signaling through the mammalian target of rapamycin. *Curr Opin Clin Nutr Metab Care* (2004), **7**:39–44.

36. Paolini CL, Marconi AM, Ronzoni S, Di Noio M, Fennessey PV, Pardi G, et al., Placental transport of leucine, phenylalanine, glycine, and proline in intrauterine growth-restricted pregnancies. *J Clin Endocrinol Metab* (2001), **86**:5427–32.

37. Glazier JD, Cetin I, Perugino G, Ronzoni S, Grey AM, Mahendran D, et al., Association between the activity of the system A amino acid transporter in the microvillous plasma membrane of the human placenta and severity of fetal compromise in intrauterine growth restriction. *Pediatr Res* (1997), **42**:514–9.

38. Mayhew TM, Manwani R, Ohadike C, Wijesekara J, and Baker PN, The placenta in pre-eclampsia and intrauterine growth restriction: studies on exchange surface areas, diffusion distances and villous membrane diffusive conductances. *Placenta* (2007), **28**:233–8.

39. Barker DJ, Adult consequences of fetal growth restriction. *Clin Obstet Gynecol* (2006), **49**:270–83.

40. Hay WW Jr., Nutrition and development of the fetus: carbohydrate and lipid metabolism. In: Nutrition in Pediatrics, eds. Walker WA, Watkins JB, and Duggan CP (Basic Science and Clinical Applications), 4th edn (Hamilton, Canada: BC Decker, in press, 2008).

41. Magnusson-Olsson AL, Hamark B, Ericsson A, Wennergren M, Jansson T, Powell TL, Gestational and hormonal regulation of human placental lipoprotein lipase. *J Lipid Res* (2006), **47**:2551–61.

42. Coleman RA, Placental metabolism and transport of lipid. *Fed Proc* (1986), **45**:2519–23.

43. Rice GE, Wong MH, Farrugia W, and Scott KF, Contribution of type II phospholipase A2 to in vitro phospholipase A2 enzymatic activity in human term placenta. *J Endocrinol* (1998), **157**:25–31.

44. Diderholm B, Stridsberg M, Norden-Lindeberg S, and Gustafsson J, Decreased maternal lipolysis in intrauterine growth restriction in the third trimester. *BJOG* (2006), **113**:159–64.

45. Glatz JFC and vanderVusse GJ, Cellular fatty acid-binding proteins: their function and physiological significance. *Prog Lipid Res* (1996), **35**:243–82.

46. Herrera E, Implications of dietary fatty acids during pregnancy on placental, fetal and postnatal development – a review. *Trophoblast Res* (2002), **16**: S9–19.

47. Hornstra G, Al MD, Van Houwelingen AC, and Foreman-van Drongelen MM, Essential fatty acids in pregnancy and early human development. *Eur J Obstet Gynecol Reprod Biol* (1995), **61**:57–62.

48. Jumpsen J, Van Aerde J, and Clandinin MT, Fetal lipid requirements: implications in fetal growth retardation. In: Placental Function and Fetal Nutrition, ed. Battaglia FC (Philadelphia: Nesttec, Vevey/Lippincott-Raven, 1997), pp. 157–65.

49. Woltil HA, Van Beusekom CM, Schaafsma A, Muskiet FA, Okken A, Long-chain polyunsaturated fatty acid status and early growth of low birth weight infants. *Eur J Pediatr* (1998), **157**:146–52.

50. Whelan J, Antagonistic effects of dietary arachidonic acid and ω-3 polyunsaturated fatty acids, *J Nutr* (1996), **126**:1086S–91S.

51. Helland IB, Smith L, Saarem K, Saugstad OD, and Drevon CA, Maternal supplementation with very-long-chain n-3 fatty acids during pregnancy and lactation augments children's IQ at 4 years of age. *Pediatrics* (2003), **111**:e39–44.

52. Uauy R, Mena P, Wegher B, Nieto S, and Salem N Jr., Long chain polyunsaturated fatty acid formation in neonates: effect of gestational age and intrauterine growth. *Pediatr Res* (2000), **47**:127–35.

53. Carlson SE, Cook RJ, Werkman SH, and Tolley EA., First year growth of preterm infants fed standard compared to marine oil ω-3 supplemented formula. *Lipids* (1992), **27**:901–7.

54. Carlson SE, Werkman SH, Rhodes PG, and Tolley EA, Visual acuity development in healthy preterm infants: effect of marine oil supplementation. *Am J Clin Nutr* (1993), **58**:35–42.

55. Hoggard N, Hunter L, Lea RG, Trayhurn P, and Mercer JG, Ontogeny of the expression of leptin and its receptor in the murine fetus and placenta. *Br J Nutr* (2000), **83**:317–26.

Nutritional regulation and requirements for pregnancy and fetal growth

Mineral requirements of the mother and conceptus

Lorraine Gambling and Harry J. McArdle

Introduction

During development, the fetus is entirely dependent on the mother for the supply of minerals. Although the dietary level required is relatively small, they are essential because they play central roles in all stages of growth and development. Minerals are both central components of catalytic sites and stabilizing factors in many enzymes and transcription factors. Therefore, they play a role in almost every cellular function, from protein translation to intracellular signalling. Clearly, any limitation in the supply will have profound effects, both short- and long-term, for the mother, fetus, and newborn. For the fetus, these damaging effects can become apparent before, or even in the absence of, any clinical signs of deficiency in the mother. The range and extent of the detrimental effects seen in the developing fetus are dependent on the severity of the deficiency, whether it occurs only for a single mineral, and the gestational age at which the deficiency occurs. Mineral supplementation during pregnancy is commonplace, but supplementation late in gestation or in postnatal life may not overcome the damage caused by the earlier restriction.

Minerals essential for pregnancy

Because of the difficulties, both ethical and practical, of studying the effect of maternal mineral status in humans, our current level of understanding has been derived mainly from observational and intervention studies in which maternal intakes, low or high, are associated with adverse or favorable pregnancy outcomes [1] and from extrapolation from animal studies [2].

Minerals known to be of major importance during pregnancy include calcium, copper, iodine, iron, magnesium, selenium, and zinc. Deficiencies in these minerals have been associated with complications of pregnancy, childbirth, or fetal development. In this review, we consider each, briefly examining their physiological roles, discussing how the symptoms of deficiency overlap, and what the short- and long-term consequences may be. For convenience, we have arranged the paragraphs on their physiological roles alphabetically, but this should not be taken as an indication of their relative importance to normal growth and development.

Calcium is the most abundant mineral in the human body. More than 99% of total body calcium is stored in the bones and teeth, where it functions to support their structure. The remaining 1% is found throughout the body in blood, muscle, and interstitial fluids [3]. Calcium also has an important regulatory role. The 1000-fold gradient between extracellular and intracellular ionic calcium concentration is fundamental to cellular signal transduction and amplification. An induced influx of calcium triggers and activates a variety of cellular physical and metabolic events, including muscle contraction, neurotransmission, enzyme and hormone secretion, and muscle and blood vessel contraction and relaxation [4].

Copper can act as an electron acceptor or donor. As such, it is central to many redox-active enzymes. For example, it is a central component of many enzymes involved in metabolic reactions including angiogenesis and oxygen transport [5]. Synthesis of a range of essential compounds, such as neurotransmitters and the proteins of connective tissue, is dependent on copper-containing enzymes, lysyl oxidase and dopamine β-monooxygenase, respectively. It is a central part of the cytochrome complexes involved in energy metabolism.

Iodine is a nonmetallic trace element; approximately 75% of the body's iodine is located in the thyroid gland. The only role known for iodine in the human body is in the synthesis of thyroid hormones by the thyroid gland, and all biological actions of iodine are ascribed to the thyroid hormones. The major thyroid hormone secreted by the thyroid gland is thyroxine, which is taken up by cells and converted into triiodithyrone. These two enzymes are required for the maintenance of metabolic rate, cellular metabolism, and integrity of connective tissue [6].

Almost two thirds of iron in the body is found in the red blood cells as hemoglobin, the protein that carries oxygen to tissues. Myoglobin, the oxygen reserve in muscle, amounts to approximately 10% of the body iron. The remaining iron is ubiquitously present throughout the body. There are four major classes of iron-containing proteins: hem proteins, iron-sulphur proteins, iron storage and transport proteins, and iron-containing enzymes. Iron is an integral part of several classes of enzymes, including cytochromes, the role of which in oxidative metabolism is to transfer energy within the mitochondria. Other iron-containing enzymes are involved in the synthesis of steroid hormones and of bile acids, detoxification of foreign substances in the liver, and synthesis of neurotransmitters, such as dopamine and serotonin in the brain.

Magnesium is the fourth most abundant mineral in the body. Approximately 50% of it is found in bone and 40% in muscles and soft tissues. Only 1% of magnesium is found in blood. The physiological importance of magnesium lies in its role in skeletal development and in the maintenance of electrical potential in nerve and muscle membranes. In bone, magnesium forms a surface constituent of the hydroxyapatite mineral component. Tissue magnesium also functions as a cofactor for enzymes requiring adenosine triphosphate (ATP), enzymes involved in energy metabolism, protein synthesis, and RNA and DNA synthesis. Calcium homeostasis is controlled in part by a magnesium-requiring mechanism.

The selenium content of normal adult humans can vary widely, reflecting the profound influence of the environment on the selenium contents of soils, crops, and human tissues. Approximately 30% of tissue selenium is contained in the liver, 15% in the kidney, 30% in muscle, and 10% in blood plasma [7]. Selenium is an integral part of many enzymes, and during stress, infection, or tissue injury, a number of these enzymes may act to protect against oxidative damage and are essential for the metabolism of thyroid hormones [8].

Zinc is a component of more than 300 enzymes, where it has structural, regulatory, or catalytic roles. Zinc-containing enzymes are involved in the synthesis and degradation of carbohydrates, lipids, proteins, and nucleic acids, as well as in the metabolism of other micronutrients. In addition, zinc acts to stabilize the molecular structures of a variety of DNA-binding proteins that contain zinc fingers [9]. This role for zinc ensures that it is vital for successful RNA synthesis and hormone responses.

Mineral deficiencies

Mineral deficiencies are a global problem, affecting both the developed and developing worlds [10]. Populations significantly at risk are the elderly, infants, growing children, and pregnant women. It is clear that a deficiency in one or more of these essential minerals will affect all major physiological functions because these deficiencies will result in alteration in cell division, cellular differentiation, and the normal pattern of protein synthesis. Years of medical and scientific studies have shown the significant and far-reaching consequences of mineral deficiencies on the population, ranging from fatigue to impaired cognitive function. Mineral deficiencies also lead to immune dysfunction, impaired brain and nervous system development, the development and function of skeletal muscle, gastrointestinal problems, and compromised bone metabolism [10]. In this section, we discuss the consequences of deficiencies using both animal and human models and consider how these might be best treated, if indeed they can.

Extent of mineral deficiencies

Deficiencies in essential minerals can occur through several mechanisms, primary and secondary. Primary deficiency is simply an inadequate dietary intake of that particular mineral. Because the fetal supply of minerals from the mother is mediated through the placenta, in the specific case of the fetus, a primary mineral deficiency can occur as a result of insufficient placental transfer. Secondary mineral deficiencies can occur through several means, including genetic disease, drug interactions, and disease-associated alterations in mineral metabolism.

Primary deficiencies – some examples

The main cause of mineral deficiencies is a poor-quality diet, often due to an inadequate intake of animal source foods, especially in vegetarians, low socioeconomic groups, and developing countries. It is unlikely that a mineral deficiency would occur in isolation. The average daily intakes for women are presented in Table 3.1. Even in the United Kingdom and the United States, daily intake of half of these minerals is significantly lower than the recommended

Table 3.1 Effects of maternal mineral deficiencies during pregnancy

	Maternal	Fetal	Neonatal
Calcium	Preeclampsia	Premature delivery Abnormal fetal development	Hypertension Increased risk of adult disease
Copper	Miscarriage	Anencephaly Abnormal fetal development	Low neonatal stores
Iodine	Miscarriage	Premature delivery Anencephaly Abnormal fetal development	Mental retardation
Iron	Preeclampsia Hemorrhage Postnatal depression	Premature delivery Spina bifida Low birth weight	Low neonatal stores Anemia Delayed neurological development Increased risk of adult disease
Magnesium	Preeclampsia	Premature delivery Spina bifida Low birth weight	Increased risk of adult disease
Selenium	Preeclampsia Miscarriage	Premature delivery Spina bifida	
Zinc	Preeclampsia	Premature delivery Anencephaly Spina bifida Low birth weight	Low neonatal stores

levels. National differences are also apparent, which is important when setting reference values and developing strategies to tackle deficiencies.

Dietary-induced mineral deficiencies are caused by a combination of total intake and bioavailability of the mineral in the diet. Iodine and selenium are generally efficiently absorbed by humans with more than 80% to 100% of that available in the diet being absorbed. However, the content differs with geochemical, soil, and cultural conditions [11]. The bioavailability of calcium from dietary components is generally less important than the overall calcium content of the diet. However, the calcium component of the diet has a significant inhibitory effect on the absorption of other minerals [11].

There are two kinds of dietary iron: hem- and nonhem iron. Hem iron is found in meat, poultry, and fish, whereas nonhem iron is obtained from cereal, pulses, legumes, fruits, and vegetables. The average absorption of hem iron is approximately 25% [12]. The absorption of nonhem iron, copper, magnesium, and zinc is influenced by several factors in the diet, including the concentration of other minerals, phytates, and protein.

Secondary deficiencies – some examples

Genetic disorders of dietary deficiencies are relatively uncommon, probably because most are prenatally lethal. Menkes syndrome is an X-linked genetic disease

Table 3.2 Average daily intakes

Mineral	United Kingdom	United States
Calcium	107	74
Copper	86	127
Iodine	108	
Iron	74	69
Magnesium	81	78
Selenium	71	185
Zinc	100	120

This table shows average daily intake for women between the ages of 19 and 50 years of age in the United Kingdom [59, 60] and the United States [61, 62]. Intake is expressed as a percentage of their national reference intakes.

that affects the placental transfer of a micronutrient because of a defect in a copper-transporting ATPase gene [13]. Babies born with this disorder have numerous problems. They are dystonic and ataxic and have a distinctive "kinky hair" phenotype. They will normally die within the first few years of life, usually from aortic aneurysms. Maternal mineral intake can also be affected by genetic diseases. For example, acrodermatitis enteropathica is an inherited disease that causes insufficient zinc absorption, and mothers with this disease deliver babies with congenital abnormalities (see Table 3.2) [14].

Table 3.3 Recommended dietary allowance

	Females aged 19–50 years	Pregnancy	Lactation
*Calcium (mg/d)	1000	1000	1000
Copper (μg/d)	900	1000	1300
Iodine (μg/d)	150	220	290
Iron (mg/d)	18	27	9
Magnesium (mg/d)	320	360	320
Selenium (μg/d)	55	60	70
Zinc (mg/d)	8	11	12

The values are stated as recommended dietary allowance, * except for calcium, which is stated as "adequate intake" for women between the ages of 19 and 50 years [11].

Therapeutic drugs can also affect maternal mineral status through altered uptake or metabolism. Several drugs chelate micronutrients, thereby reducing circulating concentrations, including D-penicillamine. Infants born to women who have received D-penicillamine during pregnancy exhibit symptoms consistent with copper deficiency, similar to those described earlier for babies with Menkes syndrome [15]. Even everyday drugs such as diuretics and laxatives can have an effect on mineral status.

Several disease states, including chronic diarrhea, diabetes, alcoholism, and hypertension, also alter mineral metabolism [16]. The teratogenesis associated with maternal diabetes and alcoholism is associated, in part, with the adverse affects of mineral deficiency [17]. Diseases such as malaria, as well as infection with intestinal parasites, also impair and alter the metabolism of multiple micronutrients [16].

Extent of mineral deficiencies

Iron and iodine are the two most common nutritional disorders in the world. Nearly half of the pregnant women in the world are thought to be iron deficient: Even in industrialized countries, most pregnant women suffer from some degree of iron deficiency. For example, 75% of pregnant women in Paris show evidence of depleted iron stores, and only 5% of women of childbearing age have adequate iron intakes [18].

Magnesium deficiency is also thought to be common; approximately 20% of the population consumes less than two thirds of the recommended dietary allowance [19] (Table 3.3). Clinical levels of deficiencies in copper, selenium, and zinc may be rare; however, mild deficiencies are likely due to the estimated levels of low intake. With the increased demands of pregnancy added to this, it is likely that many pregnant women, even in industrialized countries, will have suboptimal micronutrient status.

Effects of deficiencies

Mineral deficiencies have varied effects because of the wide range of roles they play. In pregnancy, the effects can be seen in both the mother and her fetus (Table 3.1). The mother can suffer from pregnancy-induced hypertension, anemia, preeclampsia, labor complications, and death [20].

Fetal growth and development follow a specific timeline, and therefore the susceptibility to mineral deficiency will be altered throughout pregnancy. Severe micronutrient deficiencies during pregnancy can lead to high rates of spontaneous abortion, to congenital abnormalities, and to stillbirth. More moderate reductions in mineral supply can lead to placental dysfunction, premature birth, and low birth weight. Early postnatal development is also affected with impaired neurological and immunological function. There is now growing evidence that nutrient deficiency, including minerals, during fetal development, can put the child at greater risk of adult-onset diseases such as cardiovascular disease, obesity, and Type II diabetes [21].

Maternal well-being

Iron deficiency during pregnancy increases maternal mortality. In fact, up to 40% of maternal perinatal deaths may be linked to iron-deficiency anemia [22]. It is associated with an increased risk from maternal hemorrhage, and peripartum blood loss has more severe consequences for an iron-deficient mother. In addition to maternal iron deficiency, clinical investigations have linked low maternal serum levels of calcium, magnesium, and selenium to preeclampsia (e.g. [23]). One possible hypothesis for these findings is that deficiencies in such minerals may inhibit the placenta's antioxidant defenses.

Maternal blood selenium levels are low in women who experience a first-trimester miscarriage, compared with women at the same stage of pregnancy who carry to term [24]. Similar evidence implicates low levels of copper and iodine in miscarriage [25].

Mothers who were iron deficient during pregnancy are likely to remain deficient into the postnatal period, which increases the risk of postnatal depression [26].

Fetal outcome

In the United States, approximately 3% of children are born with serious malformations, and an additional 1% die within a year from birth defects, premature birth, or low birth weight [27]. Evidence continues to mount for the role of suboptimal maternal nutrition, before and during pregnancy, in these effects. Much of our knowledge about the role of minerals in fetal development has been acquired from animal studies [2], and these studies continue to be essential for establishing the mechanisms behind these effects [28].

Premature delivery is the major cause of perinatal morbidity and mortality in the developed world. There is extensive evidence linking low maternal iron levels with an increased risk of premature birth [29], and deficiencies in calcium, iodine, magnesium, selenium, and zinc have now all been associated with preterm delivery [30].

Neural tube defects (NTDs) are one of the most common birth defects, occurring in approximately one in 1000 live births in the United States. Spina bifida and anencephaly are examples of these defects, with the most severe, anencephaly, being incompatible with life. It has been estimated that up to 70% of NTDs can be prevented by supplementation with the vitamin folate [31]. It is likely that mineral deficiencies play a role in the remaining 30% of NTDs. Evidence has now linked low maternal intakes and serum levels of iron, magnesium, selenium, and zinc with an increased risk of spina bifida [31]; in the cases of iron and magnesium this increased risk can be as great as fivefold [32]. It has also been noted that offspring born to women who suffered from acrodermatitis enteropathica, a genetic zinc deficiency disease, had a high incidence of malformations – in particular, anencephaly. Epidemiological evidence to support the role of zinc deficiency in anencephaly came from studies in the Middle East, which related a high incidence of the fetal abnormality with maternal zinc deficiency [33]. The interactions of these minerals with folate may also have a significant impact on the incidence of NTDs and pregnancy outcome. In fact, it has long been noted that pregnancy outcome is significantly improved when folate and iron supplementation is provided together [34]. A molecular connection has been established between these two critical micronutrients, with a protein identified, SLC46A1, which acts as both a folate and hem transporter [35].

Investigations into two severe genetic disorders in humans, Menkes and occipital horn syndromes, have provided clear evidence for the essential role of copper in fetal development. These two X-linked diseases are caused by mutations in the copper-transporting ATPase gene, *ATP7A*. Infants with Menkes syndrome are characterized by progressive degeneration of the brain and spinal cord, hypothermia, connective tissue abnormalities, and failure to thrive. These abnormalities can all be linked to decreased activity of a number of copper-dependent enzymes [13].

Neonatal nutrition

Exclusive breast-feeding is now recommended by all international agencies for the first 6 months of life because of the benefits for infant health. The importance of the mother's nutritional status has been highlighted [36] but it is not routinely monitored. This is particularly important in the case of minerals such as iodine and selenium, for which the concentration in milk has been shown to be sensitive to changes in the maternal diet during lactation [37]. In contrast, maternal diet has no effect on the milk content of copper, iron, magnesium, or zinc [38]. It has been shown that the transport of copper, iron, and zinc into breast milk is tightly controlled by transporters in the mammary gland [39]. Interestingly, although the calcium content of breast milk is not dependent on maternal intake during lactation, it does seem to relate to maternal calcium intake during the last third of pregnancy [40].

The mineral supply present in milk is believed to be in highly bioavailable forms [39]. For example, it is estimated that infants can use more than 50% of the iron in breast milk compared with less than 12% of the iron in infant formula. The concentrations of minerals in breast milk decrease during the first 6 months, resulting eventually in an insufficient supply of minerals from breast milk later in infancy [41]. This decreasing level of nutrient supply brings into focus the importance of mineral stores accumulated by the infant during pregnancy.

The infant's gestational age and birth weight strongly affect the size of stores at birth, with the last fifth of gestation being critical [42]. Therefore, preterm infants may not have accumulated the required amount of mineral stores to sustain growth through the period in which they are exclusively breast-fed [43]. This is also likely to be the case for full-term infants born to mineral-deficient mothers. Several studies have shown that a normal birth weight infant born to an anemic mother is more likely to develop anemia during the first 6 months of life than a normal birth weight infant born to a mother with adequate iron status [44]. There is also recent information that extending the breast-feeding period from 4 to 6 months, even in infants of normal iron status, may result in iron deficiency, because the mother cannot give sufficient iron from her breast milk [45].

Offspring development

The effects of maternal mineral deficiency persist well beyond gestation and parturition. For humans, the current evidence indicates that the brain is the organ most sensitive to these prolonged effects. One of the most devastating consequences of maternal iodine deficiency is irreversible mental retardation in the offspring. These effects occur because iodine is required for the synthesis of thyroid hormones, which in turn regulate the metabolic pattern of most organs, especially the brain. Even mild or subclinical maternal hypothyroidism during pregnancy may have subtle effects on neuropsychological development of the offspring [46]. The window of sensitivity also extends into the neonatal period because iodine deficiency in lactating women may result in insufficient iodine to the infant.

Infants who were subject to iron deficiency in the womb also display symptoms of impaired brain development. Unfortunately, the effects are long-lasting and may be irreversible. Children who had a low iron status at birth have significantly worse language ability, fine-motor skills, and emotional control (47).

In the past 2 decades, epidemiological studies have shown, even within the normal range for birth weight, that there is an inverse correlation between weight at birth and adult risk of disease and development of specific degenerative conditions, including obesity, coronary heart disease, stroke, Type II diabetes, cancer, and depression [21]. Maternal nutrition is an important factor in determining birth weight; therefore, it is now believed that inappropriate nutrition during gestation may affect the offspring's risk of developing certain diseases in adulthood, a phenomenon know as *fetal programming*. The mechanism(s) through which inappropriate nutrition during gestation exerts its effects is currently unclear. To this end, several animal models have been established, using global caloric restriction or alteration in a specific dietary component [48].

Models of maternal mineral deficiency are among those models clearly mimicking the human situation. Offspring subjected to iron deficiency during gestation develop hypertension, dyslipidemia, and obesity [49]. As yet no other model of maternal mineral deficiency has shown all of these particular symptoms, but maternal calcium deficiency has induced hypertension in the offspring [50], and perinatal magnesium restriction predisposes the offspring to insulin resistance and glucose intolerance [51].

Adaptations during pregnancy and lactation

To meet the increased demand for the essential minerals during pregnancy and lactation, maternal physiology undergoes several alterations. Maternal intestinal uptake is increased, excretion is decreased, and minerals are mobilized and reutilized from various body stores. In recognition of the increased requirements, many government-recommended daily allowances (RDAs) are higher for pregnant and lactating women than for the general population.

Absorption

Most minerals of those discussed here are absorbed from the small intestine through both an active, saturable mechanism and simple diffusion [11].

As the demand for iron increases in the second trimester, absorption increases by about 50%, and in the last trimester it may increase by up to approximately 4 times (7). Pregnancy has also been shown to increase the efficiency of absorption of calcium, copper, and zinc, although to a lesser extent than demonstrated for iron [52, 53].

Excretion

Selenium bioavailability and absorption are high even in the nonpregnant state; therefore, to conserve more selenium, pregnancy induces a decrease in urinary selenium excretion [52]. A similar mechanism also improves copper retention, but only by approximately 4% [53].

Utilization and redistribution of body stores

To meet the increased demands during pregnancy and lactation, maternal stores are mobilized, and other maternal sources of minerals are redistributed. Some minerals, such as iron, have extensive stores in the body, as ferritin in the liver. It is estimated that a pre-pregnancy store level of 500 mg is required for the mother and fetus to remain iron sufficient throughout gestation [7]. Unfortunately, it is uncommon for women today to have iron stores of this size, which at least partly accounts for the high incidence of iron deficiency in pregnancy.

Unlike iron, there are no easily accessible stores of calcium, magnesium, and zinc. For these minerals, the skeleton acts as a "store," and during pregnancy and lactation, these minerals are mobilized [54]. Bone turnover is elevated during pregnancy and lactation. Additionally, selenium, some magnesium, and zinc can be released through tissue catabolism and reutilized for the needs of the fetus [55].

Placental transfer

The greatest period of fetal mineral accumulation takes place from mid-gestation and is maximal during the third trimester. Minerals are transported across the placenta by both passive diffusion and active transport. Selenium is passively transported across the placenta [56], and hence the fetus is critically dependent on maternal levels. The active transport mechanisms, especially those operating for iron, ensure that the fetus has an adequate supply of nutrients – if necessary, at the expense of the maternal stores or even functional pools [57]. The fact that during the third trimester, fetal concentrations of calcium are greater than those in the mother indicates active transport of calcium [58]. Evidence has been put forward for both passive and active placental transfer of copper, possibly related to the stage of gestation [5].

Recommended daily intake

An increased RDA is recommended during pregnancy for all but one of the minerals discussed in this chapter (Table 3.3). Information on what is thought to be the required dietary requirement for each individual mineral is provided by many agencies acting for national governments, the European Commission, and the World Health Organization. Because there is considerable variation in nutrient requirements throughout a person's lifetime, values are given for specific life stages, including pregnancy and lactation. The values are regularly updated, taking into account new scientific knowledge regarding the links among nutrition, health, and disease. Currently the most up-to-date dietary reference values are provided

by the United States and Canada (Table 3.3). The RDA is the average daily nutrient intake level that is required to meet the nutrient requirements of almost all – 97% – of healthy individuals in a particular life stage and sex group. Historically, dietary reference values for pregnancy were estimated by a factorial method, combining total maternal and fetal demand. The more recent reference values, including those listed here, take into account the known physiological adaptations to pregnancy that occur in the mother. The recommendations now also take into account the age of the mother, because in adolescent pregnancies, intakes need to be increased by an amount proportional to the incomplete maternal growth at conception.

The nutritional demands of lactation are considerably greater than those of pregnancy. Newborns double their birth weight within the first 4 to 6 months of life. For breast milk to provide all the nutritional requirements underpinning this growth rate, it must provide an amount of energy equivalent to the total energy cost of pregnancy. Therefore, along with the continued maternal physiological adaptation, a further increase in daily dietary intake is recommended for most of the minerals.

Conclusions

In conclusion, we have discussed the variety and complexity of mineral requirements during pregnancy. We have not included many aspects. For example, we have not discussed interactions between the micronutrients. In itself, this is a complex and multifaceted area, and there are many interactions we do not understand. We know that iron and copper metabolism are tightly interlinked and are beginning to comprehend the mechanisms. Zinc, iron, and copper are also linked, but we know little about how the interactions are mediated. Calcium and iron, iodine and selenium, also show mutual regulation. We have not examined many studies that have tested supplementation strategies, because the literature is vast, complex, and inconclusive. Neither have we considered the consequences of dietary overload of minerals, mainly because this is a rare problem in pregnancy. For these, more detailed discussions, the reader is referred to the many excellent reviews published in the *British Journal of Nutrition*, among others. We hope, however, we have provided an overview of the fascinating and clinically essential roles that minerals play during development, gestation, and lactation.

References

1. Picciano MF, Pregnancy and lactation: physiological adjustments, nutritional requirements and the role of dietary supplements. *J Nutr* (2003), **133**:1997S–2002S.

2. Widdowson EM, Trace elements in foetal and early postnatal development. *Proc Nutr Soc* (1974), **33**:275–84.

3. Nordin B, ed., *Calcium, Phosphate and Magnesium Metabolism* (Edinburgh: Churchill Livingstone, 1976).

4. Bootman MD, Collins TJ, Peppiatt CM, Prothero LS, MacKenzie L, De Smet P, et al., Calcium signalling – an overview. *Semin Cell Dev Biol* (2001), **12**:3–10.

5. Ralph A and McArdle H, *Copper Metabolism and Requirements in the Pregnant Mother, Her Fetus, and Children* (New York: International Copper Association, 2001).

6. Delange F, The disorders induced by iodine deficiency. *Thyroid* (1994) **4**:107–28.

7. Organisation FaAOotUSaWH, *Vitamin and Mineral Requirements in Human Nutrition* (Bangkok, Thailand: Joint FAO/WHO Expert Consultation, 2004, pp. 21–30).

8. Arthur JR, Nicol F, and Beckett GJ, The role of selenium in thyroid hormone metabolism and effects of selenium deficiency on thyroid hormone and iodine metabolism. *Biol Trace Elem Res* (1992), **34**:321–5.

9. Berg JM and Shi Y, The galvanization of biology: a growing appreciation for the roles of zinc. *Science* (1996), **271**:1081–5.

10. Sanghvi T, Van Ameringen M, Baker J, Fiedler J, Borwankar R, Phillips M, et al., Vitamin and mineral deficiencies technical situation analysis: a report for the Ten Year Strategy for the Reduction of Vitamin and Mineral Deficiencies. *Food Nutr Bull* (2007), **28**(Suppl 1):S160–219.

11. Academies IoMotN, *Dietary Reference Intakes. The Essential Guide to Nutrient Requirements* (Washington, DC: National Academies Press, 2006).

12. Hallberg L, Bioavailability of dietary iron in man. *Annu Rev Nutr* (1981), **1**:123–47.

13. Kaler SG, Menkes disease. *Adv Pediatr* (1994), **41**:263–304.

14. Verburg DJ, Burd LI, Hoxtell EO, and Merrill LK, Acrodermatitis enteropathica and pregnancy. *Obstet Gynecol* (1974), **44**:233–7.

15. Rosa FW, Teratogen update: penicillamine. *Teratology* (1986), **33**:127–31.

16. Bo S, Lezo A, Menato G, Gallo ML, Bardelli C, Signorile A, et al., Gestational hyperglycemia, zinc, selenium, and antioxidant vitamins. *Nutrition* (2005), **21**:186–91.

17. Uriu-Hare JY, Stern JS, and Keen CL, Influence of maternal dietary Zn intake on expression of diabetes-induced teratogenicity in rats. *Diabetes* (1989), **38**:1282–90.

18. Galan P, Hercberg S, Soustre Y, Dop MC, and Dupin H, Factors affecting iron stores in French female students. *Hum Nutr Clin Nutr* (1985), **39**:279–87.

19. Durlach J, New data on the importance of gestational Mg deficiency. *J Am Coll Nutr* (2004), **23**:694S–700S.

20. Ramakrishnan U, Manjrekar R, Rivera J, Gonzalez-Cossio T, and Martorell R, Micronutrients and pregnancy outcome. *Nutr Res* (1999), **19**:103–59.

21. Barker DJ, Mothers, Babies and Health in Later Life (Edinburgh: Churchill Livingstone, 1998).

22. Scholl TO and Hediger ML, Anemia and iron-deficiency anemia: compilation of data on pregnancy outcome. *Am J Clin Nutr* (1994), **59**(Suppl 2):492S–500S, discussion S–1S.

23. Rayman MP, Bode P, Redman CW, Low selenium status is associated with the occurrence of the pregnancy disease preeclampsia in women from the United Kingdom, *Am J Obstet Gynecol* (2003), **189**:1343–9.

24. Barrington JW, Lindsay P, James D, Smith S, and Roberts A, Selenium deficiency and miscarriage: a possible link? *Br J Obstet Gynaecol* (1996), **103**:130–2.

25. Buamah PK, Russell M, Milford-Ward A, Taylor P, and Roberts DF, Serum copper concentration significantly less in abnormal pregnancies. *Clin Chem* (1984), **30**:1676–7.

26. Corwin EJ, Murray-Kolb LE, and Beard JL, Low hemoglobin level is a risk factor for postpartum depression. *J Nutr* (2003), **133**:4139–42.

27. Kimmel CA, Generoso WM, Thomas RD, and Bakshi KS, A new frontier in understanding the mechanisms of developmental abnormalities. *Toxicol Appl Pharmacol* (1993), **119**:159–65.

28. Keen CL, Clegg MS, Hanna LA, Lanoue L, Rogers JM, Daston GP, et al., The plausibility of micronutrient deficiencies being a significant contributing factor to the occurrence of pregnancy complications. *J Nutr* (2003 May); **133**(5 Suppl 2):1597S–605S.

29. Allen LH, Biological mechanisms that might underlie iron's effects on fetal growth and preterm birth. *J Nutr* (2001), **131**(2S-2):581S–9S.

30. Aggett PJ, Trace elements of the micropremie. *Clin Perinatol* (2000), **27**:119–29, vi.

31. Czeizel AE and Dudas I, Prevention of the first occurrence of neural-tube defects by periconceptual vitamin supplementation. *N Engl J Med* (1992), **327**:1832–5.

32. Groenen PM, van Rooij IA, Peer PG, Ocke MC, Zielhuis GA, and Steegers-Theunissen RP, Low maternal dietary intakes of iron, magnesium, and niacin are associated with spina bifida in the offspring. *J Nutr* (2004), **134**:1516–22.

33. Cavdar AO, Arcasoy A, Baycu T, and Himmetoglu O, Zinc deficiency and anencephaly in Turkey. *Teratology* (1980), **22**:141.

34. Mahomed K, Iron and folate supplementation in pregnancy. *Cochrane Database of Systematic Reviews* (2006), 3:CD001135.

35. Laftah AH, Latunde-Dada GO, Fakih S, Hider RC, Simpson RJ, and McKie AT, Haem and folate transport by proton-coupled folate transporter/haem carrier protein 1 (SLC46A1). *Br J Nutr* (2008), **10**:1–7.

36. World Health Organization, The Optimum Duration of Exclusive Breastfeeding (2001). Available at: http://www.who.int/nutrition/publications/optimal_duration_of_exc_bfeeding_report_eng.pdf.

37. World Health Organization, Selenium (Geneva: World Health Organization, 1987).

38. Dorea JG, Iron and copper in human milk. *Nutrition* (2000), **16**:209–20.

39. Lonnerdal B, Trace element transport in the mammary gland. *Annu Rev Nutr* (2007), **27**:165–77.

40. Ortega RM, Martinez RM, Quintas ME, Lopez-Sobaler AM, and Andres P, Calcium levels in maternal milk: relationships with calcium intake during the third trimester of pregnancy. *Br J Nutr* (1998), **79**:501–7.

41. Krebs NF and Hambidge KM, Zinc requirements and zinc intakes of breast-fed infants. *Am J Clin Nutr* (1986), **43**:288–92.

42. Dewey KG and Chaparro CM, Session 4: Mineral metabolism and body composition iron status of breast-fed infants. *Proc Nutr Soc* (2007), **66**:412–22.

43. Lonnerdal B, Copper nutrition during infancy and childhood. *Am J Clin Nutr* (1998), **67**(Suppl 5):1046S–53S.

44. De Pee S, Bloem MW, Sari M, Kiess L, Yip R, and Kosen S, The high prevalence of low hemoglobin concentration among Indonesian infants aged 3–5 months is related to maternal anemia. *J Nutr* (2002), **132**:2215–21.

45. Chantry CJ, Howard CR, and Auinger P, Full breastfeeding duration and risk for iron deficiency in U.S. infants. *Breastfeed Med* (2007), **2**:63–73.

46. Vermiglio F, Lo Presti VP, Moleti M, Sidoti M, Tortorella G, Scaffidi G, et al., Attention deficit and hyperactivity disorders in the offspring of mothers exposed to mild-moderate iodine deficiency: a possible novel iodine deficiency disorder in developed countries. *J Clin Endocrinol Metab* (2004), **89**:6054–60.

47. Tamura T, Goldenberg RL, Hou J, Johnston KE, Cliver SP, and Ramey SL, et al., Cord serum ferritin concentrations and mental and psychomotor development of children at five years of age. *J Pediatr* (2002), **140**:165–70.

48. Armitage JA, Khan IY, Taylor PD, Nathanielsz PW, and Poston L, Developmental programming of the metabolic syndrome by maternal nutritional imbalance: how strong is the evidence from experimental models in mammals? *J Physiol* (2004), **561**:355–77.

49. Gambling L, Dunford S, Wallace DI, Zuur G, Solanky N, Srai SK, et al., Iron deficiency during pregnancy affects postnatal blood pressure in the rat. *J Physiol* (2003), **552**:603–10.

50. Bergel E and Belizan JM, A deficient maternal calcium intake during pregnancy increases blood pressure of the offspring in adult rats. *BJOG* (2002), **109**:540–5.

51. Venu L, Kishore YD, and Raghunath M, Maternal and perinatal magnesium restriction predisposes rat pups to insulin resistance and glucose intolerance. *J Nutr* (2005), **135**:1353–8.

52. King JC, Effect of reproduction on the bioavailability of calcium, zinc and selenium. *J Nutr* (2001), **131**(Suppl 4):1355S–8S.

53. Turnlund JR, Swanson CA, and King JC, Copper absorption and retention in pregnant women fed diets based on animal and plant proteins. *J Nutr* (1983), **113**:2346–52.

54. Krebs NF, Reidinger CJ, Robertson AD, and Brenner M, Bone mineral density changes during lactation: maternal, dietary, and biochemical correlates. *Am J Clin Nutr* (1997), **65**:1738–46.

55. World Health Organization, Trace Elements in Human Health and Nutrition (Geneva: World Health Organization, 1996).

56. Nandakumaran M, Dashti HM, Al-Saleh E, and Al-Zaid NS, Transport kinetics of zinc, copper, selenium, and iron in perfused human placental lobule in vitro. *Mol Cell Biochem* (2003), **252**:91–6.

57. Gambling L, Charania Z, Hannah L, Antipatis C, Lea RG, and McArdle HJ, Effect of iron deficiency on placental cytokine expression and fetal growth in the pregnant rat. *Biol Reprod* (2002), **66**:516–23.

58. Namgung R and Tsang RC, Bone in the pregnant mother and newborn at birth. *Clin Chim Acta* (2003), **333**:1–11.

59. Henderson L, Irving K, Gregory J, Bates C, Prentice A, Perks J, et al., Vitamin and mineral intake and urinary analytes. In: The National Diet & Nutrition Survey: Adults Aged 19 to 64 Years (London: Her Majesty's Stationary Office, 2004).

60. Ministry of Agriculture, Faculty of Agriculture and Forestry. Total diet survey – aluminium, arsenic, cadmium, chromium, copper, lead, mercury, nickel, selenium, tin and zinc. Food Surveillance Information Sheet No. 191 (London: Her Majesty's Stationary Office, 1999).

61. Alaimo K, McDowell MA, Briefel RR, Bischof AM, Caughman CR, Loria CM, et al., Dietary intake of vitamins, minerals, and fiber of persons ages 2 months and over in the United States: Third National Health and Nutrition Examination Survey, Phase 1, 1988–91. *Adv Data* (1994), **14**:1–28.

62. Board IoMFaN. Dietary Reference Intakes for Vitamin C, Vitamin E, Selenium and Carotenoids (Washington, DC: The National Academy of Sciences, 2000). Available at: http://books.nap. edu/ openbook.php?record_id= 9810&page=R1.

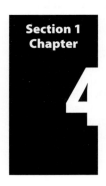
Nutritional regulation and requirements for pregnancy and fetal growth

Individualized growth curves and size at birth

Eve Blair

Measuring appropriateness of fetal growth

Growth is the rate of increase in a dimension per unit time. Mass is the dimension traditionally considered for fetal growth because it is the most easily and accurately measured dimension at birth, but with prenatal imaging, prenatal growth of body parts can be monitored. Recognition of the importance of fetal growth is implicit in the importance traditionally accorded birth weight as an indicator of pregnancy success. With increasing survival of preterm births and increasing sources of evidence from which to estimate gestational duration, Lubchenco et al. [1] estimated appropriateness of intrauterine growth from the position on a chart of birth weight by duration of gestational age (GA). This introduced the concept of time to the consideration of size at birth and initiated the study of fetal growth. An example of the now-familiar sigmoid plots of observed birth weight against GA is shown in Figure 4.1.

The importance of accurate data for gestational duration

The belated introduction of the time dimension is doubtless associated with the difficulty of accurately measuring gestational duration, given its usually occult initiation. The traditional method of estimating GA from maternal recall of the date of commencement of the last normal menstrual period (LNMP) relies on assumptions concerning the accuracy of recall, length of menstrual cycle and the position of ovulation therein, menstrual regularity, and an absence of hormonal perturbations (e.g. prior conceptions, hormone therapies). The evidence required to support these assumptions is frequently lacking. The reliability of the LNMP method can be enhanced by early pregnancy testing and clinical examination, but the

introduction of ultrasound fetometry provided a further valuable source of evidence. Estimating GA from fetal size assumes a uniform rate and pattern of growth between fetuses. This assumption holds precisely in the hours after conception but becomes less tenable as pregnancy progresses. The time at which the most accurate estimates of GA can be made by fetometry is a compromise between being before discernible variation in growth rate develops between fetuses but after a well-defined dimension is sufficiently large compared with the errors in making the measurement. Measurement of maximum embryonal length at approximately 10 weeks gestation, before the spine has started to flex, has been suggested as the best compromise [2]. At this time, gestation can be estimated to within 5 days. However, many women have not presented for antenatal care by 10 weeks post-LNMP. After 12 weeks gestation, the smaller biparietal diameter of the head is the dimension utilized for gestational dating by ultrasound fetometry, so the measurement error can be proportionally greater, decreasing the precision of the GA estimate.

Much effort has been expended in improving the accuracy of neonatal assessment of GA, but even the most accurate measures [3, 4], which require both time and training to perform, are rather imprecise with systematic biases away from term [5] and may require adjustment for ethnic origins [6]. However, in contrast to antenatal estimates, neonatal GA is estimated directly as a number of weeks, rather than a date (of LNMP) or a fetal dimension on a given date, minimizing the risk of recording errors, so neonatal estimates tend to be reliably recorded. Thus neonatal estimates provide a valuable check on antenatal estimates, recording errors in the data that have been demonstrated to be responsible for a substantial proportion of the recorded GAs that were incompatible with recorded birth weight [7] in pregnancies resulting from extrauterine fertilization for which gestational

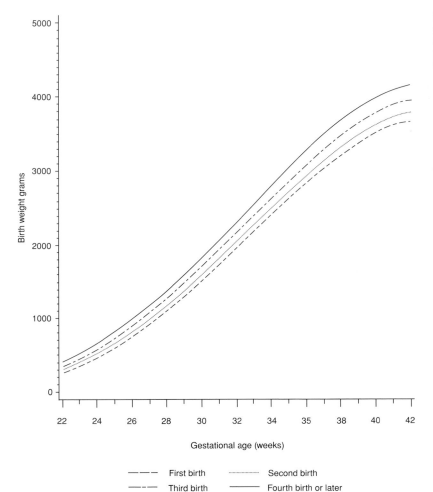

Figure 4.1 Mean of male and female optimal birth weight by gestational age at delivery and parity, estimated for births to women of height 162 cm. (Redrawn from Blair et al. [16].)

duration is accurately known. Neonatal estimates therefore serve primarily to indicate gross errors in recorded antenatal estimates [8].

However achieved, an accurate estimate of GA is the first requirement for estimating the appropriateness of fetal growth. With GA available, growth can be assessed by comparing the measured gestation-specific anthropometric dimension with a standard. Therefore, the second requirement is an appropriate standard, and the third is selection of how the comparison should be made.

Selecting a standard of fetal growth

Lubchenco's charts were derived from a population residing in Denver, Colorado, altitude 1610 m (5280 feet), where lower atmospheric oxygen tension slows rates of fetal growth. Comparison with these charts therefore overestimated the appropriateness of growth of neonates born at lower altitudes. Altitude is only one of the factors responsible for differences in interfetal growth rates; for example, the same GA girls tend to weigh less than boys, taller parents tend to have larger babies, and primiparous women and women carrying multiple pregnancies tend to have smaller babies. When such determinants are taken into account the standard is said to be *individualized*.

Obstetricians may be interested in predicting actual birth weight if they want to make timely decisions concerning the method of delivery. In this case, it is appropriate to consider all known determinants of fetal growth along with gestational duration to achieve the most accurate prediction. Factors known to be associated with fetal growth include infant gender and other genetically endowed traits, ethnicity, maternal size, maternal weight gain, paternal size, maternal parity, plurality of the pregnancy, maternal lifestyle factors including nutritional status, exposure to tobacco smoke and other toxins, altitude of residence, maternal medical factors including diabetes, hypertensive disease (with or without proteinuria), and infections, particularly TORCH (toxoplasma, other viruses, rubella, cytomegalovirus, herpesvirus) infections and those of the genitourinary tract. Individualized predicted fetal growth curves can be derived by statistical modeling that accounts for as many factors for which good data are available in representative samples [9].

Because it is appropriate for different fetuses to grow at different rates, the estimation of fetal growth may be considered in terms of appropriateness of growth given the circumstances of that particular fetus. Inappropriate growth may reflect an underlying pathology, which, if recognized, can be treated, ameliorated, indicate the need for further observations, or predict outcome. Furthermore, appropriateness of growth is frequently considered as a factor in epidemiological research. To identify appropriateness of growth, an obvious standard for comparison is the optimal growth trajectory, how the fetus would grow in the absence of any pathological factors affecting its growth. In such circumstances, the only factors determining the rate of growth would be nonpathological.

Nonpathological determinants of fetal growth

Fetal sex is perhaps the only incontrovertibly nonpathological factor, but many others are usually nonpathological or unalterable, particularly once fetal growth is being assessed.

Chromosomal anomalies, genetic anomalies, and factors resulting in other birth defects may affect fetal growth, and it is safest to exclude all births with birth defects from the population from which optimal growth trajectories are derived. Parental growth potential dictates the growth potential of their offspring. This is usually reflected in parental stature, unless the parents' genetic potential for growth has not been realized, as may occur, for example, following exposure to nutritional deprivation in childhood. In developed countries, childhood nutritional deprivation is unusual, and parental heights may be considered a surrogate measure of the inherited potential for growth to adulthood in their offspring. Bodybuilders

aside, lean body weight may also be considered a surrogate for the genetic potential for body size, but the more usually available measure of body weight during the pregnancy is also influenced by the highly variable fat mass, and for the mother, by the increasing weight of the products of conception.

If appropriateness of growth is to be estimated from fetal dimensions, then duration of growth (GA) must be considered. In the absence of mistaken induction (or pregnancy termination), very low GA at delivery has a pathological cause; however, time itself cannot be considered a pathological factor. Thus, GA at delivery is not a pathological determinant of weight, although certain values of GA are associated with growth-restricting pathologies.

Maternal weight gain during pregnancy is associated with birth weight primarily because it includes the mass of the fetus. It is therefore a measure of fetal growth (imperfect on account of including weights of maternal fluid volume expansion and products of conception other than the fetus) rather than a determinant.

The maternal contribution to fetal growth includes both her genetic contribution to the fetus' growth potential and her ability to provide fetal nutrition. The latter will be limited by the uterine area available for placentation, for which maternal height may also be considered a surrogate. Thus, maternal size is a stronger determinant of fetal growth than is paternal size, particularly because, at least in population studies, the identity of the father is seldom confirmed.

Birth weight has frequently been observed to vary with ethnicity [10]. However, mean maternal size, gestational duration, and social, economic, and nutritional status can vary significantly between ethnic groups, as can the frequency of growth-determining pathology. All these factors should be considered when comparing optimal growth trajectories between ethnic groups, particularly those with the strongest effects on birth weight – namely, gestational duration, maternal size, and frequency of growth-restricting pathologies. When these are adjusted for, differences in growth trajectory tend to diminish. For example, the consistently lower weights of births to Aboriginal women in Western Australia have been shown to be almost entirely explained by a slightly shorter mean GA, a higher burden of recognized growth-restricting pathology, and tobacco smoke exposure. With the unquantifiable contribution attributable to social disadvantage, it was concluded that these factors were responsible for the

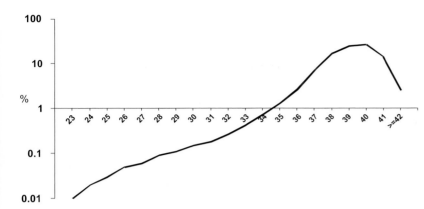

Figure 4.2 Distribution of gestational duration at delivery for singleton neonatal survivors: Western Australia, 1980–2000.

lower birth weights rather than any ethnic difference in optimal fetal growth rate [9]. Obviously, maternal lifestyles and medical pathologies adversely affecting fetal growth must be considered pathological.

The increasing fetal growth rate with increasing parity (Figure 1) has been attributed to what has been termed *priming of the uterus* or *irreparable damage to the epithelium of the spiral arteries*. This facilitates nutrient transfer through uterine blood vessels in subsequent pregnancies. At which parity does optimal growth occur? The best pregnancy outcomes are associated with second and third births, but selection by social and medical factors may be more responsible for this observation than any effects attributable to variations in fetal growth. Because first pregnancy is unavoidable if there is to be a second or third, parity is usually considered a nonpathological determinant of fetal growth, although biologically fetal growth in the first pregnancy may be considered restricted. Similarly, fetal growth is curtailed in a multiple pregnancy when the sum of fetal demands approaches the maternal limits of supply. Naturally this occurs earlier in pregnancy as the number of fetuses increases. This may account for at least some part of the less optimal outcomes of multiples born after the onset of multiplicity-related growth restriction than those of singletons born at the same gestations. However, because pregnancy reduction, at least of twin pregnancies, is seldom desired nor are the hazards warranted, it is reasonable to compare growth with a standard optimal for a given multiplicity, thus treating multiplicity as a nonpathological determinant of growth.

The optimal growth curve should therefore be individualized to the individual's sex, multiplicity of the pregnancy, maternal height and parity, and, when paternity is known with certainty, paternal height. Pregnancies affected by any of the pathological determinants of fetal growth should be excluded from the population from which the optimal standards are derived (e.g. Blair 2005).

Birth weight versus estimated fetal weights and statistically modelled trajectories

Growth charts were initially constructed from the observed median birth weight of infants born in each gestational week. Problems with this method include:

1. The decreasing number of births with decreasing GA; see Figure 4.2.
2. The bi- or multimodal distribution of birth weight observed at low gestations.
3. The observed increase in dispersion of weights about the mean weight with decreasing gestation.
4. The pathological causes of preterm birth may impair fetal growth, and preterm born infants tend to be systematically growth restricted relative to infants of the same gestational age whose pregnancies continue to term.

The nonuniform GA distribution could be addressed by selecting several preterm birth cohorts to each term cohort, the sampling multiple increasing with decreasing GA. However, to achieve a sample with a similar number of births before 28 weeks as at term, the sampling multiple for births less than 28 weeks would approximate an unachievable ~110-fold.

The second and third observations are biologically counterintuitive and arise primarily as a result

37

of errors in the recorded GA. Some errors are systematic on account of breakthrough bleeding at 4-week intervals early in pregnancy, the frequency of which decreases rapidly at each 4-week interval. If this bleeding is mistaken for a normal menstrual period, GA estimated from LNMP dates, even if certain and accurately recorded, will be systematically underestimated by 4 weeks or, less frequently, by 8 weeks [11, 12]. Even though only a small proportion of births are likely to have such systematically underestimated gestations, because the vast majority of births occur at term or near term (Figure 4.2), the small proportion of term and near-term births with systematically underestimated GAs contributes a significant proportion of those recorded as being born 4 or 8 weeks earlier, creating multimodal distributions. The extremely nonuniform GA distribution also means that random errors increase the distribution of birth weights at less frequently occurring GAs to a greater degree than the more frequently occurring. GA errors, particularly the systematic 4- and 8-week gestational overestimations, can be largely eliminated when they most affect median birth weight by setting upper limits to acceptable birth weights in the GA range at which growth is sufficiently rapid for there to be little overlap between weight distributions 4 gestational weeks apart [13, 14].

The fourth problem, the tendency of preterm births to be growth restricted, initially recognized by Lubchenco et al. [1], is the most intransigent. In response, intrauterine growth charts have been constructed from fetal weights estimated from fetometric measurements taken throughout gestation on infants subsequently born at term. The problem with these lies in the accuracy of the estimating equations. Systematic weight overestimation is likely because the equations relating fetal weight to fetometric dimensions are derived from births that must necessarily occur *after*, usually up to 7 days after, the measurements were made. It also assumes that the shape of preterm born infants will reflect those of infants at the same gestation who are subsequently born at term. Dudley, systematically reviewing the performance of such equations [15], concluded that random errors were large, with systematic overestimation of low- and underestimation of high-weight fetuses and questioned the validity of such equations, even without taking into account the delay in weight measurement in the data from which the equations are derived.

Do all preterm born infants grow abnormally relative to their gestational peers subsequently born at term, or is it possible to select normally grown preterm born infants? From the 1998–2002 cohort of Western Australian Caucasian singleton neonatal survivors, pregnancies affected by the factors most frequently associated with pathological deviations in growth were excluded. These factors were maternal smoking, vascular disease or diabetes, birth defects, or TORCH infections [16]. These criteria excluded 37.6% of the population that were born at term, 54.4% of those born 33–36 weeks GA, and 76.6% of those born <33 weeks GA, confirming that the frequency of growth-deviating pathology is associated with gestation of delivery. However, we had no reason to believe that the remaining 23.4% of those born <33 weeks ($n = 334$), 45.6% of those born 33–36 weeks ($n = 2522$), and 62.4% of term births ($n = 59 557$) would be abnormally grown and used the characteristics of these births to derive equations for *optimal* growth curves that included terms for fetal sex, maternal height, and parity.

The development of individualized growth curves has been made possible by the increasing sophistication of computer software that fits statistical models (equations) relating a continuous outcome (e.g. birth weight) to many variables. These may be plotted as in Figure 4.1 for specific sets of circumstances, but an equation is both more flexible and robust because it represents all possible circumstances. Therefore, individualized growth curves are usually presented by equations for median weight rather than graphs.

How to "measure" appropriateness of growth

Lubchenco et al.'s growth charts [1] presented a series of percentile positions on the birth weight distribution observed in each gestational stratum, the 10th being the lowest percentile presented and the 90th being the highest. Much clinical practice involves making decisions – for example, differentiating normal from abnormal, so observations tend to be categorized. This occurred in the study of fetal growth, and traditionally those with weights below some cutoff point, often the 10th percentile position, occasionally 3rd percentile or two standard deviations from mean, are categorized as small for their gestational age (SGA) and those above the 90th as large for gestational age (LGA), implying that these weights are less appropriate than intermediate weights. However, these cutoff points are arbitrary: births identified by lower cutoff points are more likely to be pathologically growth restricted, but a greater proportion of pathologically growth-restricted infants will be excluded than with higher cutoff points. It is frequently desirable to have a measure of the degree of inappropriateness, and percentile position has significant drawbacks as a quantitative variable and is suboptimal even as a categorical variable because:

- Percentiles are ordered, but not interval, measures in which the difference in the dimension between adjacent percentiles at the extremes is very much greater than those in the middle of the distribution, presenting limited valid analytical possibilities and a great potential for misinterpretation.
- Extreme percentile positions (those frequently of most interest) are at the extremes of an approximately Gaussian distribution where observations are sparse and most subject to error. They are therefore the least precise and the most sensitive to data quality.
- Extreme percentiles are the most sensitive to the incidence of growth-disturbing pathologies in the population and vary most with the health of the population used as the standard [16].

Percentile positions should therefore be abandoned in favor of a more generalizable, continuous measure of which the ratio of observed dimension to an individualized value of the dimension at peak observation density is an obvious example. For birth weight, this ratio has been termed the *birth weight ratio* [17], the individualized birth weight ratio [18], or, more descriptively, the proportion of optimal birth weight [16]. Birth weight is often considered because, for many pregnancies, the sole assessment of growth is made at birth. However, a better appreciation of growth can be obtained by comparing the growth trajectory of specific fetal dimensions throughout gestation with an individualized standard. This allows the differentiation of fetuses for whom the dimension follows a similar trajectory to that of fetuses without growth-restricting pathology (for whom the proportion of optimal ratio will remain constant) from fetuses with a faltering of the initial trajectory, for whom the proportion of optimal will drop. After the possibility of measurement error has been eliminated (by replicating observations), the later are growth restricted, whatever their birth weight. The dimensions most often measured fetometrically for this purpose are the head circumference, its diameters, femur length, and, most sensitively in the third trimester, abdominal circumference.

The role of maternal nutrition in fetal growth

The conceptus is initially nourished in a low-oxygen environment by polyols secreted from the uterine walls. This appears to be quite immune to external manipulation in naturally occurring conceptuses, but after a placental supply has been established, maternal nutritional status has a complex relationship with fetal growth, much researched in the interests of animal husbandry. However, the relevance of animal research to human pregnancy and diets is questionable, and only human data are discussed here. A significant proportion of the human literature reports observational data from which it is not possible to differentiate cause, effect, or merely noncausal associations mediated by factors such as social class. Such studies serve primarily to suggest nutritional hypotheses that should be tested in randomized controlled trials before dietary interventions can be recommended. The evidence reported here is therefore confined to randomized controlled trials or other experimental settings where the nutritional interventions were not self-selected.

There are methodological challenges in the study of nutritional supplementation in human populations associated primarily with the initial nutritional status of subjects. Neglect of these challenges may account for the confusion in the literature, spawning many systematic reviews and even a review of systematic reviews [19]. A nutritional supplement is of benefit only if the supplement is a biological requirement and not already present in sufficient quantities. Additional supplementation may even be detrimental. Therefore, if the initial status of research subjects is heterogeneous with respect to the nutrient, the results of its supplementation can also vary. Nonetheless, a few comments can be made.

Under famine or near-famine conditions, fetal growth appears increasingly restrained by a lack of maternal energy supply as pregnancy progresses. Observations made following the unique event of the short-term Dutch famine during World War II indicate that birth weight was most affected when famine was experienced only in the second half of pregnancy [20]. In developing countries, maternal macronutritional deficiencies can occur frequently and have been successfully addressed by balanced protein/energy supplementation [19, 21]. The effects on birth weight tend to be small, and the benefits may be better measured by perinatal mortality [22, 23]. High protein supplementation (>20% of energy provided as protein) has repeatedly been shown to reduce fetal growth in both the developed and developing world, although protein-induced birth weight reduction may not be accompanied by the anticipated increase in perinatal mortality [22]. Maternal macronutritional deprivation is rare in the developed world, and efforts to increase the reduced birth weight seen in underprivileged women in the developed world by macronutrient supplementation tend to be unsuccessful.

In the developed world, the major causes of fetal growth pathology are maternal vascular disease, particularly preeclampsia, maternal infections, particularly of the genitourinary tract, chromosomal and genetic anomalies, and, increasingly, syndrome X, the metabolic anomaly that includes diabetes and insulin resistance. There is some evidence that these may respond to micronutritional therapy. However, as with macronutrient therapy, micronutrient therapy is beneficial only if the specific nutrients being supplied are lacking initially and are supplied in a timely fashion.

Nutrient supplementation and fetal growth

The literature related to preeclampsia is given as an example. Preeclampsia affects up to 5% of all pregnancies, depending on its definition. It is associated with raised maternal blood pressure, proteinuria, and fetal growth restriction; if severe, it can be life-threatening to both mother and child. It is more likely to occur in primiparae and in women with a family history of preeclampsia or a history of preeclampsia in previous pregnancies. It has been variously suggested that vitamin D [24], marine oils [25], vitamins C plus E [26], and calcium [27] can each protect against preeclampsia, but the results of randomized controlled supplementation trials have been confusing. Two Cochrane systematic reviews published in 2005 suggested that vitamin C (five trials and 766 women)[28] and vitamin E (four trials, 566 women)[29] may alone or in combination reduce the incidence of preeclampsia with relative risks approaching statistical significance. The authors concluded that insufficient data were available and conducted a much larger trial in which supple-

mentation with 1000 mg vitamin C plus 400 IU vitamin E was associated with a small, statistically insignificant increase in the frequency of preeclampsia. These differences could have been due to chance because all trials had similar levels of vitamin supplementation and much higher than recommended daily intakes, and most subjects lived in developed countries. However, they varied with respect to subject selection criteria. The latest, largest trial selected primiparae between 14 and 22 weeks in whom more than 90% of both intervention and control groups had adequate vitamin C intake, and approximately 43% had adequate vitamin E intake before supplementation. The trials included in the earlier systematic reviews selected women at higher a priori risk of preeclampsia, and their vitamin status before supplementation was not known.

Whether the initial vitamin status of subjects can explain the observed differences for vitamin C and E supplementation, the systematic review of the calcium supplementation to prevent preeclampsia [27] makes it clear that calcium supplementation is beneficial only to women with low initial calcium intake.

If nutritional supplements can be beneficial only if they are lacking, the question is whether any essential vitamins and minerals are routinely lacking in pregnant women in developed countries. There is a significant minority of women who appear to require more folate than is obtained from their diet to avoid neural tube defects, and many women are chronically short of iron because of menstruation. Thus, their routine supplementation appears defensible. Randomized controlled trials have shown that iron supplementation can increase birth weight in Zimbabwe [30], and a systematic review concluded that the decrease in proportion of low birth weight and SGA babies following multivitamin supplementation was attributable entirely to the iron and folate components [31], although a randomized controlled trial from Nepal observed a mean gain in birth weight of 77 g when 13 micronutrients were added to iron and folate supplementation, somewhat more than might have been anticipated from the 1.2-day increase in gestational duration. However, such trials tend to be conducted in developing countries, and Milman [32] sounded a word of caution, pointing out that iron negatively influences the absorption of other divalent metals (which includes calcium) and should not be supplemented if ferritin is present at more than 70 μg/l.

It has been argued that because the diet afforded by modern mass market agricultural methods is depleted in many vitamins and minerals relative to diets produced at a more leisurely pace [33], and because health promotion messages to minimize exposure to sunlight in the interests of avoiding skin cancers have resulted in a population tendency to vitamin D deficiency [24], it may be advisable even for women with apparently adequate diets to take a balanced multivitamin supplement before and during pregnancy. However, the possibility of detrimental effects with oversupplementation (as with iron or protein) and the likelihood of inappropriate supplementation, demonstrated to be common in Finland [34], suggest that the conclusion arrived at by Ramachandran [35] in India, who stated that each women should be assessed individually before appropriate dietetic advice can be given, is universally applicable.

Fetal growth has a tightly programmed schedule. After a stage has passed, it cannot be revisited. Therefore, when deviation from an established fetal growth trajectory is recognized, it is too late to correct that deviation by addressing any nutritional imbalance that may have caused it. Any recognized nutritional deficiency should of course be rectified because this may prevent further disadvantage and will assist the woman in recovering from the pregnancy, but for optimum fetal growth, women must enter pregnancy in a nutritionally optimal state. The use of individualized growth curves cannot do much to direct nutritional advice for the index pregnancy, although it can inform such advice for subsequent pregnancies and for the woman's recovery.

Conclusion

Individualized fetal growth curves can be used to assess the appropriateness of fetal growth given the nonpathological characteristics or predict size at birth given all growth-determining characteristics of the pregnancy. Fetal growth may be affected by the mother's nutrition throughout her life. In developed countries, adequate micronutrition before conception and avoidance of teratogens in early pregnancy are the nutritional factors most relevant to optimal fetal growth. In developing countries, it may be necessary to add adequate balanced macronutrition throughout pregnancy, but this is an unusual problem in developed countries where an oversupply of macronutrients leading to obesity and diabetes poses greater problems.

Summary Table

Obtaining an individualized growth curve

- Decide whether you want to (a) identify optimal size or (b) predict actual size.
- Choose the fetal or newborn dimension of interest.
- Choose the variables on which you wish to individualize: (a) nonpathological determinants of fetal growth, (b) all known and measurable determinants of fetal growth.
- Choose from the literature or derive a standard that addresses the variables on which you wish to individualize or is derived from a population with characteristics similar to the index individual.

Estimating appropriateness of growth

- Estimate GA of the index individual as accurately as possible.
- Obtain the optimal dimension estimated for the individual by solving the chosen standard equation for the values of the determinants appropriate to the individual, including GA.
- Divide the observed value of the dimension by the optimal value, multiply by 100 to give a percentage; 100% indicates that the newborn is optimally grown, and the further from 100%, the less appropriate the individual's growth.
- For birth weight, ratio values between 85% and 115% are generally considered normal.
- For longitudinal fetometric measurements, note the ratio at each assessment. A constant ratio indicates an appropriate growth trajectory.

Predicting actual size

- Solve the chosen standard equation for the values of the determinants appropriate to the individual, where GA takes the value at which delivery is anticipated.

References

1. Lubchenco LO, Hansman C, Dressler M, and Boyd E, Intrauterine growth as estimated from liveborn birth weight data at 24 to 42 weeks gestation. *Pediatrics* (1963), **32**:793–800.

2. Wisser J, Dirschedl P, and Krone S, Estimation of gestational age by transvaginal sonographic measurement of greatest embryonic length in dated human embryos. *Ultrasound Obstetr Gynecol* (1994), **4**:457–62.

3. Dubowitz L, Dubowitz V, and Goldberg C, Clinical assessment of gestational age in the bewborn infant. *J Pediatr* (1970), **77**:1–10.

4. Ballard J, Novak K, and Driver M, A simplified score for diagnosis of gestational age in the newborn infant. *J Pediatr* (1979), **95**:769–74.

5. Alexander G, Hulsey T, Smeriglio V, Comfort M, and Levkoff A, Factors influencing the relationship between a newborn assessment of gestational maturity and the gestational age interval. *Paediatr Perinat Epidemiol* (1990), **4**:133–46.

6. Sayers S, Estimation of Gestational Age in Aboriginal Neonates (Darwin, Australia: Menzies School of Health Research Annual Report 1988–89, 1989).

7. Callaghan W, Schieve L, and Dietz P, Gestational age estimates from singleton births conceived using assisted reproductive technology. *Pediatr Perinat Epidemiol* (2007), **21**(Suppl 2):79–85.

8. Blair E, Liu Y, and Cosgrove P, Choosing the best estimate of gestational age from routinely collected population-based perinatal data. *Pediatr Perinat Epidemiol* (2004), **18**:270–6.

9. Blair E, Why do Aboriginal neonates weigh less? II. Determinants of birthweight for gestation. *J Paediatr Child Health* (1996), **32**:498–503.

10. Gardosi J, Ethnic differences in fetal growth. *Ultrasound Obstetr Gynecol* (1995), **6**:73–4.

11. Blair E and Stanley FJ, Intrauterine Growth Charts for Singleton Liveborn West Australian Infants (Canberra: Australian Government Printer, 1985).

12. Ananth C, Menstrual versus clinical estimate of gestational age dating in the United States: temporal trends and variability in indices of perinatal outcomes, *Pediatr Perinat Epidemiol* (2007), **21**(Suppl 2):22–30.

13. Liu YC and Blair EM, Predicted birthweight for singletons and twins. *Twin Res* (2002), **5**:529–37.

14. Qin C, Dietz P, England L, Martin J, and Callaghan W, Effects of different data-editing methods on trends in race-specific preterm delivery rates, United States,1990–2002. *Pediatr Perinat Epidemiol* (2007), **21**(Suppl 2):41–9.

15. Dudley N, A systematic review of the ultrasound estimation of fetal weight. *Ultrasound Obstetr Gynecol* (2005), **25**:80–9.

16. Blair E, Liu Y, de Klerk N, and Lawrence D, Optimal fetal growth for the Caucasian singleton and assessment of appropriateness of fetal growth: analysis of a total population perinatal database. *BMC Pediatr* (2005), **5**(13).

17. Morley R, Brooke O, Cole T, Powell R, and Lucas A, Birthweight ratio and outcome in preterm infants. *Arch Dis Child* (1990), **65**:30–4.

18. Wilcox M, Johnson I, Maynard P, Smith S, and Chilvers C, The individualised birthweight ratio: a more logical outcome measure of pregnancy than birthweight alone. *Br J Obstetr Gynaecol* (1993), **100**:342–7.

19. Merialdi M, Carroli G, Villar J, Abalos E, Gulmezoglu A, Kulier R, et al., Nutritional interventions during pregnancy for the prevention or treatment of impaired fetal growth: an overview of randomized controlled trials. *J Nutr* (2003), **155**(Suppl 2):1626S–31S.

20. Morley R, Owens J, Blair E, and Dwyer T. Is birthweight a good marker for gestational exposures that increase the risk of adult disease? *Paediatr Perinat Epidemiol* (2002), **16**:194–9.

21. Kramer M, Energy and protein intake in pregnancy. *Cochrane Database of Systematic Reviews* (2003), **4**:CD000032.

22. Rush D, Maternal nutrition and perinatal survival. *Nutr Rev* (2001), **59**:315–26.

23. Di Mario S, Say L, and Lincetto O, Risk factors for stillbirth in developing countries: a systematic review of the literature. *Sex Transm Dis* (2007), **34**:S11–21.

24. Perez-Lopez F, Vitamin D: the secosteroid hormone and human reproduction. *Gynecol Endocrinol* (2007), **23**:13–24.

25. Makrides M, Dudley L, and Olsen S, Marine oils and other prostaglandin precursor, supplementation for pregnancy uncomplicated by pre-eclampsia or intrauterine growth restriction (2006). Available at: http://www.cochrane.org/reviews/en/ab003402.html.

26. Rumbold A, Crowther C, Haslam R, Dekker G, and Robinson J, Vitamins C and E and the risks of preeclampsia and perinatal complications. *N Engl J Med* (2006), **354**:1796–806.

27. Hofmeyr G, Roodt A, Atallah A, and Duley L, Calcium supplementation to prevent pre-eclampsia – a systematic review. *S Afr Med J* (2003), **93**:224–8.

28. Rumbold A and Crowther C, Vitamin C supplementation in pregnancy (2005). Available at: http://www.cochrane.org/reviews/en/ab004072.html.

29. Rumbold A and Crowther C. Vitamin E supplementation in pregnancy (2005). Available at: http://www.cochrane.org/reviews/en/ab004069.html.

30. Mishra V, Thapa S, Retherford R, and Dai X, Effect of iron supplementation during pregnancy on birthweight: evidence from Zimbabwe. *Food Nutr Bull* (2005), **26**: 338–47.

31. Haider B, and Bhutta Z, Multiple-micronutrient supplementation for women during pregnancy (2006). Available at: http://www.cochrane.org/reviews/en/ab004905.html.

32. Milman N, Iron prophylaxis in pregnancy – general or individual and in which dose? *Ann Hematol* (2006), **85**:821–8.

33. Glenville M, Nutritional supplements in pregnancy: commercial push or evidence based? *Curr Opin Obstetr Gynecol* (2006), **18**:642–7.

34. Arkkola U, Uusitalo U, Pietikainen M, Metsala J, Kronberg-Kippila C, Erkkola M, et al., Dietary intake and use of dietary supplements in relation to demographic variables among pregnant Finnish women. *Br J Nutr* (2006), **96**:913–20.

35. Ramachandran P, Maternal nutrition – effect on fetal growth and outcome of pregnancy. *Nutr Rev* (2002), **60**:S26–34.

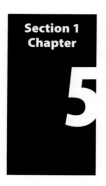

5 Maternal diets in the developing world

Shobha Rao and Chittaranjan Yajnik

- Poor fetal growth in the developing world is largely attributed to widespread maternal undernutrition.
- In most developing countries in Asia and Africa, the rates of low birth weight are above 20%, calling for Public Health action.
- Low birth weight is prone to reduced growth, altered body proportions, and a number of metabolic and cardiovascular changes.
- In addition to a woman's good nutrition throughout life, a sociodemographic environment that is conducive to sustaining optimal fetal growth is necessary.
- Maternal diets in the developing world are inadequate in major macronutrients. Moreover, cultural beliefs, practices, and food taboos greatly influence maternal intake.
- Multiple micronutrient deficiencies exist because of inadequate food intake, poor dietary quality, poor bioavailability, or a combination of these factors.
- Systematic research is essential to identify micronutrients of potential interest, examine whether intervention at the preconceptional stage could have an impact on fetal growth, explore food-based interventions and test their efficacy, and so on.

Introduction

In recent years, several developing countries, especially in Southeast Asia, have seen relative prosperity, middle-class affluence, and unprecedented economic development. It is uncertain, however, whether this has been associated with improvements in health, especially that of women and children, and whether the underlying determinants of ill health have changed [1], for in many Asian countries, childhood malnutrition continues to be a major public health problem. High prevalence of low birth weight (LBW) continues to be a major nutritional concern. Eighty percent of all newborns with LBW at term are born in Asia; approximately 15% and 11% are born in middle and western Africa, respectively; and 7% are born in the Latin American and Caribbean regions [2]. The majority of LBW in developing countries is due to intrauterine growth restriction (IUGR), whereas most LBW in industrialized countries results from preterm birth. High prevalence of LBW in developing countries is therefore a reflection of a more severe problem related to maternal undernutrition.

Poor fetal growth in the developing world is largely attributed to widespread maternal undernutrition. In fact, poor nutritional status at conception, low gestational weight gain due to inadequate dietary intake, and short maternal stature due to mother's own childhood undernutrition or infection are believed to be the major determinants for LBW in developing countries [3]. Infants born with LBW suffer from extremely high rates of morbidity and mortality, underweight, stunting, or wasting through childhood. Moreover, recent studies provide evidence for the association of intrauterine undernutrition with increased risks of adult disease. The implication is that even before eliminating the long-standing problem of undernutrition, developing countries such as India face epidemics of diabetes, hypertension, and coronary heart disease. Maternal nutrition is thus of paramount importance and requires critical understanding to plan effective strategies. In particular, identifying effective time windows for nutritional interventions to adolescents or pregnant women, understanding the role of macro- and micronutrients in fetal growth, and considering the importance of various nonnutritional factors are some of the major issues that require urgent attention.

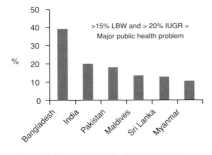

Source: de Onis et al. (1998) *Eur J Cl Nutr* 52(S1):S5.

Figure 5.1 Incidence of low birth weight at term in selected Asian countries . (From de Onis M, Blössner M, and Villar J, Levels and patterns of intrauterine growth retardation in developing countries. *European Journal of Clinical Nutrition* [1998], 52[Suppl 1]:S5–15.)

Prevalence of LBW in developing world

The geographical incidences of LBW at term in selected Asian countries show that Bangladesh has the highest incidence (~40%), followed by India and Pakistan (between 20% and 25%; Figure 5.1). In most developing countries in Asia and Africa, the rates are above 20%, calling for public health action.

The majority of LBW in developing countries is due to IUGR, the causes of which are complex and multiple, depending primarily on the mother, placenta, fetus, and combinations of all three. The countries where high proportions of LBW are seen are also the countries where women have low body mass index indicating maternal undernutrition. Although poor maternal nutritional status is a major determinant of LBW, the factors responsible range from sociodemographic to genetic, illustrating a wide spectrum of underlying causes. To arrive at effective strategies to combat the problem of LBW, it may be necessary to first look into the short- and long-term implications of LBW. For example, maternal nutritional interventions could be short-term remedies, whereas education, gender discrimination, and poverty must be dealt with through long-term strategies.

The risk of neonatal death for infants who weigh between 2000 and 2499 g at birth is estimated to be 4 times higher compared with those weighing 2500 to 2999 g and 10 times higher compared with those weighing 3000 to 3499 g [4]. Apart from high mortality risk, various studies have shown the relation of LBW with risk of morbidity. In India and Bangladesh, more than half of the deaths due to pneumonia could be prevented if LBW were eliminated. In fact, LBW is also implicated as a contributor to impaired immune

function, which may be sustained throughout childhood [5–7].

Among survivors of LBW, another important problem is childhood growth. Most LBW children remain shorter and lighter as adults. Similarly, the impact on neurological function is yet another adverse effect that LBW babies face, and it is not clear whether existing interventions directed toward these infants will improve their cognitive outcome. In developing countries where children are exposed to poor nutrition, high levels of infection, and other conditions of poverty, the long-term development is dependent on the quality of their environment. Because LBW occurs more often in deprived environments, it can serve as a marker of associated poor outcomes throughout life.

The recent hypothesis on fetal origins of adult diseases suggests that fetal undernutrition at critical periods of development in utero and during infancy leads to permanent changes in body structure and metabolism [8–11]. Adults born with LBW suffer an increased risk of high blood pressure, obstructive lung disease, high blood cholesterol, and renal damage. In short, those of LBW are prone to reduced growth, altered body proportions, and a number of metabolic and cardiovascular changes. The hypothesis not only has brought a paradigm shift from genetic explanations of noncommunicable disease to phenotypic ones but has also emphasized the overwhelming importance of maternal nutrition. It further implies that improving nutrition of young girls and women is probably the important step toward the prevention of LBW and its accompanying disease burden to break the cycle of intergenerational undernutrition and LBW.

Maternal undernutrition before conception

Although large-scale food shortages and famines are now uncommon, rates of maternal malnutrition in the developing countries are among the highest in the world. Countries with a higher percentage of LBW generally have a higher percentage of women with low body mass index (BMI). Several studies have reported a positive correlation between maternal anthropometry (weight/height/BMI) and birth weight [12, 13]. Undernutrition evident by decreased maternal height (stunting) and below normal prepregnancy body weight and pregnancy weight gain are among the strongest predictors of LBW. Pre-pregnancy body weight and gestational weight gain have an

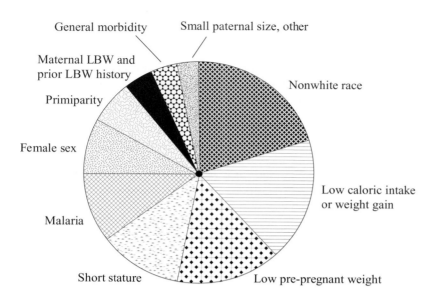

Figure 5.2 Relative importance of established factors with direct causal impact on intrauterine growth retardation (IUGR) in rural developing countries. (From Kramer,[3] figure 1, P.2.)

independent but cumulative influence on birth weight (Figure 5.2).

A better understanding of the relationship of birth size to maternal nutrition is critical for planning effective interventions to improve birth weight. However, the relationship is not yet clearly understood. Studies that investigated the relationship are scarce, and those that are available are inconsistent [14]. This relationship is influenced by many biological and socioeconomic factors that vary widely among different populations. For example, it differs among adolescents [15], among women from low socioeconomic class [16] who have poor nutritional status before conception, and even in most developed countries such as Austria, where women have cosmetic undernutrition [17]. India's poor fetal growth is at least partly caused by maternal chronic energy deficiency and stunting [18]. A study from rural Maharashtra, India, reported that size at birth was strongly predicted by maternal pre-pregnancy nutritional status [19]. Inadequate maternal nutrition around the time of conception is reported to be associated with nongenetic congenital abnormalities and LBW [20]. Maternal weight is a composite of the mother's own intrauterine, infant, childhood, and pubertal growth, as well as of energy and protein balance in adult life. Her nutritional experiences at these different times are reflected in her head circumference, height, fat, and muscle mass. A striking new finding of the Pune Maternal Nutrition Study (PMNS) was that maternal head circumference was the measurement most strongly related to overall fetal growth and neonatal abdominal and mid upper arm circumference [19].

Studies in Jamaica have in fact indicated that in humans, poor dietary status before conception may be a risk factor for LBW and also for elevated blood pressure in offspring [21]. Additionally, our work on Wistar rats has clearly demonstrated that poor nutritional status before conception may show influence on functioning of vital organs by way of inflated glucose and cholesterol levels in offspring at later ages [22].

The populations in which proportions of mothers with low BMI are high are also the populations in which several sociodemographic factors have a significant impact. For example, in countries such as India where son preference is high, most girls experience undernutrition from childhood. It is known that a girl child is less likely to be breast-fed and receives less medical treatment during illness because of gender bias. In fact, it has been reported that beyond the age of 5 years, the nutritional intakes of female children are lower than male children in every age group [23]. A review of Indian studies shows that girls have greater mortality rates in infancy, shorter periods of breast-feeding, less varied diet during preschool and school age, and less attention paid to their health compared with boys [24]. Continuation of slow and gradual height growth even beyond 18 years has been reported in undernourished children from poor communities. The continuation of growth at later ages raises significant concerns, especially in the case of rural girls who marry at an early age and have early conception.

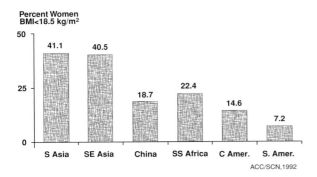

Figure 5.3 Chronic energy deficiency in women aged 15 to 49 years.

Adolescent pregnancy is known to increase risk for pregnancy wastage and LBW [15], even in Western populations. The case becomes worse for rural undernourished girls, for whom nutritional stress begins in childhood and continues through adolescence into adulthood. Low dietary intake and participation in farming activities demanding higher energy lead to sustained energy deficits. A majority of young married girls from developing countries thus have poor nutritional status before conception and need urgent attention (Figure 5.3).

One of the social factors that has been shown to have a significant impact is maternal literacy. Maternal education is shown to be significantly associated with age at marriage, age at first delivery, seeking antenatal care, and having hospitalized care, all of which are known to have an effect on birth weight [25]. These observations not only highlight the importance of good nutrition throughout a woman's life time but also indicate the need for a sociodemographic environment that is conducive to sustaining optimal fetal growth.

Maternal nutrition – macronutrients

Maternal malnutrition has been shown to be associated with fetal malnutrition, and estimates of IUGR in the less developed countries, especially those in South Asia, range from 25% to 50%. Nutritional deficiencies are common in women of reproductive age in developing countries, with epidemiological and biological studies suggesting that specific nutritional deficiencies can contribute to maternal morbidity and in turn affect the pregnancy outcome. Similarly, nutritional insults during different periods of gestation have differing effects on birth. Early work of McCance and Widdowson [26] showed that undernutrition in early

intrauterine life tends to produce small but normally proportional animals, whereas undernutrition later in development leads to selective organ damage and disproportionate growth. A major difference in developed and developing countries is that proportional growth retardation is common in developing countries, whereas disproportionate growth retardation is common in developed countries. Asymmetrical IUGR infants have better prognoses for long-term growth and development than do symmetrical IUGR infants.

Poverty is a basic underlying cause of maternal malnutrition in most poor communities of the developing countries. Maternal diets are therefore mainly lacking in major macronutrients. In India too, despite large differences in habitual dietary patterns in different States of India, several studies report low dietary intakes of energy and protein [27–29]. Many of the earlier maternal interventions were therefore concentrated on supplying energy and proteins. However, studies of energy protein supplementation during pregnancy have produced varying and sometimes conflicting results [30], although the most recent RCT trial from the Gambia has reported that a high energy, antenatal dietary supplement can increase maternal weight gain, reduce LBW by 35%, and significantly reduce stillbirth and neonatal deaths by 55% and 40%, respectively [31, 32].

Cultural beliefs, practices, and food taboos also play a role to some extent in determining maternal intakes in some of the populations in developing countries. For example, in rural populations in India, foods such as chicken, meat, eggs, banana, or papaya are considered to be "hot" foods that cause abortion and are prohibited during pregnancy. Similarly, social beliefs such as that the desire for more sleep during pregnancy is a sign of female fetus or that working until late gestation results in easy delivery in fact have adverse influences on pregnancy outcome. Further, in the absence of medical facilities in rural areas, especially in remote or tribal areas, maternal intakes are intentionally kept low to prevent a baby from becoming big and thus reducing difficulties at the time of delivery. All such beliefs and practices clearly contribute to the problem of LBW.

In many poor communities in the developing world where LBW is a major problem, women are often involved in hard work such as farming activities throughout gestation. The impact of maternal activities on birth size, combined with low nutritional intake, cannot be overlooked. Among rural mothers enrolled in the PMNS, it was observed that maternal activity was inversely related to birth size even after adjusting for maternal confounding variables. In particular, a strenuous activity such as fetching water from the well was associated with lower birth weight [33]. Reported studies [34] show that farming communities often are exposed to seasonal energy stress because of slack and harvest periods that greatly affect the maternal intakes. In fact, it has been shown that prevalence of LBW differed significantly in these seasons. Further, it was observed that reduction in activity can influence birth size, especially during harvest season, when more food is available. The implication is that maternal activity can be a modifiable factor to improve birth size in farming communities.

Maternal nutrition – micronutrients

In most populations, maternal diets are inadequate in both macronutrients and micronutrients. However, it cannot be denied that macronutrient deficiency has received by far the most attention, and as a result energy/protein-rich interventions are under way in many developing countries. Among reasonably well-nourished women of industrialized countries, maternal diet has at most a small impact on placental and birth weights, but it may be an important determinant of fetal growth in developing countries [35]. Maternal micronutrient deficiencies are less recognized. However, available data on the relationship between maternal micronutrient status with actual pregnancy outcome is scarce. In India, more than 60% of women suffer from folate deficiency, and those deficiencies are greater in magnitude during pregnancy. Subclinical vitamin deficiencies suffer from subtle functional deficits. It has been shown using animal models that pups born to dams fed a 50% vitamin-restricted diet had significantly higher body fat and altered lipid metabolism at 6 months of age, suggesting a predisposition to insulin resistance in later life [36]. Similarly, in a prospective study on urban women from South India, the most notable finding was that low maternal vitamin B_{12} concentration throughout pregnancy was independently associated with increased risk of IUGR even after controlling for all possible maternal factors [37].

It is also true with regard to deficiencies of minerals such as iron, zinc, and calcium, which are known to have an important role in fetal growth. In a comparative study on women who delivered LBW babies

with those who delivered normal weight babies, it was observed that the maternal diets in the former group were deficient in folate, iron, and calcium [38]. Although nutrient requirements in the first trimester are quantitatively small, nutritional deprivation during this period can adversely affect placental structure and indirectly ultimately the birth weight. Deficiencies of vitamin A, folate, and iron may be associated with growth retardation, whereas supplementation with calcium and manganese may increase birth weight and length [39]. Placental and fetal growth is thus most vulnerable to maternal nutrition (protein and micronutrients) status in the early pregnancy (first trimester), a period of peri-implantation and of rapid placental development [40]. This has been also supported by an observational study showing that onset of coronary artery disease was earlier among persons conceived during the Dutch Famine [41].

Although maternal undernutrition in developing countries is often in the form of multiple micronutrient deficiencies, the literature linking maternal micronutrient status with birth size is dominated by studies of single micronutrients [42]. One of the major findings of the PMNS was that consumption of micronutrient-rich foods such as green leafy vegetables, fruit, and milk was significantly associated with fetal growth (Table 5.1) [43], even after adjusting for maternal confounding factors. Furthermore, this association was even stronger among undernourished women (<40 kg, i.e. below the lowest tertile of maternal pre-pregnancy weight). In this population, birth size was not associated with energy or protein intake but was associated with consumption of these micronutrient-rich foods. These observations suggest that micronutrients play an important role when macronutrients in the maternal diet are inadequate.

Micronutrients can affect birth weight directly, indirectly, or both by their interaction with each other. Deficiency in one or more micronutrients is due to inadequate food intake, poor dietary quality, poor bioavailability, or a combination of these factors. Thus, quite often in developing countries where LBW is prevalent, multiple micronutrient deficiencies coexist, and the reductionist approach seems illogical. There is no such thing as a key micronutrient and a single micronutrient supplement would be expected to produce an effect only if it were the sole nutrient limiting fetal growth. A systematic review on micronutrients and fetal growth shows that there is no good evidence that single-micronutrient supplements lead to

Table 5.1 Relation between frequency of maternal intake of green leafy vegetables and fruits at 28 weeks gestation and milk at 18 weeks gestation and neonatal anthropometry among rural mothers

Food group	Frequency	N	Birth weight (g)	Length (cm)	Head[a] (cm)	Mid upper arm[a] (cm)	Abdominal[a] (cm)	Triceps skinfold, mm	Sub-scapular skinfold (mm)	Placental weight (g)
						Neonatal measurements				
Green Leafy Vegetables, wk 28	Never	60	2571 ± 356	47.0 ± 2.0	32.6 ± 1.2	9.6 ± 1.0	28.2 ± 1.8	3.9 ± 1.4	3.9 ± 1.2	347 ± 69
	<Once/wk	175	2601 ± 341	47.5 ± 1.9	32.9 ± 1.2	9.6 ± 0.8	28.2 ± 2.0	4.0 ± 1.2	4.1 ± 1.2	354 ± 66
	Once/wk+	225	2675 ± 363	48.0 ± 2.0	33.2 ± 1.2	9.7 ± 0.9	28.6 ± 1.9	4.1 ± 1.2	4.0 ± 1.2	358 ± 82
	≥ Alternate days	149	2742 ± 350	47.9 ± 1.9	33.3 ± 1.2	9.9 ± 0.9	29.1 ± 1.7	4.4 ± 1.2	4.3 ± 1.2	371 ± 81
	p^1		<0.001	<0.01	<0.001	<0.05	<0.001	<0.001	<0.05	<0.05
	p^2		<0.005	<0.05	<0.005	<0.05	<0.005	<0.001	<0.05	0.41
Fruits, wk 28	<Once/wk	44	2598 ± 340	47.5 ± 1.7	32.7 ± 1.1	9.7 ± 0.8	28.6 ± 2.0	4.1 ± 1.2	4.2 ± 1.2	352 ± 76
	Once/wk+	363	2633 ± 355	47.5 ± 2.0	32.9 ± 1.2	9.6 ± 0.9	28.5 ± 1.9	4.1 ± 1.2	4.1 ± 1.2	353 ± 75
	≥ Once/day	202	2721 ± 357	48.1 ± 1.9	33.4 ± 1.2	9.8 ± 0.8	28.8 ± 1.9	4.1 ± 1.2	4.2 ± 1.2	370 ± 79
	p^1		<0.01	<0.01	<0.001	0.09	0.15	0.44	0.67	<0.05
	p^2		0.13	0.23	<0.01	0.80	0.45	0.38	0.99	0.07
Milk products, wk 18	Never	95	2643 ± 369	47.5 ± 2.0	32.9 ± 1.2	9.6 ± 1.0	28.5 ± 2.1	4.2 ± 1.2	4.1 ± 1.2	354 ± 78
	<0nce/wk	134	2618 ± 356	47.6 ± 2.0	33.0 ± 1.2	9.7 ± 0.9	28.6 ± 1.7	4.1 ± 1.2	4.1 ± 1.2	348 ± 79
	Once/wk+	116	2639 ± 344	47.6 ± 2.0	33.0 ± 1.1	9.5 ± 0.8	28.5 ± 1.9	4.1 ± 1.2	4.1 ± 1.2	352 ± 71
	≥ Alternate days	281	2704 ± 361	48.0 ± 2.0	33.2 ± 1.3	9.8 ± 0.9	28.8 ± 2.0	4.1 ± 1.2	4.1 ± 1.2	371 ± 77
	p^1		<0.05	<0.05	<0.01	<0.05	0.15	0.90	0.41	<0.01
	p^2		0.14	0.13	<0.01	0.11	0.52	0.48	0.46	<0.01

[a] Circumference.

Values are mean ± SD.

p^1 values after adjustment for sex, parity, and gestational age at delivery; p^2 values after additional adjustment for pre-pregnant weight, energy intake, activity, social class, weight gain up to 28 weeks, and relevant micro- and macronutrients – namely, erythrocyte folate concentration for green leafy vegetables, serum vitamin C concentration for fruits, and fat intake for milk products.

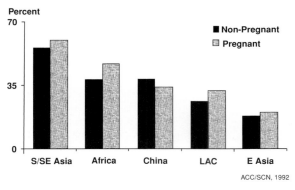

ACC/SCN, 1992

Figure 5.4 Prevalence of anemia in women aged 15 to 49 years.

improvement in fetal growth and survival in under-nourished populations. The more logical approach of multiple-micronutrient supplements has been inadequately tested [42]. Randomized control trials examining the impact of multiple vitamin and mineral supplementation during gestation on birth weight, although scarce, have shown significant effects [44, 45].

In view of the widespread prevalence of anemia (Figure 5.4) and the unequivocal benefits of folic acid in preventing neural tube defects, the most popular maternal intervention with micronutrients that is under way in many developing countries is that of iron and folic acid. However, it cannot be denied that despite implementation of this maternal intervention over 2 decades, it has hardly improved the pregnancy outcome in India. It is worthwhile to mention here that this supplementation is often given in the last 100 days of pregnancy, although in fact it is required in early pregnancy. Secondly, the dose of folic acid given in this intervention is high, approximately 4 times the requirements of a nonpregnant woman. Increasing concern has been raised for high levels of folic acid supplementation in regions where vitamin B_{12} deficiency is endemic [46]. In particular, imbalance between folate and vitamin B_{12} may be associated with adverse neurological effects in vulnerable sectors of the population such as pregnant and lactating women and their infants [47]. A recent finding from the PMNS has shown that children born to mothers with lowest vitamin B_{12} but highest folate status had the most adipose tissue and the highest insulin resistance at age 6 years [48].

Reappraisal of maternal interventions

The current research thus underscores the importance of maternal nutrition in the short-term – that is, with respect to improving birth outcome – and in the long-term, given that fetal adaptations to maternal undernutrition increase risks of adult disease in later life. Reappraisal of maternal interventions is essential not only to improve existing interventions but also to explore future possibilities through systematic research.

First, it is necessary to investigate whether the addition of a few micronutrients to existing interventions with iron and folic acid is necessary to improve birth outcome. For example, vitamin A, calcium, or zinc could be of potential interest given their association with fetal growth. Thus, well-conducted trials to determine whether there are benefits of supplementation with multiple micronutrients compared with a single micronutrient in populations at high risk of micronutrient deficiency and LBW are essential. The second important issue is that of the timing of intervention. In rural communities in the developing world, where poor nutritional status of young girls before conception poses high risk for LBW, it is important to examine whether preconceptional nutritional supplementation would yield greater effects on birth outcome. Third, considering the limited resources available in such countries, it is worthwhile to explore the possibility of planning food-based rather than pharmaceutical interventions and study their efficacy along with their implications for health policy.

More detailed studies in subgroups of mothers to examine mechanisms including the effects of micronutrients on the maternofetal supply line, maternal metabolism and body composition, and adaptation to pregnancy and infection are needed. Studies that look into interactions between micronutrients and their bioavailability are also necessary. Finally, nutrition intervention cannot be a permanent solution, especially in countries with limited resources. In many poor communities, improving environment, knowledge, and awareness through social actions would be an ultimate answer to yield sustainable benefits. Thus, the combined efforts of scientists, clinicians, and policy makers in different countries are needed to evaluate the relevance and appropriateness of the existing guidelines on maternal interventions in their own populations.

References

1. Bhutta ZA, Gupta I, De'Silva H, Manandhar D, Awasthi S, Hussain SMM, Salam MA, Maternal and child health: is South Asia ready for change? *BMJ* (2004), **328**: 816–19.

2. Pojda J and Kelley L, 2000. ACC/SCN Nutrition Policy Paper #18. Geneva: United Nations Administrative Committee on Coordination/Subcommittee on Nutrition.

3. Kramer M, Determinants of low birth weight: methodological assessment and meta-analysis. *Bull WHO* (1987), **65**:663–737.

4. Ashworth A, Effects of intrauterine growth retardation on mortality and morbidity in infants and young children. *Eur J Clin Nutr* (1998), 52 (Suppl 1): S34–S42.

5. Chandra RK, Nutrition and the immune system: an introduction. *Am J Clin Nutr* (1997), **66**(2): 460S–463S.

6. Chandra RK, Nutrition and immunology: from the clinic to cellular biology and back again. *Proc Nutr Soc* (1999), **58**(3): 681–683.

7. Victora C, Smith P, Vaughan J, Nobre L, Lombardi C, Teixeria A, et al. Influence of birth weight on mortality from infectious diseases: a case-control study. *Pediatrics* (1988), **81**:807–811.

8. Law CM, Initiation of hypertension in utero and its amplification throughout. *BMJ* (1993), **306**:24–27.

9. Fall CHD, Weight in infancy and prevalence of coronary heart disease in early life. *BMJ* (1995), **310**:17–19.

10. Lithell HO, McKeigue PM, Berglund L, Mohsen R, Lithell UB, and Leon DA. Relation of size at birth to noninsulin dependent diabetes and insulin concentration in men aged 50–60 years. *BMJ* (1996), **312**:406–410.

11. Barker DJP, Mothers, Babies and Health in Later Life (Edinburgh: Churchill Livingstone, 1998).

12. Rao, M, Diet and nutritional status of pregnant women in rural Dharwad. *Ecol Food Nutr* (1986), **18**:125–133.

13. Bhatia BD, Tyagi NK, and Sur AM. Nutritional indicators during pregnancy. *India Pediatr* (1988), **25**:952–959.

14. Susser M, Maternal weight gain, infant birth weight and diet: casual consequences. *Am J Clin Nutr* (1991), **53**:1384–1396.

15. Scholl TO, Hediger ML, Schall JT, Khoo CS, and Fischer RL, Maternal growth during pregnancy and the competition for nutrients. *Am J Clin Nutr* (1994), **60**:183–188.

16. Hediger ML, School TO, Schall JI, Healey MF, and Fischer RL, Changes in maternal upper arm fat stores are predictors of variation in infant birth weight. *J Nutr* (1994), **124**:24–30.

17. Krichengast S and Hartmann B, Maternal pre-pregnancy weight status and pregnancy weight gain as major determinants for new born weight and size. *Ann Hum Biol* (1998), **25**:17–28.

18. Gopalan C, Low birth weight: Significance and implications. In: Nutrition in Children, Developing Country Concerns, ed. HPS Sachdev and P Chaudhury (New Delhi: Imprint Publications, 1994).

19. Fall CHD, Yajnik CS, Rao S, Coyaji KJ, and Shier RP, The effects of maternal body composition before pregnancy on fetal growth: The Pune Maternal Nutrition and Fetal Growth Study. In: Fetal Programming Influences on Development and Disease in Later Life, ed. by PM Shaughn O'Brien, T Wheeler, and DJP Barker (London: RCOG Press, 1999).

20. Doyle W, Crawford MA, Srivastava A, and Costeloe KL. Inter pregnancy nutrition intervention with mothers of low birth weight babies living in an inner city area – a feasibility study. *J Hum Nutr Diet* (1999), **12**:517–27.

21. Godfrey KM, Forrester T, Barker DJP, Jackson AA, Landman JP, Hall JS, et al., Maternal nutritional status in pregnancy and blood pressure in childhood. *BJOG* (1994), **101**:398–403.

22. Joshi S, Garole V, Daware M, Girigosdavi S, and Rao S, Maternal protein restrictions before pregnancy affects vital organs of offspring in Wistar rats. *Metabolism* (2003), **52**:13–18.

23. Devdas RP, and Easwaran PP, Intra family food intake of selected rural households and food consumption patterns of pregnant women. *Indian J Nutr Diet* (1986), **23**:343–6.

24. Ghosh S, The female child in India – a struggle for survival. *Nutrition Foundation of India Bulletin* (1987), **8**:1–4.

25. Gokhale MK, Kanade AN, Rao S, Kelkar RS, Joshi SB, and Girigosavi ST, Female literacy: the multifactorial influence on child health in India. *Ecol Food Nutr* (2004), **43**:257–78.

26. McCance RA, and Widdowson EM, The determinants of growth and form. *Proc Roy Soc London (Biol)* (1974), **185**:1–17.

27. Hutter I, Reduction of food intake during pregnancy in rural South India. *Trop Med Int Health* (1996), 1:399–405.

28. Ratwani L, and Varma M, A study of nutritional status and food practices of the pregnant and lactating women residing in selected desert areas of Jodhpur. *Indian J Nutr Diet* (1989), **26**:304–10.

29. Vijayalaxmi P, Kuputhai U, and Meenakshi Devi N, Nutritional profile of selected expectant mothers and the cost of

pregnancy. *Indian J Nutr Diet* (1988), **25**:247–53.

30. Kramer M, Effects of energy and protein intakes on pregnancy outcome: an overview of the research evidence from controlled clinical trials. *Am J Clin Nutr* (1993), **58**:627–35.

31. Ceesay SM, Prentice AM, Cole TJ, Foord F, Poskitt EME, et al. Effect on stillbirths and perinatal mortality: West Kiang Trial only. *BMJ* (1997), **315**:786–90.

32. Ceesay SM, Prentice AM, Cole TJ, Foord F, Weaver LT, Poskitt EM, et al., Effects on birth weight and perinatal mortality of maternal dietary supplements in rural Gambia: 5 year randomised controlled trial. *BMJ* (1997), **315**:786–90.

33. Rao S, Kanade A, Margetts BM, Yajnik CS, Lubree H, Rege S, Desai S, Jackson A, Fall CHD, Maternal activity in relation to birth size in rural India. The Pune Maternal Nutrition Study. *Eur J Clin Nutr* (2003), **57**:531–42.

34. Prentice AM, Cole TJ, Foord FA, Lamb WH, and Whitehead RG, Increased birth weight after prenatal dietary supplementation of rural African women. *Am J Clin Nutr* (1987), **46**:912–25.

35. Mathews F, Yudkin P, and Neil A, Influence of maternal nutrition on outcome of pregnancy: prospective cohort study. *BMJ* (2000), **320**:941–2.

36. Venu L, Harishankar N, Prasanna Krishna T, and Raghunath M, Maternal dietary vitamin restriction increases body fat contact but not insulin resistance in WNIN rat offspring up to 6 months of age. *Diabetologia* (2004), **47**:1493–1501.

37. Muthayya S, Kurpad AV, Duggan CP, Bosch RJ, Dwarkanath P, Mhaskar A, et al., Low maternal vitamin B12 status is associated with intrauterine growth retardation in urban South Indians. *Eur J Clin Nutr* (2006), **60**:791–801.

38. Rees GA, Doyle W, Srivastava A, Brooke ZM, Crawford MA, and Costealae KL, The nutrient intakes of mothers of low birth weight babies – a comparison of ethnic groups in East London, U.K. *Matern Child Nutr* (2005), **1**:91–9.

39. Luke B, Nutritional influences on fetal growth. *Clin Obstet Gynecol* (1994), **37**:530–49.

40. Wu G, Bazer FW, Cudd TA, Meininger CJ, and Spencer TE, Maternal nutrition and fetal development. *J Nutr* (2004), **134**:2169–72.

41. Painter RC, Rooij SRDE, Bossuyt PM, Semmers TA, Osonond C, Barker DJ, et al., Early onset of coronary artery disease after prenatal exposure to the Dutch famine. *Am J Clin Nutr* (2006), **84**:322–7.

42. Fall CHD, Yajnik CS, Rao S, Devies AA, Brown N, and Farrant JW. Fetus and infant: micronutrient and fetal growth. *J Nutr* (2003), **133**:1747S–56S.

43. Rao S, Yajnik CS, Kanade AN, Fall CHD, Margetts BM, Jackson AA, et al., Intake of micronutrient-rich foods in rural Indian mothers and size of their babies at birth (Pune Maternal Nutrition Study). *J Nutr* (2001), **131**:1217–24.

44. Gupta P, Ray M, Dua T, Radhakrishnan G, Kumar R, and Sachdev HPS, Multimicronutrient supplementation for undernourished pregnant women and the birth size of their offspring: a double blind, randomized, placebo-controlled trial. *Arch Pediatr Adolesc Med* (2007), **161**:58–64.

45. Osrin D, Vaidya A, and Shrestha Y, Effects of antenatal multiple micronutrient supplementation on birth weight and gestational duration in Nepal: double blind, randomized controlled trial. *Lancet* (2005), **365**:955–62.

46. Refsum H, Folate, vitamin B12 and homocysteine in relation to birth defects and pregnancy outcome. *Br J Nutr* (2001), **85**(Suppl 2):S109–13.

47. Smith AD, Folic acid fortification: the good, the bad and the puzzle of vitamin B12. *Am J Clin Nutr* (2007), **85**:3–5.

48. Yajnik CS, Deshpande SS, Jackson AA, Refsum SH, Rao S, Fisher DJ, et al., Vitamin B12 and folate concentration during pregnancy and insulin resistance in the offspring: the Pune Maternal Nutrition Study. *Diabetologia* (2008), **51**:29–38.

Nutritional regulation and requirements for pregnancy and fetal growth

6 Preeclampsia

Fergus McCarthy and Louise Kenny

Definition of preeclampsia

Preeclampsia is defined by the International Society for the Study of Hypertension in Pregnancy as gestational hypertension of at least 140/90 mmHg on two separate occasions 4 or more hours apart accompanied by significant proteinuria of at least 300 mg in a 24-hour collection of urine, arising de novo after the 20th week of gestation in a previously normotensive woman and resolving completely by the 6th postpartum week [1]. It usually occurs during the second half of pregnancy and complicates 2% to 8% of pregnancies. Some women are considered to be at higher risk of developing preeclampsia than the general female population, and some of these are listed in Table 6.1. For example, women with antiphospholipid syndrome have a risk approximately 9 times greater than that of the general population of developing preeclampsia.

Implications of preeclampsia

Preeclampsia is a major cause of maternal and perinatal mortality and morbidity worldwide, causing 15% of all direct maternal deaths in the United Kingdom [2] and a fivefold increase in perinatal mortality with iatrogenic prematurity being the main culprit [3]. The Confidential Enquiry into Stillbirths and Deaths in Infancy report cites one in six stillbirths as occurring in pregnancies complicated by maternal hypertension [4]. Preeclampsia also carries implications in adult life, with offspring of affected preterm pregnancies demonstrating poor growth in childhood [5] and an increased risk of hypertension, heart disease, and diabetes [6].

Pathogenesis of preeclampsia

The individual stages in the pathogenesis of preeclampsia are generally well accepted. However, debate continues regarding the primary precipitating factor. Two theories, the two-stage process and the continuum theory, have emerged to explain the primary precipitating factor. The continuum theory proposes that preeclampsia is an exaggerated form of the inflammatory response of normal pregnancy. It is suggested that this occurs in response to a relative increase in trophoblastic debris, which is released from a poorly perfused placenta. The exaggerated inflammatory response can also be triggered by a normal amount of trophoblastic debris in susceptible women [7]. The second theory, the two-stage process, associates the primary event for the development of preeclampsia appears as a failure of the second wave of trophoblast invasion from 16 to 20 weeks gestation with failure to destroy the muscularis layer of the spiral arterioles. This causes shallow endovascular cytotrophoblast invasion with enhanced inflammatory response and endothelial cell dysfunction as key features in the pathogenesis of preeclampsia [8]. This endothelial dysfunction appears to occur as a result of oxidative stress and is mediated by high levels of free radicals and low levels of antioxidants as supported by the observation that markers of oxidative stress are present in the maternal circulation of affected women [9].

Potential contribution by specific nutritional deficiencies

Many vitamins and food supplements have been advocated for the prevention of preeclampsia, and others, in excess or in deficiency, have been implicated in the pathogenesis of the disease. However, because the precise mechanisms underlying the etiology of preeclampsia at a cellular and molecular level are incompletely understood, it is largely unknown whether the correction of nutritional deficiencies or other forms of dietary manipulation may play a part in primary prevention of this disease. Similarly, it is not known whether dietary intervention would be most effective if commenced preconceptually or antenatally. In this chapter, we discuss the role of maternal

Table 6.1 Risk factors for the development of preeclampsia

Risk factor	Unadjusted relative risk (95% confidence interval)
Age ≥ 40 years, primiparae	1.68 (1.23–2.29)
Age ≥ 40 years, multiparae	1.96 (1.34–2.87)
Family history	2.90 (1.70–4.93)
Nulliparity	2.91 (1.28–6.61)
Multiple pregnancy	2.93 (2.04–4.21)
Preexisting diabetes	3.56 (2.54–4.99)
Pre-pregnancy body mass index ≥ 35	4.29 (3.52–5.49)
Previous preeclampsia	7.19 (5.85–8.83)
Antiphospholipid syndrome	9.72 (4.34–21.75)

Table 6.2 Summary of role of dietary supplements in the prevention or treatment of preeclampsia

Dietary agent	Role in treatment/prevention of preeclampsia
Antioxidants	Reduction in relative risk of developing preeclampsia, reduction of incidence of small for gestational age but an increase in the incidence of preterm labor
	Vitamins C and E have conflicting evidence but do not appear to be beneficial; their use may be associated with adverse outcomes
L-arginine	Insufficient evidence to recommend its use
Calcium	Significant reduction in occurrence of preeclampsia particularly in high-risk groups
	Associated with increased risk of HELLP syndrome (hemolysis, elevated liver enzymes, low platelets)
Chinese herbal medicine	Insufficient evidence to recommend its use
Fish oil	No evidence of any benefit
Folic acid	Insufficient evidence to recommend its use
Garlic	No evidence of any benefit
Iron	May worsen predisposition to developing preeclampsia
Japanese herbal medicine	Insufficient evidence to recommend its use
Magnesium	No evidence of any benefit
Multivitamin supplementation	Insufficient evidence to recommend its use
Salt intake	No evidence of any benefit
Zinc	No evidence of any benefit

nutrition in the prevention and development of preeclampsia.

Antioxidants

Antioxidants protect proteins and enzymes from oxidation and destruction by free radicals and help to maintain cellular membrane integrity. Antioxidants can be categorized as either free radical scavengers that trap or decompose existing free radicals, or cellular and extracellular enzymes that inhibit peroxidase reactions involved in the production of free radicals [10]. Free radical scavengers include vitamin C (ascorbate), vitamin E (tocopherols), carotenoids, and glutathione. Antioxidant enzymes include glutathione peroxidase, superoxide dismutase, and catalase, which are dependent on the presence of cofactors such as selenium, zinc, and iron. Although antioxidant enzymes are important for intracellular defenses, nonenzymatic antioxidants are the major defense mechanism in the extracellular compartment.

Many studies have been performed to investigate the link between a variety of antioxidants and the development of preeclampsia. Many of these were of poor quality with inconclusive results. Therefore, a Cochrane review was performed. In its final analysis, this included seven trials involving more than 6000 women and assessed the effectiveness of any antioxidant supplement during pregnancy for prevention of preeclampsia [11]. Supplements included various doses and combinations of vitamin C, vitamin E, selenium, halibut liver oil (containing vitamin A), fish oil, and lycopene, sometimes with other interventions (e.g. aspirin). Supplementation with any antioxidants during pregnancy compared with control or placebo was associated with a 39% reduction in the relative risk of preeclampsia, which corresponds to an absolute risk reduction of 3%. There was also a reduction in the incidence of small-for-gestational-age infants, but a slight increase in preterm birth. However, most of the data came from poor quality and/or quasi-randomized studies. Data were insufficient to allow reliable conclusions about the possible impact of this therapy in subgroups of high- or low-risk women or to provide guidance on the optimal type and dosage of antioxidants or timing of supplementation.

Vitamins C and E have been studied because of their perceived function as antioxidants. In one randomized trial, vitamin C (1000 mg/day) and vitamin E (400 IU/day) were administered to women at high risk of developing preeclampsia during the second and third trimesters [12]. Vitamin supplementation was associated with a significant reduction in the frequency of preeclampsia. However, subsequent trials have not confirmed these findings. A larger, multicenter trial in a diverse group of women at high risk of developing preeclampsia, conducted by the investigators of the original study, found that the incidence of preeclampsia was similar for women given vitamin C and E supplementation and those given placebo [13]. This study also reported that the number of low birth weight neonates was slightly higher in treated women. This may have been related to a trend toward slightly earlier onset and more severe disease in treated patients. Post hoc analysis showed that vitamin supplementation was associated with increased frequency of gestational hypertension and stillbirth. Another multicenter trial randomly assigned nulliparous women without medical or obstetrical complications to receive daily supplementation with vitamin C plus vitamin E or placebo from the second trimester until delivery [14]. The incidence of preeclampsia was similar for both groups. There were no significant differences in the incidence of small-for-gestational-age neonates, death/serious neonatal complications, or preterm birth. The difference in prevalence of preeclampsia between these two trials may be attributed to differences in the populations studied. Certainly it seems that antioxidant supplementation does not prevent preeclampsia. Furthermore, there is a possibility that the therapy increases the risk of adverse effects in women with specific risk factors for the disease.

Two studies have addressed the issue of whether antioxidants alter the course of established preeclampsia [15, 16]. Neither reported a clinical benefit.

A recent systematic review of trials evaluating vitamin E supplementation in a variety of clinical settings [17] demonstrated harmful effects associated with supplementation. A recently published case-control study investigated the association between maternal dietary and supplement intake of the antioxidants vitamin E, retinol, and congenital heart defects [18]. This study demonstrated an association between high maternal vitamin E intake by diet and supplements and an increased risk of congenital heart disease in the mother's offspring. These findings highlight the need for controlled evaluation of vitamin E and other antioxidant supplementation in pregnancy. Therefore, at present, antioxidant supplementation in the form of vitamin C and vitamin E cannot be recommended for the prevention or treatment of preeclampsia.

Arginine

Arginine is an alpha amino acid that is synthesized by adults through the urea cycle. Arginine is the immediate precursor of nitrous oxide, urea, ornithine, and agmatine. Nitrous oxide is a potent vasodilator; therefore, arginine supplementation has been suggested as a potential treatment in a condition in which vasodilatation may be beneficial. Administration of organic nitrates or L-arginine has been shown to improve uterine-placental circulation and to lower maternal blood pressure [19–22]. A recent pilot study by Facchinetti et al. [23] shows promising results in prolonging the latent period to the development of preeclampsia in patients with gestational hypertension by means of arginine supplementation. However, this benefit needs to be confirmed in larger studies with adequate power to evaluate the effectiveness of L-arginine in preventing the development to preeclampsia. Currently, arginine supplementation cannot be recommended for the prevention or treatment of preeclampsia [24].

Calcium

The relationship between calcium intake and hypertension in pregnancy was first described in 1980, when epidemiological studies suggested that women who lived in areas with high dietary calcium intake had a lower incidence of preeclampsia. A Cochrane systematic review including 12 studies of more than 15 000 women compared the use of at least 1 g of calcium daily during pregnancy with placebo [25]. Preeclampsia was significantly reduced with calcium supplementation compared with placebo. A similar effect was observed in nonproteinuric hypertension. The effect was greatest for women at high risk of developing preeclampsia and for those with low baseline calcium intake. Calcium supplementation was also associated with a significant reduction in the incidence of maternal death or serious morbidity, but somewhat perplexingly, it increased the incidence of HELLP syndrome. HELLP syndrome refers to a clinical syndrome characterized by hemolysis, elevated liver enzymes, and low platelets that may occur in pregnancy. It is thought to represent a variant of preeclampsia. The benefit from calcium supplementation appears to be maternal as there was no effect on the risk of preterm birth or perinatal death. There were no reports of adverse events related to calcium supplementation but long-term follow-up was minimal. Overall, the benefits of less preeclampsia, fewer maternal deaths, and reduced severe morbidity support the use of calcium supplementation during pregnancy for women with low dietary intake of calcium.

Chinese herbal medicine

Traditional Chinese medicine is a theoretical and methodological system that incorporates concepts of cause, diagnosis, and treatment. Several traditional Chinese medicines are thought to protect the maternal spleen, liver, and kidneys in preeclampsia by encouraging vasodilatation, increasing blood flow, and decreasing platelet aggregation. Some of these medicines have been reported to be effective in the treatment of preeclampsia [26]. However, in a systematic Cochrane review, no appropriate good-quality randomized controlled trials were found for analysis [27]. Therefore, Chinese herbal medicine cannot be recommended for the prevention or treatment of preeclampsia.

Fish oil

It has been proposed that fish oil supplements may have a variety of protective vascular effects including reductions in systemic blood pressure and in the incidence of preeclampsia and pregnancy-induced hypertension [28, 29]. One randomized double-blind placebo controlled trial randomized 253 pregnant women at high risk of developing proteinuric or non-proteinuric pregnancy-induced hypertension or asymmetrical intrauterine growth retardation to 2.7 g of MaxEpa daily (1.62 g of eicosapentaenoic acid and 1.08 g of docosahexaenoic acid) or placebo. There was no difference in an intention-to-treat analysis between the placebo and active treatment groups for occurrence of any of the primary outcomes [30]. A second prospective trial enrolled 386 pregnant women with a history of pregnancy-induced hypertension in a previous pregnancy and randomly assigned them to a fish oil or olive oil supplement, beginning after 16 weeks of gestation [31]. These and two subsequent trials [32, 33] found that fish oil supplementation had no effect on the incidence or development of hypertension. Meta-

analysis of these trials also failed to show a reduction in the risk of preeclampsia [34].

Folic acid

Homocysteine has been reported to be increased in the plasma of women who subsequently develop preeclampsia. Elevated homocysteine levels may damage the lining of blood vessels resulting in the signs and symptoms of preeclampsia. Folic acid supplementation has been studied in women with hyperhomocysteinemia because homocysteine levels have been weakly and negatively correlated with plasma folate concentrations. Leeda et al. [35] supplemented a high-risk group of women with hyperhomocysteinemia and a history of previous preeclampsia or intrauterine growth restriction with 5 mg folic acid and 250 mg of vitamin B_6. The supplementation resulted in a normalized methionine loading test in all patients in the study and showed a favorable perinatal outcome. The study had very small numbers and was not randomized to placebo. Folic acid may have a role to play in this high-risk group, but in the general population, it is not known whether folic acid has a role to play in the prevention or treatment of preeclampsia.

Garlic

Garlic is part of the *Allium* or onion, family. The suggestions that garlic may lower blood pressure, reduce oxidative stress, inhibit lipid oxidation, and/or inhibit platelet aggregation have led to the hypothesis that garlic may have a role in prevention of preeclampsia [36–38]. Experimental studies have demonstrated that garlic may also increase the production of nitric oxide [39], which is itself a platelet inhibitor and vasodilator. A Cochrane review looked at the use of garlic for preventing preeclampsia and its complications [40]. Only one trial of 100 women met inclusion criteria, and it showed no difference between dried garlic and placebo in the prevention of preeclampsia [41]. There is insufficient evidence to recommend increased garlic intake for preventing preeclampsia and its complications. However, because there are now many varieties of garlic available and there is a lack of appropriately powered studies, further research is warranted.

Iron

The placental ischemia and malperfused placenta that occur in preeclampsia result in the production of free radicals, which may cause oxidative stress [8]. These free radicals such as superoxide and hydrogen peroxide are unlikely to initiate cellular damage directly. However, in the presence of metal ions, particularly iron and copper, they can generate hydroxyl radical, which can result in endothelial cell damage [42, 43]. Iron is already present in large amounts in the placenta, and levels may further increase in the ischemic placenta by destruction of red blood cells from thrombotic, necrotic, and hemorrhagic areas [44]. No trials have demonstrated that the routine use of iron supplementation in pregnancy can prevent the development of preeclampsia. Iron supplementation, unlike many of the other dietary components discussed in this chapter, may also have a detrimental effect when used in excess in pregnancy by promoting oxidative stress by decreasing serum antioxidant capacity.

Japanese herbal medicine

In Japan, certain traditional herbal medicines (Kampo medicines) are used clinically with standardized quantities and quality of ingredients. One of these medicines, Tokishakuyaku-san (TS), is used to alleviate symptoms of menopause and as a tocolytic in the treatment of preterm labor. One animal study performed investigated the effect of TS on pregnant rats in which a preeclampsia-like syndrome had been induced [45]. The authors concluded that TS may have a beneficial effect in preeclampsia, but further studies are needed.

Magnesium

Magnesium is one of the essential minerals required by humans in relatively large amounts. Magnesium works with many enzymes to regulate body temperature and synthesize proteins as well as to maintain electrical potentials in nerves and muscle membranes. The MAGPIE (Magnesium Sulphate for the Treatment of Pre-eclampsia) trial demonstrated the importance of magnesium in the treatment of preeclampsia and the prevention of eclampsia [46]. Many women, especially those from disadvantaged backgrounds, have intakes of magnesium below average. Makrides and Crowther [47] systematically reviewed the use of magnesium supplementation in pregnancy before 25 weeks gestation. However, of the seven studies included in the systematic analysis, only one study met the prespecified criteria for a high-quality trial. This one high-quality study randomized 400 normotensive primigravid women aged 13 to 25 years to receive 365 mg elemental magnesium or placebo daily from 13 to 24 weeks gestation. The authors concluded that the poor quality of many of the trials was likely to have resulted in a bias favoring magnesium supplementation, but there is not enough high-quality evidence to show that dietary magnesium supplementation during pregnancy is beneficial in reducing the incidence or severity of preeclampsia. There were also no differences between the magnesium and placebo groups for the frequency of preterm birth (<37 weeks), gestational age at birth, birth weight, small for gestational age, the frequency of admission to a neonatal unit, miscarriage, and neonatal death [48].

Multiple micronutrient supplementations

Micronutrients are vitamins and minerals required in minute amounts for normal functioning, growth, and development. Micronutrients include vitamin A, zinc, iron, and beta carotene. The resulting micronutrient deficiencies are exacerbated in pregnancy, leading to potentially adverse effects on the mother such as anemia, hypertension, complications of labor, and death. A Cochrane review involving nine trials and more than 15 000 women showed insufficient data to demonstrate a reduction in the development of preeclampsia by routine use of micronutrients [49].

Salt intake

Controlled salt intake has long been recommended for the control of essential hypertension. On this basis, salt restriction was widely recommended during pregnancy for the prevention and treatment of preeclampsia. However, the literature has mixed opinions, and at one stage in the 1960s, high salt intake was recommended to prevent preeclampsia [50]. Duley et al. [51] performed a Cochrane review that included two trials involving 603 women. Neither trial proved a reduced incidence of preeclampsia in the presence of salt [52]. Therefore, in the absence of further evidence, salt intake during pregnancy remains a personal preference [53].

Zinc

Zinc is one of the mediators of the antioxidant enzymes such as glutathione peroxidase, superoxide dismutase, and catalase. A low maternal serum zinc concentration has been reported in pregnancies complicated by preeclampsia [54, 55], and it has been suggested that the incidence of preeclampsia may be reduced by zinc supplementation [56]. One double-blind randomized control trial investigated the effect of zinc supplementation on a healthy middle-class population of more than 1000 women and concluded that zinc supplementation does not appear to have any role in the prevention or treatment of preeclampsia [57]. It may have a role to play in improving birth weight and preventing prematurity in populations at high risk of poor pregnancy outcomes.

The role of diet and lifestyle factors

Rest

Restriction of activity and prolonged resting have traditionally been advocated for the prevention and treatment of many of the ailments of pregnancy, including the prevention and treatment of hypertension [58]. This was based on a belief that exercise may reduce uteroplacental blood flow and therefore rest would increase it. Women with preeclampsia suffer from reduced uteroplacental blood, and therefore it was hypothesized that rest might prevent or reduce the severity of preeclampsia. Two studies met inclusion criteria for a Cochrane review [59, 60]. These two studies, although included, were themselves substandard, raising more questions than they answered. There is insufficient evidence to support recommending rest or reduced activity to women for preventing preeclampsia and its complications [61]. It is also unclear whether rest and the resulting immobilization may predispose pregnant women to increased risks of thromboembolic disease in the hypercoagulable setting of pregnancy.

Exercise

The evidence linking the promotion of regular exercise and a reduction in the risk of hypertension in the nonpregnant person is well established. However, it remains unclear whether the promotion of exercise in a pregnant woman will reduce her risk of developing or reduce the severity of preeclampsia. Exercise during pregnancy may not be without risks with several observational studies linking exercise during pregnancy with small-for-gestational-age babies, preterm birth, and maternal injury [62, 63]. Two studies met the requirements for a Cochrane review [64]. However, these trials had small numbers and were unable to provide reliable conclusions regarding the role of exercise in the prevention of preeclampsia [65].

Vegans

Veganism is a philosophy and lifestyle that seeks to exclude the use of animal derived products for food, clothing, or any other purpose. Vegans do not use or consume animal products of any kind. Carter et al. [66] examined the incidence of preeclampsia and reproductive outcomes in a community of vegan mothers. The study included 775 women, 240 of whom were primigravidas. This retrospective observational study revealed only one case of preeclampsia occurring in this cohort of women suggesting that a vegan diet, a diet that is low in arachadonic acid, may be protective against the development of preeclampsia. Other possible explanations for the low incidence of preeclampsia in this population include the retrospective nature of the study, which may have resulted in bias, low levels of smoking and stress, a "healthy" diet, and high levels of aerobic exercise.

Obesity

An association between obesity and hypertensive disorders during pregnancy has been consistently reported. In particular, maternal weight and body mass index (BMI) are independent risk factors for preeclampsia, as well as other hypertensive disorders [67–69]. A review of 13 cohort studies comprising nearly 1.4 million women found that the risk of preeclampsia doubled with each 5 to 7 kg/m² increase in pre-pregnancy BMI [69]. This relation persisted in studies that excluded women with chronic hypertension, diabetes mellitus, or multiple gestations, or after adjustment for other confounders. The mechanism whereby obesity imparts an increased risk for preeclampsia is not known. Current hypotheses suggest that the pathophysiological changes associated with obesity-related cardiovascular risk, such as insulin resistance, hyperlipidemia, and subclinical inflammation, are also responsible for the increased incidence of preeclampsia in obese pregnant women [70–72].

What dietary advice can be given and how does this relate to those with a genetic predisposition?

The search for dietary supplements that may prevent or treat preeclampsia continues, and currently there is no good evidence to support the routine use of dietary supplements in the prevention and treatment of preeclampsia in a low-risk antenatal population. Those patients at high risk of developing preeclampsia should be considered on an individual basis. Achieving an ideal BMI relationship between a person's height and weight by weight loss before conception may be the most prudent advice in many patients. Calcium supplementation may be considered in women at high risk for developing preeclampsia but only after potential risks are discussed. Further dietary supplementation is not recommended outside of the setting of a clinical trial, and patients should be made aware that dietary supplementation may have adverse effects on the mother or fetus.

Potential future research

Unfortunately, more than anything, this chapter highlights the significant lack of quality studies from which to draw conclusions regarding the role of nutrition in the prevention or treatment of preeclampsia. Further research is needed to clarify whether potential health benefits are specific to particular preparations, constituents, or doses. Further trials should be large and should collect information about perinatal mortality and morbidity as well as maternal mortality and morbidity associated with any intervention. A particularly important topic appears to be that of determining the effects of calcium supplementation at a community level.

Key clinical points

- Preeclampsia is a common condition complicating 2% to 8% of pregnancies.
- Preeclampsia is a leading cause of severe obstetric morbidity and mortality for both mother and fetus throughout the world.
- Preeclampsia is associated with a fivefold increase in perinatal mortality and has medical implications such as the development of diabetes late into adult life.
- It is believed to be the result of an exaggerated form of the inflammatory response of normal pregnancy.
- The mechanisms underlying this etiology are poorly understood, and therefore it is difficult to speculate whether the correction of nutritional deficiencies may play a part in primary prevention.
- Many dietary agents and lifestyle factors have been implicated in its occurrence. However, good-quality randomized trials comparing these agents against placebo are generally not available. It is therefore not possible to recommend the use of many of these agents in the prevention and treatment of preeclampsia.
- Some dietary interventions used such as iron supplementation may be detrimental and further predispose women to developing preeclampsia.
- Dietary advice with the aim of achieving an ideal BMI is one of the few dietary interventions known to reduce the risk of developing preeclampsia.

References

1. Davey DA and Macgillivray I, The classification and definition of the hypertensive disorders of pregnancy. *Am J Obstet Gynecol* (1988), **158**:892–8.

2. Confidential Enquiries into Maternal and Child Health, Why Mothers Die 2000–2002. Report on confidential enquiries into maternal deaths in the United Kingdom (London: Royal College of Obstetricians and Gynaecologists, 2004).

3. Farag K, Hassan I, and Ledger WL, Prediction of preeclampsia: can it be achieved? *Obstet Gynecol Surv* (2004), **59**:464–82; quiz 485.

4. Confidential Enquiry into Stillbirths and Death in Infancy, 5th Annual Report. (London: Maternal and Child Health Research Consortium, 1998).

5. Mccowan L, Harding J, Barker S, and Ford C, Perinatal predictors of growth at six months in small for gestational age babies. *Early Hum Dev* (1999), **56**:205–16.

6. Barker DJ, Gluckman PD, Godfrey KM, Harding JE, Owens JF, and Robinson JS, Fetal nutrition and cardiovascular disease in adult life. *Lancet* (1993), **341**:938–41.

7. Redman CW and Sargent IL, Placental debris, oxidative stress and pre-eclampsia. *Placenta* (2000), **21**:597–602.

8. Roberts JM and Hubel CA, Is oxidative stress the link in the two-stage model of pre-eclampsia? *Lancet* (1999), **354**:788–9.

9. Roberts JM and Speer P, Antioxidant therapy to prevent preeclampsia. *Semin Nephrol* (2004), **24**:557–64.

10. Diplock AT, Charleux JL, Crozier-Willi G, Kok FJ, and Rice-Evans C, et al., Functional food science and defence against reactive oxidative species. *Br J Nutr* (1998), **80**(Suppl 1):S77–112.

11. Rumbold A, Duley L, Crowther C, and Haslam R, Antioxidants for preventing pre-eclampsia. *Cochrane Database Syst Rev* (2005), **4**:CD004227.

12. Chappell LC, Seed PT, Briley AL, Kelly FJ, Lee R, Hunt BJ, et al., Effect of antioxidants on the occurrence of preeclampsia in women at increased risk: a randomised trial. *Lancet* (1999), **354**:810–6.

13. Poston, L, Briley, AL, Seed, PT, Kelly, FJ, and Shennan AH, Vitamin C and vitamin E in pregnant women at risk for preeclampsia (VIP trial): randomised placebo-controlled trial. *Lancet* (2006), **367**:1145–54.

14. Rumbold AR, Crowther CA, Haslam RR, Dekker GA, and Robinson JS, Vitamins C and E and the risks of preeclampsia and perinatal complications. *N Engl J Med* (2006), **354**:1796–806.

15. Stratta P, Canavese C, Porcu M, Dogliani M, Todros T, Garbo E, et al., Vitamin E supplementation in preeclampsia. *Gynecol Obstet Investig* (1994), **37**:246–9.

16. Gulmezoglu AM, Hofmeyr GJ, and Oosthuisen MM, Antioxidants in the treatment of severe pre-eclampsia: an explanatory randomised controlled trial. *BJOG* (1997), **104**:689–96.

17. Miller ER 3rd, Pastor-Barriuso R, Dalal D, Riemersma RA, Appel LJ, and Guallar E, Meta-analysis: high-dosage vitamin E supplementation may increase all-cause mortality. *Ann Intern Med* (2005), **142**:37–46.

18. Smedts HP, de Vries JH, Rakhshandehroo M, Wildhagen MF, Verkleij-Hagoort AC, Steegers EA, and Steegers-Theunissen RP, High maternal vitamin E intake by diet or supplements is associated with congenital heart defects in the offspring. *BJOG* (2009), **116**: 416–23.

19. Ramsay B, De Belder A, Campbell S, Moncada S, and Martin JF, A nitric oxide donor improves uterine artery diastolic blood flow in normal early pregnancy and in women at high risk of pre-eclampsia. *Eur J Clin Investig* (1994), **24**:76–8.

20. Grunewald C, Kublickas M, Carlstrom K, Lunell NO, and Nisell H, Effects of nitroglycerin on the uterine and umbilical circulation in severe preeclampsia. *Obstet Gynecol* (1995), **86**:600–4.

21. Neri I, Di Renzo GC, Caserta G, Gallinelli A, and Facchinetti F, Impact of the L-arginine/nitric oxide system in pregnancy. *Obstet Gynecol Surv* (1995), **50**:851–8.

22. Facchinetti F, Longo M, Piccinini F, Neri I, and Volpe A, L-arginine infusion reduces blood pressure in preeclamptic women through nitric oxide release. *J Soc Gynecol Investig* (1999), **6**:202–7.

23. Facchinetti F, Saade, GR Neri I, Pizzi C, Longo M, and Volpe A, L-arginine supplementation in patients with gestational hypertension: a pilot study. *Hypertens Pregn* (2007), **26**:121–30.

24. Ekerhovd E, Dietary supplementation with L-arginine in women with preeclampsia. *Acta Obstet Gynecol Scand* (2004), **83**:871; author reply 872.

25. Hofmeyr GJ, Duley L, and Atallah A, Dietary calcium supplementation for prevention of preeclampsia and related problems: a systematic review and commentary. *BJOG*, **114**:933–43.

26. Liu SY, Xu YY, and Zhu JY (1994) [The effects of Salvia miltiorrhizae Bge and Ligustrazine on thromboxane A2 and prostacyclin in pregnancy induced hypertension]. *Zhonghua Fu Chan Ke Za Zhi* (2007), **29**:648–50, 697.

27. Zhang J, Wu TX, and Liu GJ, Chinese herbal medicine for the treatment of pre-eclampsia.

Cochrane Database Syst Rev (2006), (**2**):CD005126.

28. Secher NJ and Olsen SF, Fish-oil and pre-eclampsia. *BJOG* (1990), **97**:1077–9.

29. Sorensen JD, Olsen SF, Pedersen AK, Boris J, Secher NJ, and Fitzgerald GA, Effects of fish oil supplementation in the third trimester of pregnancy on prostacyclin and thromboxane production. *Am J Obstet Gynecol* (1993), **168**:915–22.

30. Onwude JL, Lilford RJ, Hjartardottir H, Staines A, and Tuffnell D, A randomised double blind placebo controlled trial of fish oil in high risk pregnancy. *BJOG* (1995), **102**:95–100.

31. Olsen SF, Secher NJ, Tabor A, Weber T, Walker JJ, and Gluud C, Randomised clinical trials of fish oil supplementation in high risk pregnancies. Fish Oil Trials In Pregnancy (FOTIP) Team. *BJOG* (2000), **107**:382–95.

32. Smuts CM, Huang M, Mundy D, Plasse T, Major S, and Carlson SE, A randomized trial of docosahexaenoic acid supplementation during the third trimester of pregnancy. *Obstet Gynecol* (2003), **101**:469–79.

33. Villar J, Abalos E, Nardin JM, Merialdi M, and Carroli G, Strategies to prevent and treat preeclampsia: evidence from randomized controlled trials. *Semin Nephrol* (2004), **24**:607–15.

34. Makrides M, Duley L, and Olsen SF, Marine oil, and other prostaglandin precursor, supplementation for pregnancy uncomplicated by preeclampsia or intrauterine growth restriction. *Cochrane Database Syst Rev* (2006), **3**:CD003402.

35. Leeda M, Riyazi N, De Vries JI, Jakobs C, Van Geijn HP, and Dekker GA, Effects of folic acid and vitamin B6 supplementation on women with hyperhomocysteinemia and a history of preeclampsia or fetal growth restriction. *Am J Obstet Gynecol* (1998), **179**:135–9.

36. Ide N, Nelson AB, and Lau BH, Aged garlic extract and its constituents inhibit Cu(2+)-induced oxidative modification of low density lipoprotein. *Plant Med* (1997), **63**:263–4.

37. Borek C, Antioxidant health effects of aged garlic extract. *J Nutr* (2001), **131**:1010S–5S.

38. Lau BH, Suppression of LDL oxidation by garlic. *J Nutr* (2001), **131**:985S–8S.

39. Das I, Khan NS, and Sooranna SR, Potent activation of nitric oxide synthase by garlic: a basis for its therapeutic applications. *Curr Med Res Opin* (1995), **13**:257–63.

40. Meher S and Duley L, Garlic for preventing preeclampsia and its complications. *Cochrane Database Syst Rev* (2006b), **3**:CD006065.

41. Ziaei S, Hantoshzadeh S, Rezasoltani P, and Lamyian M, The effect of garlic tablet on plasma lipids and platelet aggregation in nulliparous pregnants at high risk of preeclampsia. *Eur J Obstet Gynecol Reprod Biol* (2001), **99**:201–6.

42. Arosio P and Levi S, Ferritin, iron homeostasis, and oxidative damage. *Free Radical Biol Med* (2002), **33**:457–63.

43. Fang YZ, Yang S, and Wu G, Free radicals, antioxidants, and nutrition. *Nutrition* (2002), **18**:872–9.

44. Entman SS, Kambam JR, Bradley CA, and Cousar JB, Increased levels of carboxyhemoglobin and serum iron as an indicator of increased red cell turnover in preeclampsia. *Am J Obstet Gynecol* (1987), **156**:1169–73.

45. Takei H, Iizuka S, Yamamoto M, Takeda S, Yamamoto M, and Arishima K, The herbal medicine Tokishakuyakusan increases fetal blood glucose concentrations and growth hormone levels and improves intrauterine growth retardation induced by N(omega)-nitro-L-arginine methyl ester. *J Pharmacol Sci* (2007), **104**:319–28.

46. Altman D, Carroli G, Duley L, Farrell B, Moodley J, Neilson J, and Smith D, Do women with pre-eclampsia, and their babies, benefit from magnesium sulphate? The Magpie Trial: a randomised placebo-controlled trial. *Lancet* (2002), **359**: 1877–90.

47. Makrides M and Crowther CA, Magnesium supplementation in pregnancy. *Cochrane Database Syst Rev* (2001), CD000937.

48. Sibai BM, Villar MA, and Bray E, (1989) Magnesium supplementation during pregnancy: a double-blind randomized controlled clinical trial. *Am J Obstet Gynecol*, **161**:115–9.

49. Haider BA and Bhutta ZA, Multiple-micronutrient supplementation for women during pregnancy. *Cochrane Database Syst Rev* (2006), **4**:CD004905.

50. Bower D, The influence of dietary salt intake on pre-eclampsia. *J Obstet Gynaecol Brit Commonw* (1964), **71**:123–5.

51. Duley L, Henderson-Smart D, and Meher S, Altered dietary salt for preventing pre-eclampsia, and its complications. *Cochrane Database Syst Rev* (2005), **4**:CD005548.

52. Knuist M, Bonsel GJ, Zondervan HA, and Treffers PE, Low sodium diet and pregnancy-induced hypertension: a multi-centre randomised controlled trial. *BJOG* (1998), **105**:430–4.

53. Steegers EA, Eskes TK, Jongsma HW, and Hein PR, Dietary sodium restriction during pregnancy; a historical review. *Eur J Obstet Gynecol Reprod Biol* (1991), **40**:83–90.

54. Kiilholma P, Paul R, Pakarinen P, and Gronroos M, Copper and

61

zinc in pre-eclampsia. *Acta Obstet Gynecol Scand* (1984), **63**:629–31.

55. Mukherjee MD, Sandstead HH, Ratnaparkhi MV, Johnson LK, Milne DB, and Stelling HP, Maternal zinc, iron, folic acid, and protein nutriture and outcome of human pregnancy. *Am J Clin Nutr* (1984), **40**:496–507.

56. Caulfield LE, Zavaleta N, Shankar AH, and Merialdi M, Potential contribution of maternal zinc supplementation during pregnancy to maternal and child survival. *Am J Clin Nutr* (1998), **68**:499S–508S.

57. Jonsson B, Hauge B, Larsen MF, and Hald F (1996) Zinc supplementation during pregnancy: a double blind randomised controlled trial. *Acta Obstet Gynecol Scand* **75**:725–9.

58. Goldenberg RL, Cliver SP, Bronstein J, Cutter GR, Andrews WW, and Mennemeyer ST. (1994) Bed rest in pregnancy. *Obstet Gynecol* **84**:131–6.

59. Spinapolice RX, Feld S, and Harrigan JT, Effective prevention of gestational hypertension in nulliparous women at high risk as identified by the rollover test. *Am J Obstet Gynecol* (1983), **146**:166–8.

60. Herrera JA, Nutritional factors and rest reduce pregnancy-induced hypertension and preeclampsia in positive roll-over test primigravidas. *Int J Gynaecol Obstet* (1993), **41**:31–5.

61. Meher S and Duley L, Rest during pregnancy for preventing preeclampsia and its complications in women with normal blood pressure. *Cochrane Database Syste Rev* (2006), **2**:CD005939.

62. Launer LJ, Villar J, Kestler E, and De Onis M, The effect of maternal work on fetal growth and duration of pregnancy: a prospective study. *BJOG* (1990), **97**:62–70.

63. Henriksen TB, Hedegaard M, and Secher NJ, Standing and walking at work and birthweight. *Acta Obstet Gynecol Scand* (1995), **74**:509–16.

64. Meher S and Duley L, Exercise or other physical activity for preventing preeclampsia and its complications. *Cochrane Database Syst Rev* (2006), **2**:CD005942.

65. Yeo S, Steele NM, Chang MC, Leclaire SM, Ronis DL, and Hayashi R, Effect of exercise on blood pressure in pregnant women with a high risk of gestational hypertensive disorders. *J Reprod Med* (2000), **45**:293–8.

66. Carter JP, Furman T, and Hutcheson HR, Preeclampsia and reproductive performance in a community of vegans. *South Med J* (1987), **80**:692–7.

67. Sibai BM, Gordon T, Thom E, Caritis SN, Klebanoff M, Mcnellis D, and Paul RH, Risk factors for preeclampsia in healthy nulliparous women: a prospective multicenter study. The National Institute of Child Health and Human Development Network of Maternal-Fetal Medicine Units. *Am J Obstet Gynecol* (1995), **172**:642–8.

68. Sibai BM, Ewell M, Levine RJ, Klebanoff MA, Esterlitz J, Catalano PM, et al., Risk factors associated with preeclampsia in healthy nulliparous women. The Calcium for Preeclampsia Prevention (CPEP) Study Group. *Am J Obstet and Gynecol* (1997), **177**:1003–10.

69. O'Brien TE, Ray JG, and Chan WS, Maternal body mass index and the risk of preeclampsia: a systematic overview. *Epidemiology* (2003), **14**:368–74.

70. Wolf M, Kettyle E, Sandler L, Ecker JL, Roberts J, and Thadhani R, Obesity and preeclampsia: the potential role of inflammation. *Obstet Gynecol* (2001), **98**:757–62.

71. Bodnar LM, Ness RB, Harger GF, and Roberts JM, Inflammation and triglycerides partially mediate the effect of prepregnancy body mass index on the risk of preeclampsia. *Am J Epidemiol* (2005), **162**:1198–206.

72. Bodnar LM, Ness RB, Markovic N, and Roberts JM, The risk of preeclampsia rises with increasing prepregnancy body mass index. *Ann Epidemiol* (2005), **15**:475–82.

7 Macronutrients for lactation and infant growth

Thibault Senterre and Jacques Rigo

Mammary growth

Pregnancy results in many transformations and adaptations of the woman's body that continue after delivery. Each species has developed its own strategies to meet the nutritional needs of its offspring. Systemic hormones, including pituitary prolactin, ovarian estrogen and progesterone, placental lactogen, and metabolic hormones, influence breast development. Initial changes observed during pregnancy include an increase in ductal branching and the formation of alveolar buds. Expansion of alveolar buds occurs to form clusters of lobuloalveolar units, followed by the differentiation of these structures into presecretory structures [1–3].

Lactogenesis begins during pregnancy and secretory material accumulates in the acini from the third month of gestation. This prepartum milk is mainly formed of proteins and glycoproteins. Large lipid droplets are also present in alveolar cells and in luminal spaces. After delivery, lactogenesis is stimulated by a fall in plasma progesterone, while prolactin level remains high. This phenomenon is independent of suckling and declines after a few days if the breast is not stimulated. Histological examination of the mammary gland during lactation reveals prominent luminal structures and ducts. Few adipocytes are visible, reflecting their delipidation rather than a decrease in their number. Change in the size and cellular distribution of lipid droplets is the more obvious histological transition from pregnancy to lactation [1, 3, 4].

Human milk production and composition

There is remarkable similarity in women's milk production throughout the world, independent of lifestyle and nutritional status. Colostrum is the first milk produced just after delivery; this thick and yellow milk contains a mixture of residual materials present in mammary gland and ducts. Colostrum is progressively replaced by newly secreted milk, called transitional milk. The initial physiological changes on the first day after delivery are independent of suckling or milk expression, but breast-feeding frequency on the second day of life is positively correlated with milk volume on Day 5. Thereafter, milk volume depends on infant demand, and potential milk available at each feeding is comparable. The maintenance of established milk secretion is mainly dependent on the hypothalamic-pituitary axis, which regulates prolactin and ocytocin secretion secondary to suckling stimulation [1, 4, 5].

Initial volumes of colostrum vary between 2 and 20 ml per feeding. Two to three days after delivery, transitional milk appears and is characterized by an increase in volume and by major changes in composition until the second week of life. Immunoglobulins and protein content decrease, whereas fat and lactose content increase the caloric content. Milk volume is associated with lactose secretion and water dilution. Volume of milk increases from less than 100 ml/day on the first day to about 600 ml/day after 96 hours. The mean amount of milk produced by mothers from developed countries is quite similar to women from developing countries. Parity has a positive influence on the onset of milk volume. Milk production is stable during the first months of lactation, but there is a wide range of milk intake among healthy breast-fed term infants, averaging 750 to 800 ml per day but ranging from 450 to 1200 ml/day because of infant demands (Table 7.1). If exclusive breast-feeding is continued after 6 months of age, milk production continues to increase. When complementary feedings are introduced, milk production decreases because of the infant's demand regulation and is usually between 400 and 600 ml in developed countries and between 600 and 700 ml in developing countries. Several studies reported a potential capacity of milk production up to 3 to 3.5 l/day. Any factor influencing frequency, intensity, or duration of suckling influences the volume. Exercise,

Table 7.1 Human milk (HM) composition (first 6 months)

Volume	750–800 ml/day	(range, 450–1200 ml/day)
Energy	2800 kj/l	670 kcal/L
Fats	37–40 g/l	50%–55% of HM energy
Carbohydrates	70–74 g/l	40%–45% of HM energy
Proteins	8–12 g/l	5%–6% of HM energy

manual labor, and losing weight do not usually alter an established milk volume secretion because of energy-sparing adaptations. Milk volume diminishes only in extreme malnutrition or severe dehydration. In fact, lactose content is the main regulator of osmolality and milk volume is related to lactose synthesis, which is very stable [1, 5–7].

Energy density of human milk is related to protein, fat, and carbohydrate contents. In well-nourished populations, milk fats average about 37 to 40 g/l and contribute to half or more of the total energy: milk carbohydrates average approximately 70 to 74 g/l and 40% to 45% of total energy, and milk proteins average approximately 8 to 12 g/l and only 5% to 6% of total energy (Table 7.1). Even if milk protein concentration decreases with postnatal age, these have relatively little impact on global milk energy density. According to various studies, energy density in human milk varies from 255 kJ/dl (61 kcal/dl) to 310 kJ/dl (74 kcal/dl). The mean metabolizable energy content generally used for human milk is 280 kJ/dl (67 kcal/dl; Table 7.1) [5, 8–11].

Milk fat concentration, and thus, energy density, varies both within a feed (hind milk is higher in fat than fore milk) and during a 24-hour period (depending on diet, on meals, and thus on populations). Data from different populations indicate that milk fat concentration is positively correlated with body fatness. However, this may not have a strong impact on total milk energy intake by infants allowed to nurse on demand because mean energy intake is the main determinant of volume intake. Thus, low energy density may be compensated for by a higher volume intake [9–11].

Lactose is the principal carbohydrate of human milk and is the second major component of human milk after water. Its concentration is stable. Human milk is isotonic with plasma, and 60% to 70% of osmotic pressure is due to lactose. Lactose is synthesized by the mammary gland and is constant throughout the day between 6.2 and 7.2 g/dl. Oligosaccharides are the third largest solid constituent of milk after lac-

tose and triglycerides. A lot of oligosaccharides have been identified in human milk. They are implicated in many functional aspects of human milk [8, 12, 13].

Most proteins are specific of milk secretions. They are synthesized from free amino acids in the secretary cells of mammary glands. Human milk proteins are mainly composed by casein and whey proteins. The term *casein* includes a group of milk-specific proteins characterized by ester-bound phosphate, high in proline content, and with low solubility at pH 4–5. Caseins form particles or micelles that are complexes of calcium caseinate and calcium-phosphate, which enhance calcium/phosphorus absorption and biodisponibililty. Concentration of protein in human milk and whey protein:casein ratio vary with lactation. Human milk proteins concentrations based on nitrogen measures decline from approximately 2–3 g/dl in colostrum to about 1.3–1.5 g/dl on Day 10 after delivery, 1.0–1.2 g/l at 1 month, and 0.8–0.9 g/dl thereafter. The whey protein:casein ratio changes from 90:10 in early milk to 60:40 in mature milk and 50:50 in late lactation. Nonprotein nitrogen accounts for approximately 25% of total nitrogen in human milk (ranging from 18% to 30%). Nonprotein nitrogen is not included in the true protein content, which is equivalent to protein as determined by amino acid analysis. True protein content is equivalent to total nitrogen minus nonprotein nitrogen, multiplied by 6.25. Urea represents 30% to 50% of the nonprotein nitrogen fraction and increases from colostrum to mature milk. Urea and the remaining components of nonprotein nitrogen serve partially as a nitrogen pool available for nonessential amino acid synthesis but also have many other functions (hormones, growth factors) [8, 13, 14].

Human milk fat content is the main source of energy and its most variable constituent. Fat content is low in colostrum and increases from 2% to 5% in mature milk. Prepartum secretions contain high amounts of membrane components, such as phospholipids, cholesterol, and cholesteryl esters that decrease from colostrum to mature milk. Cholesterol and phospholipid content decreases during the first week to stabilize at approximately 10 to 20 mg/dl. Fat content increases during feeding and changes over a 24-hour period as well as through lactation (diminishing after 6 months). Maternal body fat proportion influences lipid concentration in human milk. Higher fat content has been observed in well-nourished women, especially in cases of higher weight gain during pregnancy.

Primiparous women have more fat content than multiparous women [8, 15].

Human milk lipids consist of emulsified globules in the aqueous phase. The main lipids are triacylglycerol, phospholipids, and their fatty acids. Triglycerides constitute 98% of human milk fat and are the third major constituent after water and lactose. Oleic acid is the predominant fatty acid (35%), and its concentration depends on vegetable oil consumption. The second fatty acid is palmitic acid (22%), which increases in cases of low caloric intake. Short-chain fatty acids are mainly synthesized in the mammary glands, and medium-chain fatty acids come from adipocytes. Long-chain polyunsaturated fatty acids (LCPUFA) are derived from blood plasma and thus are more dependent on maternal diet. Concentrations decrease during lactation and vary greatly according to populations and studies: 10% to 18% for linoleic acid (LA; C18:2n6), 0.4% to 1.3% for alpha-linolenic acid (ALA; C18:3n3), 0.4% to 0.8% for arachidonic acid (ARA; C20:4n6), and 0.2% to 0.5% for docosahexaenoic acid (DHA; C22:6n3). N-6 and n-3 fatty acids are essential components of the phospholipids of cell membranes. They are critical for fluidity, permeability, and activity of membrane-bound enzymes and receptors. The Western diet is progressively becoming deficient in n-3 fatty acids, and consequently so is maternal milk. Trans fatty acids are also present in milk, depending on mother's diet and fat depot [8, 15–18].

Preterm infants are usually unable to be breast-fed naturally. A breast pump is used to express milk before administration. A sterile technique is necessary to avoid contamination, but milk pasteurization is frequently required. Mothers who deliver prematurely have higher milk nitrogen content and variable fat composition. In addition, some components of milk, such as fat, are lost during collection and storage. Human milk fortification is necessary to meet the high requirements of preterm infants [19, 20].

Infant nutritional requirements

Infants' energy requirements are defined as the amount of food energy necessary to balance total energy expenditure at a normal level of activity and to support and maintain growth and development consistent with long-term health. Total infant energy requirements increase with growth but decrease with age if adjusted for body weight. They correspond to 460 kJ/kg/day (110 kcal/kg/day) during the 1st month of

Table 7.2 Infant requirements during the first year of life (World Health Organization)

Energy	1st month	460 kJ (110 kcal) /kg/day
	6th month	339 kJ (81 kcal) /kg/day
	12th month	334 kJ (80 kcal) /kg/day
Protein	1st month	1.77 g/kg/day
	6th month	1.14 g/kg/day
	12th month	0.95 g/kg/day

life, lowering to 339 kJ/kg/day (81 kcal/kg/day) during the 6th month, tending to plateau until the 12th month (Table 7.2). This decrease in energy requirements is related to the decreased energy deposition for growth from 40% of total energy requirements at 1 month to 3% at 12 months. These upgraded estimates are 10% to 32% lower than the previous recommendations [14, 21].

Infants' protein requirements can be defined as the minimum intake that will allow nitrogen equilibrium at an appropriate body composition during energy balance at moderate physical activity, in addition to the needs associated with the deposition of tissues consistent with good health. The composition of human milk provides the model for estimated total protein and essential amino acid requirements during infancy, taking into account the utilization of a portion of its nonprotein nitrogen fraction. After 6 months, estimation of the protein requirements derives from a factorial approach, considering maintenance, growth deposition, and efficiency of use. Recent reassessments of estimated requirements are 10% to 25% lower than previous ones and decrease from 1.77 g/kg/day at 1 month to 1.14 g/kg/day at 6 months, tending to plateau until 12 months [14, 22, 23] (Table 7.2).

Dietary fats are the main source of infants' energy, provide essential fatty acids, and facilitate the absorption of fat-soluble vitamins. During the first 6 months of life, an infant accumulates 1300 to 1600 g of fats. Lipids are structural components of all tissues and are indispensable for cell and plasma membrane synthesis. The brain, retina, and other neural tissues are particularly rich in LCPUFA, especially DHA. Cholesterol is an essential component of all membranes and is required for growth, replication, and maintenance. Breast-feeding induces higher plasma cholesterol in infants than formulas, and some studies suggest that it may protect against hypercholesterolemia in later life. The quality of dietary lipid supply in early childhood is a major determinant of growth, development, and long-term health. N-6 and n-3 LCPUFA are derived from LA and ALA, respectively, by the same competitive enzymatic pathway, including desaturations and elongations. LA and ALA are also precursors for eicosanoid production (prostaglandins, prostacyclins, thromboxanes, and leukotrienes). These autocrine and paracrine mediators are powerful regulators of numerous cell and tissue functions [16, 18, 24, 25].

DHA is the most abundant n-3 fatty acid in the mammalian brain. Neuronal membranes and retinal photoreceptor cells receive most of their phospholipid DHA from the diet. Several studies suggest that DHA status in early infancy is positively related to visual acuity and neurodevelopmental outcomes. Cerebrocortical gray matter concentration of DHA in infants depends on their diet supplies. Breast-fed infants accumulate more DHA than formula-fed infants who are not consuming dietary DHA. ALA is the precursor of DHA, but its synthesis may be limited by enzyme insufficiency or by enzyme competition due to an excess of n-6 fatty acids. In addition, LCPUFA synthesis appears to decrease during the first year of life. Even in breast-fed infants, DHA tissue content decreases progressively after 6 months, when complementary feeding is introduced, because of its low content of LCPUFA. This may lead to insufficient DHA intakes. Therefore, especially in developing countries, breast milk as a source of essential fatty acids is important until the end of the second year of life [16, 26–31].

Differences between breast-fed infants and formula-fed infants

Human milk is markedly different from cow's milk. The infant response to human milk and formula differs with respect to endocrine, gastrointestinal, immune, renal, and metabolic functions. Immunological and anti-infectious proprieties of human milk are of major importance compared with formulas. They are related to its cellular composition, with living leukocytes, and to many soluble proteins such as lysozyme, nucleotides, glutamine, and transferrin. Lactating mammary glands are part of an integrated mucosal immune system with local production of antibodies, mainly consisting of secretory immunoglobulin A. These antibodies reflect antigenic stimulation of mucosal-associated lymphoid tissue by common intestinal and respiratory pathogens. Antibodies in breast milk are thus highly targeted against infectious agents present in the mother's and postnatal infant's environment. The immune system protects the infant against pathogenic organisms, and highly complex pathways of recognition, response, elimination, and memory have evolved to fulfill this role. The immune system also acts to ensure self-tolerance but also tolerance to food, environmental components, and commensal bacteria. Any perturbations of these functions may lead to infectious or inflammatory diseases [13, 32, 33].

The intestine is sterile at birth, and rapid colonization occurs after delivery. Maternal gut flora, delivery environment, and diet are the major determinants of initial intestinal flora in newborns. A specificity of human milk is to select a flora rich in *Lactobacillus* and bifidobacteria. Recent studies suggest that appropriate flora promote gut maturation and the gut-associated immune system. Human milk oligosaccharides, high lactose content, milk immunological functions, and other properties of human milk are the main factors influencing the breast-fed infant's flora [12, 13, 32].

Over the past several decades, the incidence of atopic diseases has increased dramatically. Environmental factors, including early infant nutrition, may influence their development. For infants at high risk of developing atopy, there is evidence that exclusive breast-feeding for at least 4 months prevents or delays the occurrence of atopic dermatitis, cow's milk allergy, and wheezing in early childhood. Epidemiologic studies have also suggested that early exposure to certain nutrients, including LCPUFA, may be protective against immune anomalies. Relative intake of LA, the n-6 LCPUFA precursor, has increased progressively in Western diets, suggesting a positive relationship between the n-6 LCPUFA supplies and the prevalence of allergic diseases via enhanced ARA and prostaglandin E2 production [16, 34, 35].

The available evidence suggests that breast-feeding may have other long-term benefits. Infants who were breast-fed experience lower mean blood pressure and lower total cholesterol in adulthood, as well as higher performance in intelligence tests. Furthermore, the prevalence of overweight/obesity and Type II diabetes is lower among breast-fed infants. These effects are statistically significant even after adjustment for various confounding factors, but for some outcomes, the magnitude is relatively modest. The protein:energy ratio of human milk is low compared with infant formulas. It seems that a higher protein:energy ratio may be responsible for the accelerated growth of formula-fed infants compared with breast-fed infants during the first year of life, which is believed to induce metabolic imprinting with adverse later consequences of formula feeding [13, 36–39].

Exclusive breast-feeding is recommended until 6 months of age, when complementary feeding should be introduced. Industrial interests conduct many studies to improve formulas to replicate breast milk more closely. Therefore, it is important to promote the use of the most innovative formulas for infants when breast-feeding is not possible [33, 36, 39–41].

Key clinical messages

- *Breast-feeding during the first hours and days after delivery improves efficiency and persistence of breast-feeding.*
- *Breast-feeding must be adapted according to the infant's demand.*
- *Exclusive breast-feeding is recommended until 6 months of age, when complementary feeding should be introduced.*
- *Industry is improving formulas to replicate breast milk more closely. It is important to promote the use of the most innovative formulas when breast-feeding is not possible.*

Maternal needs related to lactation

Milk composition is sensitive to maternal factors, such as body composition, diet, and parity. Food supplementation during lactation in areas of high malnutrition has generally little, if any, impact on milk volume, but it improves maternal health. Throughout the world, women usually produce adequate and abundant milk, even when they have inadequate diets. When milk energy density is low, infants adapt their suckling behavior to increase volume intake to maintain adequate total energy intake [1, 5].

Lactating mothers usually describe an increase in thirst and so adapt their fluid intake during lactation. However, fluid intake has no positive influence on milk volume. In all infants, water requirements are supported by exclusive breast-feeding even in warm, humid climates. In contrast, excess fluid intake could negatively influence milk production. When water is restricted, urinary output decreases before there is any reduction in milk volume. Adapting fluid intake to thirst is probably the best advice for lactating mothers (Table 7.3) [42].

Table 7.3 Maternal nutritional recommendation during lactation

Fluid	Ad libitum
Energy	+ 2100 kJ (500 kcal) /day (0–6 months)
	+ 1900 kJ (460 kcal) /day (>6 months)
Protein	+ 19 g/day (0–6 months)
	+ 12.5 g/day (>6 months)
Lipid	+ 200 mg/day docosahexaenoic acid (fish twice a week)
High risk of atopy	No specific prevention
Postpartum weight loss	Spontaneous normal loss of 0.5–1.0 kg/month in well-nourished mother; dietary restriction not recommended

The energy requirements of a lactating woman are defined as the level of energy intake from food that will balance the energy expenditure needed to maintain her body weight and composition, level of physical activity, and breast-milk production to ensure good health for her and her child and that will allow her to perform economically necessary and socially desirable activities. Energy cost of lactation is determined by the energy content of milk produced and secreted and the efficiency of the conversion of dietary energy for milk synthesis. For exclusive breast-feeding during the first 6 months after delivery, the total mean energy cost could be estimated as follows: 800 ml milk/day × 280 kJ/dl / 0.80 for efficiency = 2800 kJ/day (675 kcal/day). After 6 months, during complementary feeding, human milk production is approximately 550 ml per day, and the energy cost decreases to 1900 kJ/day (460 kcal/day) [9–11].

Fat and other nutrients are stored during pregnancy and may cover in part the additional energy needs during the first months of lactation. Postpartum weight loss is usually highest in the first 3 months and is considered by mothers to be an advantage of breast-feeding compared with formula feeding. Potential energy mobilization during lactation depends on weight gain during gestation and nutritional status of the mother. Well-nourished women usually lose 0.5 to 1.0 kg per month, whereas undernourished mothers lose an average of only 0.1 kg per month. Assuming energy content of 27 200 kJ/kg, the rate of weight loss in well-nourished women would correspond to the mobilization of 27 200 × 0.8 kg/month = 21 800 kJ/month, or 720 kJ/day (170 kcal/day) from body energy stores. This amount of energy accounts in

67

deduction from the energy cost of lactation. Thus, during the first 6 months of lactation, the energy requirement of a lactating woman represents around 2100 kJ/day (500 kcal/day). After 6 months, the contribution of weight loss is minimal – 22 kJ/day – and does not significantly influence the energy cost for milk production – 1900 kJ/day (460 kcal/day; Table 7.3). However, undernourished women and those who did not gain adequate body weight during pregnancy must conserve as much energy as possible for their own health, and the full energy demands of lactation must be provided by an increment in dietary intake [9–11].

New recommendations have been published concerning protein requirements during lactation because previous recommendations did not take into consideration the nonprotein nitrogen fraction of human milk. A factorial approach was taken to derive the protein requirements during lactation. Mean production rates of milk of well-nourished women who breast-feed exclusively during the first 6 months and partially breast-feed during the second 6 months postpartum were used, together with the mean concentrations of protein and nonprotein nitrogen in human milk, to calculate milk protein output. The protein requirements were calculated as mean + 1.96 standard deviation. The additional safe protein intake during the first 6 months of lactation is 19 g of protein per day, falling to 12.5 g of protein per day after 6 months (Table 7.3). New estimates are 20% to 50% higher than previous ones [14, 23].

Maternal dietary preferences and the nature of her dietary fat have a great impact on milk triglyceride composition. Fatty acids from maternal diet may affect up to approximately 30% of total milk fatty acids. High carbohydrate intake is associated with an increase in endogenous synthesis of C6–C16 fatty acids. In case of insufficient diet, mother fat depositions are mobilized, and milk fatty acids tend to mimic their fatty acid composition. When excessive non-fat-caloric diet is provided, milk-saturated fatty acids increase as lipids are synthesized for tissue stores. When corn oil is the mean fat source, milk levels of C18:2 and C18:3 are higher, with a major increase in LA, compared with lard or butter fats. Synthesis of fatty acids up to 16 carbons, as well as desaturations of stearic acid into oleic acid, can take place in the mammary gland, whereas LCPUFAs come directly from plasma and are directly related to maternal diet. DHA concentrations in human milk may show great variation depending on population and diet, and the ARA:DHA ratio may change from 2.8 to 0.4. The ability to synthesize DHA from ALA exists in humans, but most evidence indicates that it is limited. Therefore, adequate intake of preformed n-3 LCPUFA, and in particular DHA, appears to be important for maintaining optimal tissue functions. Several studies have shown visual and cognitive advantages in infants after maternal supplementation with oily fish or oils providing n-3 LCPUFA during pregnancy and lactation. Supplementation of lactating women with 200 mg DHA per day increased human milk content up to a level considered desirable for infant outcomes. However, intakes of up to 1 g per day of DHA or 2.7 g per day n-3 LCPUFA have been used in randomized trials without significant adverse effects. Women can meet the recommended intakes of DHA by consuming one or two portions of sea fish per week, including oily fish such as herring, mackerel, and salmon (Table 7.3). Even if fish can contribute to the dietary exposure of contaminants, these recommendations rarely exceed the tolerable intake of environmental contaminants. Levels of bioaccumulative contaminants tend to be greater in large fish that are higher in the food chain (i.e. marlin, pike, swordfish, and shark) [16, 18, 24, 25].

Cholesterol is synthesized in part by the mammary gland, and its level in milk is not affected by maternal diet. Industrially produced trans fatty acids are frequent in modern diets, and their presence in human milk reflects mothers' dietary intake. The literature includes controversies about trans fatty acids because of their association with long-term adverse biological effects [43, 44].

Dietary food allergens can be detected in breast milk and may induce allergic reactions in infants who are known to be clinically allergic to the antigen. Rare cases of anaphylaxis to cow's milk protein present in human milk have been described, even in exclusively breast-fed infants. Previous American Academy of Pediatrics publications have advised lactating mothers with infants at high risk of developing allergy to avoid peanuts and tree nuts and to consider eliminating eggs, cow's milk, and fish from their diets while nursing. According to more recent studies, their advice was recently revised to state that in infants at high risk of developing allergy, there is no convincing evidence for a long-term preventive effect of maternal diet during lactation on atopic disease (Table 7.3) [34, 35, 45].

Maternal malnutrition and restrictions

Maternal milk protein content is preserved when lactating mothers receive short-term marginal dietary protein intake. During World War II and the Dutch famine, pregnant women developed some maternal stores in anticipation of lactation, even if their fetus had intrauterine growth restriction. This demonstrates the mother's body's strong biological commitment to preparing for lactation. When the diet is insufficient, fat deposits are mobilized and milk fat mimics the composition of fat stores. Protein content in milk from poorly nourished mothers is still in the range of normal values, and malnutrition has little impact on protein concentration. Malnutrition may decrease production and secretion of immunological system components of human milk, but this remains controversial, and further investigation is necessary. It would be useful to consider whether the lactation performance of women who do not meet their energy needs might be compromised, but testing this hypothesis poses methodological challenges. Nevertheless, some evidence suggests that in women with adequate fat reserves, postpartum gradual weight loss up to 0.5 kg/week is not likely to have any adverse consequences on lactation and nutritional supplies in term infants. Nevertheless, dietary restriction to favor postpartum weight loss should be discouraged (Table 7.3) [10, 42].

Key clinical messages

- *There is remarkable similarity in milk production throughout the world, independent of lifestyle and nutritional status. Production of adequate and abundant milk supply is usually possible even in inadequate diets.*
- *Food supplementation during lactation in areas with a high incidence of malnutrition has generally little, if any, impact on milk volume. However, it improves maternal health and is always helpful.*

- *Human milk fat content is the main source of energy and its most variable constituent.*
- *The quality of dietary lipid supply, especially DHA, in early childhood is a major determinant of infant development and long-term health. LCPUFA in human milk is derived from blood plasma and so is dependent on maternal diet. Eating fish twice a week and/or 200 mg DHA supplementation per day increases human milk content to a level considered desirable for infant outcomes.*

Conclusions

Exclusive breast-feeding is recommended during the first 6 months after delivery and should be continued after introduction of complementary feeding. There is remarkable similarity across populations with widely varying nutritional status when measuring human milk volume and nutritional supplies, but there is also a wide range of individual variability. This is related to the adaptation of milk production to infant demand. Maternal dietary stores, dietary preferences, and cultural patterns should be considered in establishing recommendations for lactating women. New recommendations have recently been published concerning both infants' and lactating mothers' requirements, but these usually make minimal adjustments to account for a woman's lifestyle. Women need to be well nourished throughout gestation and to maintain adequate nutritional intakes after delivery. Supplementing malnourished mothers is advised to promote maternal as well as infant health. Well-nourished lactating women have a net increase in energy requirements to approximately 2100 kJ (500 kcal) per day, which can be met by a small increase in a well-balanced diet. Restricted diets and medications to lose weight are unwise, and maternal stores will be used for lactation. There may be some variation in milk composition related to maternal diet, especially concerning fatty acids. N-3 polyunsaturated fatty acids have decreased in Western diets, with potentially adverse effects. A supplementation of docosahexaenoic acid during lactation is advised.

References

1. Neville MC, Anatomy and physiology of lactation. *Pediatr Clin North Am* (2001), **48**:13–34.

2. Neville MC, McFadden TB, and Forsyth I, Hormonal regulation of mammary differentiation and milk secretion. *J Mammary Gland Biol Neoplasia* (2002), **7**:49–66.

3. Anderson SM, Rudolph MC, McManaman JL, and Neville MC, Key stages in mammary gland development. Secretory activation in the mammary gland: it's not just about milk protein synthesis! *Breast Cancer Res* (2007), **9**:204.

4. Neville MC, Morton J, and Umemura S, Lactogenesis. The transition from pregnancy to lactation. *Pediatr Clin North Am* (2001), **48**:35–52.

5. Neville MC and McManaman JL. Milk secretion and composition. In Neonatal Nutrition and Metabolism, eds. Thureen PJ and Hay WW (New York: Cambridge University Press, 2006), pp. 377–89.

6. Macy IG, Hunscher HA, Donelson E, and Nims B, Human milk flow. *Am J Dis Child* (1930), **6**:492–515.

7. Saint L, Maggiore P, and Hartmann PE, Yield and nutrient content of milk in eight women breast-feeding twins and one woman breast-feeding triplets. *Br J Nutr* (1986), **56**:49–58.

8. Picciano MF, Nutrient composition of human milk. *Pediatr Clin North Am* (2001), **48**:53–67.

9. Butte NF and King JC, Energy requirements during pregnancy and lactation. *Public Health Nutr* (2005), **8**:1010–27.

10. Dewey KG, Energy and protein requirements during lactation. *Ann Rev Nutr* (1997), **17**:19–36.

11. Food and Agriculture Organization (FAO), Human Energy Requirements, FAO Food and Nutrition Technical Report Series 1 (Rome: FAO/WHO/UNU Expert Consultation, 2004).

12. Kunz C, Rudloff S, Baier W, Klein N, and Strobel S, Oligosaccharides in human milk: structural, functional, and metabolic aspects. *Ann Rev Nutr* (2000), **20**:699–722.

13. Hamosh M, Bioactive factors in human milk. *Pediatr Clin North Am* (2001), **48**:69–86.

14. World Health Organization (WHO), Energy and Protein Requirements. WHO Technical Report Series no. 724 (Geneva: Joint FAO/WHO/UNU Expert Consultation, 1985).

15. Hamosh M, Enteral lipid digestion and absorption. In Neonatal Nutrition and Metabolism, eds. Thureen PJ and Hay WW (New York: Cambridge University Press, 2006), pp. 350–68.

16. Innis SM, Human milk: maternal dietary lipids and infant development. *Proc Nutr Soc* (2007), **66**:397–404.

17. Bokor S, Koletzko B, and Decsi T, Systematic review of fatty acid composition of human milk from mothers of preterm compared to full-term infants. *Ann Nutr Metab* (2007), **51**:550–6.

18. Koletzko B, Cetin I, and Brenna JT, Dietary fat intakes for pregnant and lactating women. *Br J Nutr* (2007), **98**:873–7.

19. Schanler RJ, Fortified human milk for premature infants. In: Neonatal Nutrition and Metabolism, eds. Thureen PJ and Hay WW (New York: Cambridge University Press, 2006), pp. 401–8.

20. Schanler RJ, The use of human milk for premature infants. *Pediatr Clin North Am* (2001), **48**:207–19.

21. Butte NF, Energy requirements of infants. *Public Health Nutr* (2005), **8**:953–67.

22. Dewey KG, Beaton G, Fjeld C, Lönnerdal B, and Reeds P, Protein requirements of infants and children. *Eur J Clin Nutr* (1996), **50**(Suppl 1):S119–47; discussion S147–50.

23. World Health Organization (WHO), Protein and Amino Acid Requirements in Human Nutrition, WHO Technical Report Series no. 935. Geneva: Joint FAO/WHO/UNU Expert Consultation, 2007.

24. Innis SM, Dietary lipids in early development: relevance to obesity, immune and inflammatory disorders. *Curr Opin Endocrinol Diabetes Obes* (2007), **14**:359–64.

25. Innis SM, Essential fatty acid metabolism during early development. In: Biology of Metabolism in Growing Animals, ed. Buring DG (Amsterdam: Elsevier Science, 2005), pp. 235–74.

26. Prentice AM and Paul AA, Fat and energy needs of children in developing countries. *Am J Clin Nutr* (2000), **72**(Suppl 5):1253S–1265S.

27. Uauy R and Castillo C, Lipid requirements of infants: implications for nutrient composition of fortified complementary foods. *J Nutr* (2003), **133**:2962S–72S.

28. Innis SM, Dietary (n-3) fatty acids and brain development. *J Nutr* (2007), **137**:855–9.

29. Farquharson J, Cockburn F, Patrick WA, Jamieson EC, and Logan RW, Infant cerebral cortex phospholipid fatty-acid composition and diet. *Lancet* (1992), **340**:810–13.

30. Cunnane SC, Cunnane SC, Francescutti V, Brenna JT, and Crawford MA, Breast-fed infants achieve a higher rate of brain and whole body docosahexaenoate accumulation than formula-fed infants not consuming dietary docosahexaenoate. *Lipids* (2000), **35**:105–11.

31. Carnielli VP, Simonato M, Verlato G, Luijendijk I, De Curtis M, Sauer PJ, and Cogo PE, Synthesis of long-chain polyunsaturated

fatty acids in preterm newborns fed formula with long-chain polyunsaturated fatty acids. *Am J Clin Nutr* (2007), **86**:1323–30.

32. Calder PC, Krauss-Etschmann S, de Jong EC, Dupont C, Frick JS, Frokiaer H, et al., Early nutrition and immunity – progress and perspectives. *Br J Nutr* (2006), **96**:774–90.

33. Koletzko B, Baker S, Cleghorn G, Neto UF, Gopalan S, Hernell O, et al., Global standard for the composition of infant formula: recommendations of an ESPGHAN coordinated international expert group. *J Pediatr Gastroenterol Nutr* (2005), **41**:584–99.

34. Kramer MS and Kakuma R, Maternal dietary antigen avoidance during pregnancy or lactation, or both, for preventing or treating atopic disease in the child. *Cochrane Database Syst Rev* (2006), 3:CD000133.

35. Chouraqui JP, Dupont C, Bocquet A, Bresson JL, Briend A, Darmaun D, et al., Comité de nutrition de la Société française de pédiatrie. Feeding during the first months of life and prevention of allergy. *Arch Pediatr* (2008), **15**:431–42.

36. Fewtrell MS, Session 6: Infant nutrition: future research developments in Europe EARNEST, the early nutrition programming project: EARly Nutrition programming – long-term efficacy and safety trials and integrated epidemiological, genetic, animal, consumer and economic research. *Proc Nutr Soc* (2007), **66**:435–41.

37. Owen CG, Martin RM, Whincup PH, Smith GD, and Cook DG, Does breastfeeding influence risk of type 2 diabetes in later life? A quantitative analysis of published evidence. *Am J Clin Nutr* (2006), **84**:1043–54.

38. Owen CG, Martin RM, Whincup PH, Davey-Smith G, Gillman MW, and Cook DG, The effect of breastfeeding on mean body mass index throughout life: a quantitative review of published and unpublished observational evidence. *Am J Clin Nutr* (2005), **82**:1298–307.

39. Horta BL, Bahl R, Martinés JC, Victoria CG, Evidence on the Long-Term Effects of Breastfeeding: Systematic Reviews and Meta-Analyses (Geneva: World Health Organization, 2007).

40. World Health Organization and United Nations Children's Fund, Global Strategy for Infant and Young Child Feeding (Geneva: World Health Organization, 2003).

41. Fewtrell MS, Morgan JB, Duggan C, Gunnlaugsson G, Hibberd PL, Lucas A, and Kleinman RE, Optimal duration of exclusive breastfeeding: what is the evidence to support current recommendations? *Am J Clin Nutr* (2007), **85**:635S–638S.

42. Lawrence RA and Lawrence RM, Breastfeeding: A Guide for the Medical Profession, 6th edn (Philadelphia: Elsevier Mosby, 2005).

43. Kris-Etherton PM and Innis S, American Dietetic Association, Dietitians of Canada. Position of the American Dietetic Association and Dietitians of Canada: dietary fatty acids. *J Am Diet Assoc* (2007), **107**: 1599–611.

44. van Eijsden M, Hornstra G, Van Der Wal MF, Vrijkotte TG, and Bonsel GJ, Maternal n-3, n-6, and trans fatty acid profile early in pregnancy and term birth weight: a prospective cohort study. *Am J Clin Nutr* (2008), **87**:887–95.

45. Greer, FR, Sicherer SH, and Burks AW. Effects of early nutritional interventions on the development of atopic disease in infants and children: the role of maternal dietary restriction, breastfeeding, timing of introduction of complementary foods, and hydrolyzed formulas. *Pediatrics* (2008), **121**:183–91.

Nutritional regulation and requirements for lactation and infant growth

8 Changes in nutrient requirements with age after birth

Christopher H. Knight

Introduction

This chapter considers nutritional requirements of the neonate during the period between birth and weaning. Preterm babies are the focus of the next chapter, so for our purposes "birth" is full-term birth. The World Health Organization (WHO)[1] recommends that exclusive breast-feeding be practiced until 6 months of age, and because the weaning process is normally a gradual one, I interpret birth to weaning to mean the first half-year or so of life. This is a time of rapid growth, development, and maturation, particularly of the nervous and skeletal systems. It is also a time of fat deposition. Appropriate nutrition is essential if a healthy baby is to grow into a healthy toddler. In the developed world, the majority of full-term babies do exactly that, and attention is now focused on longer-term effects of early development, particularly associations between early development and later obesity and metabolic disease. "Appropriate" nutrition encompasses a range that lies between deficiency and excess, and, where long-term health is concerned, excess may be as damaging as deficiency. The scenario is totally different in the developing world, where malnutrition caused by dietary deficiency continues to be a major threat to the life of the young child. WHO estimates that 60% of deaths under age 5 years are attributable, directly or indirectly, to malnutrition. This chapter focuses on the developed world.

To wean is to "accustom to the loss of its mother's milk" (*Oxford English Dictionary*), hence it is implicit (strictly) that the requirements of the infants under discussion are met by breast-feeding, either exclusively or in part. Thus, there is good news and bad:

- The good news: breast milk provides all the nutrients a baby needs for healthy development in the first 6 months of life [2].
- The bad news: the baby's requirements may be viewed differently by baby, mother, and health worker; may differ between babies who have

developed well in utero and those who have not; may be different between the sexes; and may be affected by environmental factors both directly and indirectly (mother's nutrition, for instance).

The truth lies somewhere between these two situations. For many mother:young dyads, the good news prevails, for others it is totally irrelevant because "breast" is replaced by "bottle." This chapter focuses on breast-feeding. The baby probably has no more or less control over the fulfilling of his or her requirements whether breast-fed or bottle-fed, but for the mother, the difference is quite fundamental. She will feel that she has little conscious control over either the amount or quality of her breast milk. For the most part, she must trust to nature to get it right, something that is rather difficult for inexperienced mothers to do without appropriate support. In contrast, she has (or believes she has) excellent control over the quantity of bottle milk and some control over its quality. Whether we consider exclusive breast-feeding, partial breast-feeding, or bottle-feeding, there is one further piece of bad news:

- Above all, requirements will differ according to the "target" that is being set. In particular, maximizing instantaneous growth will not necessarily maximize long-term health but will consciously or unconsciously be the target for many babies and for many mothers.

Finally, it should be recognized that rigid adherence to the title would result in a rather short chapter, because, for the most part, our understanding of "requirements" during early life equates to knowing what average intake has been. Requirements comprise whatever is necessary to maintain normal healthy body functions (maintenance), daily energy expenditure above maintenance (primarily locomotion), and growth. There is relatively little locomotion component in the neonate but considerable growth. Although growth is readily apparent, precise quantification is difficult because it requires knowledge of body composition as well as weight, and definitive information on composition is lacking [3]. Dietary Reference Intakes data published by the U.S. National Academy of Sciences Institute of Medicine do not list any Estimated Average Requirements for the 0- to 6-month age group and give only one (protein) for 7 to 12 months [4]. Instead, Adequate Intakes data are provided, which are stated to be mean intakes. I use the term "requirement" to mean best knowledge of what is needed for healthy growth. A number of recent reviews of neonatal nutrition are available, and those wishing a more detailed account than that provided here are recommended to read Butte et al. [5].

Targets for requirements

The "ideal" growth path is for a healthy baby to grow into a healthy toddler and hence enjoy long-term health (Fig. 8.1). Logical as this progression might seem, it is only recently that early growth has been shown to have long-term impact. This is the concept of metabolic programming, recently reviewed by Wells et al. [6]. Relationships between birth weight and risk of obesity, metabolic disease, and coronary heart disease have been demonstrated but are not always straightforward. For instance, two cohorts of intrauterine growth-restricted babies born during the Second World War (Dutch famine and Leningrad-siege) have shown different adult outcomes, while adult obesity may be associated with both low and high birth weight. It is body composition, and particularly the extent of internal fat depots, that are most likely to influence long-term health, and body weight is not a particularly good measure of body composition. However, it is also now apparent that fetal growth is only part of the picture. Metabolic programming takes place during both fetal and neonatal life [7], and it appears that low birth weight combined with early catch-up growth gives rise to the worst possible outcome (Fig. 8.1) [8]. There can be little doubt which population is at greatest risk from this combination. Cigarette smoking is the major cause of low birth weight [9], smokers are less likely to breast-feed [10], and formula-fed babies have a higher growth rate and are more likely to become obese [11]. In setting targets, there is always a need to balance short- and long-term objectives [12]. Thus, although a recommendation to *avoid* catch-up growth may be appropriate for full-term, healthy but small babies, for premature babies, the recommendation would normally

still be to *encourage* catch-up growth to ensure normal neurological development [13].

Although the "worst path" to long-term health can be identified (Fig. 8.1), it is much less clear whether what we would currently regard as "healthy growth" is necessarily the optimum weaning-age target ("best" in Fig. 8.1). The recent reformulation of WHO Child Growth Standards represents best knowledge, but the very fact that there was a need for revision demonstrates the inherent difficulty. The old growth charts were largely based on information from formula-fed infants and are now believed to have seriously overestimated optimal growth. It is unlikely that there will be further need for revision in the foreseeable future, and I show "best" and "healthy growth" as overlapping (rather than identical) only to show that there are some things we cannot know for certain. The inappropriateness of the older growth charts has implications for the metabolic programming hypothesis. Much of the data on which the hypothesis is based will have been obtained from formula-fed infants, fed (as we would now consider) excessively. So it may be that *modest* catch-up growth is appropriate for all small babies (full-term and preterm).

In addition to inappropriate birth weight and absence of breast-feeding, another factor that will cause deviation from the optimum path is disease, of the neonate, the breast-feeding mother, or both (Fig. 8.1). Surprisingly little is known about the effects of infection on energy requirements of babies. In reviewing the field, Garza [14] concluded that resting energy expenditure "remains stable, increases minimally or is raised up to 30% above baseline" during acute illness. Historical estimates of a 13% increase for every degree Celsius of fever were supported by some observations but not others. Clearly, there is a problem. Because disease cannot be predicted in advance, measurements have been made during the illness and compared with later, presumed "normal" determinations. If disease is followed by catch-up growth, the assumption is invalid, because energy expenditure will be increased by the extra growth. The usual advice offered to breast-feeding mothers is to continue breast-feeding, offering additional or prolonged feeds if the baby desires. As discussed later in the chapter, any additional energy requirement is almost certain to be met. WHO advice for babies suffering diarrhea and dehydration is to offer additional fluid while continuing to breast-feed. The health benefits of breast-feeding are many and varied [15] and are covered in a later chapter.

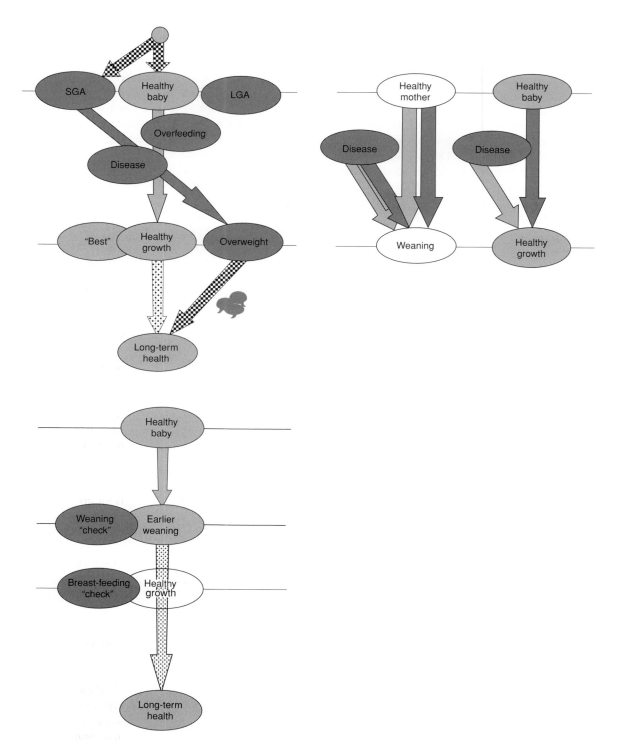

Figure 8.1 Schematic of optimal (green) and suboptimal (red) growth paths. Top left: The optimal path comprises healthy baby, healthy growth (to weaning), and long-term health. Only one of many possible suboptimal paths is shown, in which the small-for-gestational-age baby exhibits catch-up growth to become an overweight weanling. That toddler has a reduced chance of achieving long-term health. Top right: The neonate's requirements will increase with age and will probably be higher immediately after disease. Both the volume and the composition of breast milk can vary to meet those requirements. Maternal disease (mastitis, for instance) is likely to affect both volume and composition. Bottom left: There is debate over the optimum length of exclusive breast-feeding. Earlier weaning could result in a growth check, but equally breast-feeding could become inadequate and also restrict growth.

A number of studies have shown that some 20% of breast-feeding mothers will suffer mastitis [16]. The usual recommendation is to continue breast-feeding and to pay particular attention to breast emptying if possible, although in some studies (but not all), mastitis led to discontinuation of breast-feeding in a significant proportion of mothers. There is little published information on changes in breast-milk volume or composition during mastitis, but by analogy with dairy species, it is likely that both will be altered (Fig. 8.1). Volume will decrease, but effects on composition will vary depending on the pathogen and severity of infection. In the absence of evidence to the contrary, it is probably safe to assume that the baby's requirements can still be met by exclusive breast-feeding during mastitis, although it is not known what proportion of affected mothers will start to offer complementary foods.

The final panel of Figure 8.1 introduces the issue of when to wean. There has always been considerable variation in weaning practice, both within cultures across time and between cultures at the one time [12]. For babies in developing countries where hygiene is poor and the energy and protein content of supplementary foods is less than ideal, weaning represents risk. Growth faltering is commonplace. In developed countries, the great majority of babies wean successfully with no impediment to their growth and do so irrespective of exactly when or how it occurs. Nevertheless, in recent years, a debate has opened up regarding one particular aspect of exclusive breast-feeding and weaning: the 6-month debate.

- Inappropriate fetal and neonatal growth can have a negative long-term impact.
- The combination of small birth weight and rapid catch-up growth may be particularly bad.
- Mothers should be strongly advised not to smoke in pregnancy and to breast-feed rather than bottle-feed.
- Small-for-gestational-age babies should be monitored particularly carefully to ensure healthy growth while avoiding excessive catch-up growth.
- Mothers should normally be encouraged to continue breast-feeding during short-term illness of the baby.
- Similarly, mothers who develop mastitis should normally be encouraged to continue breast-feeding.

Meeting energy requirements: the 6-month debate

Energy is essential to life, and hence, if immediate energy requirements are not met in some way, other requirements become irrelevant. Because energy supply is variable in the natural world, mechanisms for depositing energy as fat and subsequently mobilizing it during times of need have evolved. Lactation is a related mechanism, whereby energetic variation is significantly diluted by the mother. Because milk has evolved as a balanced food designed to meet the nutritional requirements of the neonate, it has been argued that an amount of milk sufficient to meet energy requirements will automatically fulfill all other requirements as well [17]. It is now recommended that exclusive breast-feeding be done for the first 6 months of life [1], whereas previously the recommendation was 4 to 6 months. The advice is a global one, more designed to correct malnutrition in the developing world than to dictate to Western mothers. It also reflects the realization that earlier energy recommendations were considerable overestimates, based as they were on intake of poorly designed milk formula and the new knowledge that early overweight could have deleterious effects in the long term. The change has been controversial [18] and has prompted examination of energetic sufficiency at 6 months. In summary:

- Additional energy requirements for growth in the first few months of life mean that energy required per kilogram of body weight decreases between birth and 6 months [17].
- Because body weight increases, total energy requirement increases from around 1900 kJ/day at 1 month to around 2600 kJ/day at 6 months and is higher in boys than girls [19].
- Energy balance calculations indicate a small deficit in exclusively breast-fed babies at 6 months, suggesting that complementary feeding may be necessary [20].
- However, the same data also indicate a small deficit at 4 months, and the analysis excluded data continuing beyond 6 months, so there may be a bias against mothers committed to prolonged exclusive breast-feeding.
- Energy balance would be achieved with an intake at 6 months of around 1 kg/day.

75

- Typical human milk yield data are around 700–900 g/day, but mothers suckling twins can produce twice this amount [21].
- Milk yield is positively related to suckling frequency and efficiency [22]; mothers of twins feed 15 or more times per day.
- Mothers are accustomed to feeding frequency decreasing after the first few weeks.
- Older babies do not always have the patience to empty the breast effectively at a feed.
- Increased feeding demand is often evident at approximately 3 months and again at approximately 6 months [3].
- Social factors such as length of maternity leave will have a strong influence on the mother:young dyad at approximately 6 months.
- The limited data available indicate only small differences in health status of babies breast-fed for 4 or 6 months [18].

Taking these various pieces of information into account, I would conclude:

- Energy requirements can be met up to 6 months but require a significant level of commitment from both mother and baby, which may not always be possible.
- Mothers wishing to exclusively breast-feed to 6 months may be encouraged to do so and advised of the likely need for increased feeding frequency. The Web site of the Australian Breastfeeding Association (http://www.breastfeeding.asn.au/index.html) provides appropriate advice.
- Mothers wishing to start weaning before 6 months may be encouraged to do so and provided with appropriate advice regarding weaning foods.

For a detailed account of neonatal energy requirements in the preterm infant, the reader is recommended to read Hulzebos and Sauer [24].

Meeting protein requirements

Human milk contains considerably less protein than cow's milk and less than almost any other species [25]. However, "Dietary protein requirements are at their highest between birth and weaning to support high rates of tissue formation" [26]. These apparently contradictory statements are nothing of the sort; Dupont, drawing on an earlier review [27], made clear that exclusive breast-feeding provides for all the protein requirements of the growing baby up to weaning. As for energy, protein is provided in balance with need rather than in excess; at a typical protein content of 13 g/kg (mature human milk from standard U.K. food composition tables quoted in Emmett and Rogers [28]), 800 g/day of breast milk provides 10.4 g protein against a calculated requirement of 9.95 g (calculated from Dewey et al. [27] and revised WHO infant growth curves). Requirements for all individual amino acids can also be met by exclusive breast-feeding, by either direct supply or metabolic interconversion [26]. Relative to cow's milk, human milk contains significant amounts of nonprotein nitrogen, which may contribute to provision of nonessential amino acids but probably has no other specific dietary function. Milk protein content can fall if the maternal diet is deficient in protein and be restored by supplementation [29], but there is little evidence to indicate any problem of milk protein content in developed countries [28]. Vegans have normal protein content in their milk [29].

- Exclusive breast-feeding to 6 months meets all of the protein requirements of the healthy baby.

Meeting requirements for fat and fatty acids

Milk fat provides more than half of the neonate's dietary energy, but because energy provision has been discussed separately, this section considers the role that individual fatty acids play in growth and development. In particular, the long-chain polyunsaturated fatty acids arachidonic acid (AA) and docosahexaenoic acid (DHA) may have a special role to play in brain and retinal development [31] and are present in breast milk at low levels that are strongly influenced by maternal diet [32]. Omega-3 fatty acids (of which DHA is one) have attracted a great deal of publicity for their healthful properties, which has extended to media interest in breast-milk DHA. Cow's milk does not contain either DHA or AA, but it is added to some milk formulas. The evidence for doing so is somewhat circumstantial at present, although it is unlikely that there is any detrimental effect. Healthy term babies can synthesize both DHA and AA from their respective precursors α-linolenic acid (LNA) and linoleic acid (LA) provided they are present in the usual proportion of approximately 1.5% LNA and15% LA (an abnormal excess of either precursor would inhibit the formation of the opposite product). There is a concern that LA has been increasing in the human diet and in breast milk as dietary patterns have changed, but there is little evidence to suggest that DHA availability has been compromised. Vegan and vegetarian diets contain little or no DHA but do contain LNA and LA in the correct proportions [33]. In addition to the possibility of detrimental effects on brain development, high levels of n-6 polyunsaturated fatty acids such as AA and LA have been implicated as possible factors in inflammatory bowel disease (IBD) [34]. Once again, the evidence is somewhat circumstantial.

- The total fat content of breast milk is appropriate as an energy source.
- The fatty acid profile of breast milk is influenced by maternal diet and may have effects on brain development and IBD, but neither effect is proven.
- Breast-feeding mothers who express concern should be reassured and may be advised to increase modestly their consumption of omega-3 oils.

Meeting requirements for carbohydrate

Lactose is the principal carbohydrate in breast milk and makes a significant contribution to energy supply. Through provision of glucose, it is essential for brain and nervous tissue function. Consumption of 800 g/day of breast milk with a lactose content of 72 g/kg provides approximately 60 g of carbohydrate, from which the "adequate intake" figure is derived [4]. Apart from its energetic role, lactose also enhances calcium and magnesium absorption [35]. However, its principal function is energy provision, as discussed earlier.

- Lactose is the principal energy component of breast milk and is essential for provision of glucose and hence nervous system function.
- Exclusive breast-feeding to 6 months meets requirements for carbohydrate.

Meeting requirements for fluids

Fluid (water) requirements are stated to increase from approximately 100 ml/kg/day at birth to approximately 150 ml/kg/day at 6 months [36]. It is not clear whether this is simply breast-milk intake or an actual calculated requirement. If accurate, a 6-month-old baby weighing 8 kg would require 1200 ml of breast milk to achieve his or her fluid requirement, which is above the generally accepted breast-milk production level but well within the physiological range (discussed earlier). Studies of fluid requirements in tropical regions have indicated no need for any fluid other than breast milk to 6 months and beyond [37], an important consideration when water supplies may be contaminated.

- Water supplementation is not necessary before weaning and should be discouraged.

Meeting requirements for micronutrients

Consider the following:

"A plentiful supply of breast milk from a mother eating an adequate diet should provide all the infant's requirements of vitamins, minerals and trace elements" [28].

"All breastfed infants should receive 1.0mg of vitamin K oxide i.m. after the first feed is completed and within 6h of life. . . . All breastfed infants should receive 200 IU of oral vitamin D drops beginning during the first two months of life" [38].

The apparent contrariness can be resolved by an understanding of the rationale for vitamin K and D supplementations. Vitamin K is required for production of clotting factors and is present in breast milk only at low concentrations. There is a proven association between breast-feeding and late-onset hemorrhagic disease, sometimes called VKDB (vitamin K deficiency bleeding) [39], hence there is good reason for supplementation. In contrast to the clear advice offered by the American Association of Pediatricians [38] there is no national U.K. policy, but most neonatal units offer vitamin K as a matter of routine. Vitamin D is the one micronutrient that does not have to be supplied in the diet, because it is naturally synthesized in skin tissue by the action of sunlight (specifically ultraviolet B radiation). Deficiency causes the clinical condition of rickets in infants. Infant formula is supplemented and typically provides approximately 10 μg/l, the recommended adequate intake being 5 μg/day [4]. Breast milk provides less than one tenth of this amount. Advisory bodies are reluctant to recommend that babies be exposed to sunlight, for fear of the risk of increasing skin cancer incidence, hence the U.S. recommendation to supplement the breast-fed baby and the U.K. recommendation to supplement the breast-feeding mother (10 μg/day during pregnancy and lactation) [40]. Breast-milk levels respond to maternal supplementation but not always in an entirely consistent fashion. Detailed information on variation in breast-milk levels of micronutrients can be found in Emmett and Rogers [28]. As suggested earlier, deficiencies of vitamins and minerals are rare in full-term breast-fed babies in developed countries, but one needs to be aware of ethnic differences. Vitamin D synthesis requires greater light exposure in dark-skinned races, for instance, and there is evidence of higher incidence of rickets among Asian communities in the United Kingdom (not necessarily related to breast-feeding).

Calcium and iron deserve particular mention. Calcium, together with phosphorus, is essential for healthy skeletal development [41], as well as for normal cell functioning in most tissues. Skeletal growth is rapid during fetal life and continues postpartum but then slows. The aspects of neonatal calcium nutrition that currently receive attention are avoiding deficiencies (in developing countries) and optimizing intake for long-term development, maximizing peak bone mass, and avoiding osteoporosis. Calcium levels in breast milk are less than one third of cow's milk levels, and formula is intermediate, but the absorption of calcium from breast milk is higher than that from formula. The typical requirement of 200 to 250 mg/day is fully met by average breast-milk intake from well-nourished mothers [36] but may become marginal in mothers on poor-quality diets or those who avoid drinking milk [42]. Supplementation of the maternal diet is recommended in such circumstances.

Iron is the most abundant trace mineral in the body, and its deficiency "is probably the most frequently observed nutrient deficiency worldwide" [43]. Requirements are met partly by dietary intake but largely by internal turnover. Healthy, average-weight babies that grow at average rates generally have iron reserves that, taken together with intake from breast milk, are sufficient for the first 6 months of life, but low birth weight compromises the initial reserve, and high growth rate depletes the reserve earlier, hence supplementation may be necessary before weaning. Butte et al. [5] cited a number of references indicating normal iron status of exclusively breast-fed babies for the first 6 months of life, but others recommend supplementation after approximately 3 months [36]. Breast-milk iron content is largely unaffected by maternal iron status. The more usual time for iron deficiency to manifest is during weaning between 6 and 12 months of age, particularly if cow's milk is given [43].

- Current recommendations concerning vitamins K and D supplementation are appropriate.
- Certain ethnic populations are at particular risk for vitamin D deficiency.
- Appropriate maternal calcium intake will ensure adequate supply in breast milk.
- Iron status of exclusively breast-fed babies may become marginal before 6 months, especially in small-for-gestational-age and/or rapidly growing babies.

Requirements beyond 6 months of age

"…you may want to wean later – into your baby's second year, or later."

This quote is taken from the Australian Breast-feeding Association Web site. Different attitudes about breast-feeding are evident from comparing the weaning advice offered here (which relates almost exclusively to breast-feeding aspects) with that offered in the United Kingdom by the Food Standards Agency (which hardly mentions it). Neither approach is wrong or right, but the potential for confusion in the minds of mothers is evident. WHO advice, in contrast, is very specific: "Practice exclusive breastfeeding from birth to 6 months of age, and introduce complementary foods at six months of age (180 days) while continuing to breastfeed" [44].

It is not clear exactly what happens at 179 or 181 days. In developmental terms, there is nothing "magical" about 6 months, although energy expended on locomotion will presumably start to increase at about that time. Extension of the arguments detailed previously suggests that some mother:young dyads living in developed countries may be able to continue exclusive breast-feeding beyond 6 months and have requirements met, but for the great majority the advice to *start* weaning (introducing complementary feeds) at *around* 6 months would be sound and would recognize the tremendous individual variation in preferences of mother and baby. The Australian advice quoted almost certainly does not mean to imply that exclusive breast-feeding can readily continue to a year or beyond, although that would be one interpretation. Unfortunately, the term "to wean" is often used inaccurately to refer to either one of two specific events (the first complementary feed or the last breast-feed) when it properly refers to a lengthy and gradual process. Orthodox Jewish women breast-feed for 2 years or more, following ancient guidance given in the Talmud [45], but that advice certainly does not mention exclusive breast-feeding. There has been little scientific study of exclusive breast-feeding beyond 6 months apart from an elegant series of studies undertaken at the University of Helsinki in the 1980s [46]. Infants exclusively breast-fed to 9 months had slower growth (length, not weight), poorer iron status (but no clinical anemia), and, as recently reported, increased atopic dermatitis at age 20. Significantly, of 200 mother:young dyads recruited to this last experiment, 36 were still exclusively breast-feeding at 9 months and only 7 at 12 months. These mothers were all committed individuals (only two were lost from the experiment) and a rigid, baby-oriented protocol was applied to determine at what point exclusive breast-feeding should stop (donated human milk was offered after a breast-feed, and only when it had been needed twice were complementary feeds offered). In other words, exclusive breast-feeding to 12 months is not easy. The same conclusion can be drawn from the PROBIT (Promotion of Breast-feeding Intervention Trial) intervention trial, a large, multicenter study in Belarus designed to promote breast-feeding to WHO standards. Those still exclusively breast-feeding at and beyond 6 months numbered 251, or just 1.4% of the 17 046 recruited mother:young dyads [47]. In contrast to the Helsinki study, this trial did not find any reduction in growth of exclusively breast-fed infants, perhaps because of the less precise definition. Nonexclusive breast-feeding beyond 6 months is relatively common, but any decision to continue breast-feeding for very prolonged periods (beyond 1 year) may be made for reasons of nurture rather than nutrition – that is, it feels good for mother, baby, or both. However, in a study of long-term (12–43 months) partial breast-feeding, analysis of the rest of the diet concluded that breast milk was supplying as much as 20% to 25% of the energy intake [48], assuming that intake was at or around its recommended daily allowance.

Summary

I shall leave the final word to the European Society for Paediatric Gastroenterology, Hepatology and Nutrition's Committee on Nutrition, which recently published a commentary paper [49] and concluded (with great clarity):

- "Exclusive breast-feeding ... for about six months is a desirable goal."
- "Complementary feeding ... should not be introduced before 17 weeks and not later than 26 weeks."

From the available knowledge of neonatal requirements, I can find no basis for disagreeing with either statement.

References

1. World Health Organization, The Optimal Duration of Exclusive Breast-Feeding. Report of an Expert Consultation (Geneva: World Health Organization, 2001).

2. Food Standards Agency, Breastfeeding your baby (2008). Available at: http://www.eatwell.gov.uk/agesandstages/baby/breastfeed.

3. Fomon SJ and Nelson SE, Body composition of the male and female reference infants. *Annu Rev Nutr* (2002), **22**:1–17.

4. Institute of Medicine, Dietary reference intakes (2007). Available at: http://www.iom.edu/CMS/54133.aspx

5. Butte NF, Lopez-Alarcon G, and Garza C, Nutrient Adequacy of Exclusive Breastfeeding for the Term Infant During the First Six Months of Life (Geneva: World Health Organization, 2002).

6. Wells JCK, Chomtho S, and Fewtrell MS, Programming of body composition by early growth and nutrition. *Proc Nutr Soc* (2007), **66**:423–34.

7. Symonds ME, Integration of physiological and molecular mechanisms of the developmental origins of adult disease: new concepts and insights. *Proc Nutr Soc* (2007), **66**:442–450.

8. Dunger DB, Salgin B, and Ong KK, Early nutrition and later health. Early developmental pathways of obesity and diabetes risk. *Proc Nutr Soc* (2007), **66**:451–7.

9. Triche EW and Hossain N, Environmental factors implicated in the causation of adverse pregnancy outcome. *Semin Perinatol* (2007), **31**:240–2.

10. Scott JA and Binns CW, Factors associated with the initiation and duration of breastfeeding: a review of the literature. *Breastfeed Rev* (1999), 7:5–16.

11. Arenz S, Rückerl R, Koletzko B, and von Kries R, Breast-feeding and childhood obesity: a systematic review. *Int J Obes* (2004), **28**:1247–56.

12. Weaver LT, Rapid growth in infancy: balancing the interests of the child. *J Pediatr Gastroenterol Nutr* (2006), **43**:428–32.

13. Heird WC, Determination of nutritional requirements in preterm infants, with special reference to "catch-up" growth. *Semin Neonatol* (2001), **6**:365–75.

14. Garza C, Effect of infection on energy requirements of infants and children. *Public Health Nutr* (2005), **8**:1187–90.

15. Rosetta L and Baldi A, On the role of breast-feeding in health promotion and the prevention of allergic diseases. *Adv Exp Med Biol* (2008), **606**:467–83.

16. Vogel A, Hutchison L, and Mitchell E, Mastitis in the first year postpartum. *Birth* (1999), 26:218–25.

17. Whitehead RG and Paul AA, Long-term adequacy of exclusive breast-feeding: how scientific research has led to revised opinions. *Proc Nutr Soc* (2000), 59:17–23.

18. Fewtrell MS, Morgan JB, Duggan C, Gunnlaugsson G, Hibberd PL, Lucas A, and Kleinman RE, Optimal duration of exclusive breastfeeding: what is the evidence to support current recommendations. *Am J Clin Nutr* (2007), **85**:635S–8S.

19. Butte NF, Energy requirements of infants. *Public Health Nutr* (2005), 8:953–67.

20. Reilly JJ and Wells JCK, Duration of exclusive breast-feeding: introduction of complementary feeding may be necessary before 6 months of age. *Br J Nutr* (2005), **94**:869–72.

21. Saint L, Maggiore P, and Hartmann PE, Yield and nutrient content of milk in eight women breast-feeding twins and one woman breast-feeding triplets. *Br J Nutr* (1986), **56**:49–58.

22. Daly SEJ, Kent JC, Huynh DQ, Owens RA, Alexander BF, Ng KC, and Hartmann PE, The determination of short-term breast volume changes and the rate of synthesis of human milk using computerized breast measurement. *Exp Physiol* (1992), 77:79–87.

23. La Leche League International, Why does my baby suddenly want to nurse constantly? (2008). Available at: http://www.llli.org/FAQ/spurt.html.

24. Hulzebos CV and Sauer PJJ, Energy requirements. *Semin Fetal Neonat Med* (2007), **12**:2–10.

25. Oftedal OT, Milk composition, milk yield and energy output at peak lactation: a comparative review. *Symp Zool Soc Lond* (1984), **51**:33–85.

26. Dupont C, Protein requirements during the first year of life. *Am J Clin Nutr* (2003), 77:1544S–9S.

27. Dewey KG, Beaton G, Fjeld C, Lonnerdal B, and Reeds P, Protein requirements of infants and children. *Eur J Clin Nutr* (1996), **50**:S119–50.

28. Emmett PM and Rogers IS, Properties of human milk and their relationship with maternal nutrition. *Early Hum Dev* (1997), 49(Suppl):S7–S28.

29. Prentice AM, Roberts SB, Prentice A, Paul AA, Watkinson M, Watkinson AA, and Whitehead RG, Dietary supplementation of lactating Gambian women. I. Effect on breast-milk volume and quality. *Hum Nutr Clin Nutr* (1983), 37C:53–64.

30. Mangels AR and Messina V, Considerations in planning vegan diets: infants. *J Am Diet Assoc* (2001), **101**:670–7.

31. Guesry P, The role of nutrition in brain development. *Prev Med* (1998), **27**:189–94.

32. Innis SM, Human milk: maternal dietary lipids and infant development. *Proc Nutr Soc* (2007), **66**:397–404.

33. Sanders TA and Reddy S, The influence of a vegetarian diet on the fatty acid composition of human milk and the essential fatty acid status of the infant. *J Pediatr* (1992), **120**:S71–7.

34. Innis SM and Jacobsen K, Dietary lipids in early development and intestinal inflammatory bowel disease. *Nutr Rev* (2007), **65**:S188–93.

35. Darby MK and Loughead JL, Neonatal nutritional requirements and formula composition: a review. *J Obstet Gynecol Neonat Nurs* (1996), **25**:209–16.

36. Gregory K, Update on nutrition for preterm and full-term infants. *J Obstet Gynecol Neonat Nurs* (2004), **34**:98–108.

37. Almroth S and Bidinger PG, No need for water supplementation for exclusively breast-fed infants under hot and arid conditions. *Trans R Soc Trop Med Hyg* (1990), **84**:602–4.

38. American Association of Pediatrics, American Association of Pediatrics policy statement: breastfeeding and the use of human milk. *Pediatrics* (2005), **115**:496–506.

39. Lane PA and Hathaway WE, Vitamin K in infancy. *J Pediatr* (1985), **106**:351–9.

40. Scientific Advisory Committee on Nutrition, Infant Feeding Survey 2005: a commentary on infant feeding practices in the UK: Scientific Advisory Committee. Available at: http://www.sacn.gov.uk/reports.

41. Prentice A, Schoenmakers I, Laskey MA, de Bono S, Ginty F, and Goldberg GR, Nutrition and bone growth and development. *Proc Nutr Soc* (2006), **65**:348–60.

42. Mannion CA, Gray-Donald K, Johnson-Down L, and Koski KG, Lactating women restricting milk are low on select nutrients. *J Am Coll Nutr* (2007), **26**:149–55.

43. Thorsdottir I and Gunnarsson BS, Dietary quality and adequacy of micronutrient intakes in children. *Proc Nutr Soc* (2006), **65**:366–75.

44. Dewey KG, Guiding Principles for Complementary Feeding of the Breastfed Child (Washington, DC: Pan American Health Organization/World Health Organization, 2003).

45. Eidelman AI, The Talmud and human lactation: the cultural basis for increased frequency and duration of breastfeeding among orthodox Jewish women. *Breastfeed Med* (2006), **1**:36–40.

46. Pesonen M, Kallio MJT, Ranki A, and Siimes MA, Prolonged exclusive breastfeeding is associated with increased atopic dermatitis: a prospective follow-up study of unselected healthy newborns from birth to age 20 years. *Clin Exp Allergy* (2006), **36**:1011–18.

47. Kramer MS, Guo T, Platt RW, Shapiro S, Collet J-P, Chalmers B, et al., Breastfeeding and infant growth: biology or bias? *Pediatrics* (2002), **110**:343–7.

48. Buckley KM, Long-term breastfeeding: nourishment of nurturance. *J Hum Lact* (2001), **17**:304–12.

49. Agostoni C, Decsi T, Fewtrell M, Goulet O, Kolacek S, Koletzko B, et al., Complementary feeding: a commentary by the ESPGHAN Committee on Nutrition. *J Pediatr Gastroent Nutr* (2008), **46**:99–110.

9 Comparison between preterm and term infants

Mary Fewtrell and Sirinuch Chomtho

An infant born before 37 weeks of completed pregnancy is by definition preterm. With modern neonatal intensive care, survival is possible after as little as 23 weeks gestation. These infants present a major challenge in nutritional management because they are born during a period of extremely rapid fetal growth: the fetus normally trebles in weight between 24 and 36 weeks gestation, gaining 15–20 g/kg/day. The nutritional requirements of preterm infants therefore differ in many ways from those of healthy infants born at term. The magnitude of this difference depends on a number of factors including the degree of prematurity, events in utero that may have compromised fetal nutrition, the severity of illness during the neonatal period, and its treatment.

Fetal nutrient accretion does not occur at a uniform rate, and prematurity poses the greatest problems for nutrients for which accretion occurs predominantly during the third trimester. For example, 90% of the bone-forming minerals calcium and phosphorus are acquired during the last 12 weeks, whereas body fat content increases from 1% of body weight at 20 weeks gestation to 15% at term. Low reserves, combined with immature metabolic responses, have important consequences for the ability of preterm infants to adapt to postnatal life and withstand starvation.

Previously, the main focus in feeding preterm infants was on meeting their nutritional needs, preventing nutritional deficiencies, and promoting growth. However, evidence that early nutrition has biological effects on the individual with important implications for health has led to a conceptual change. Nutritional practice was previously underpinned largely by observational or physiological studies, or by small clinical trials designed to test for the effects of specific products on nutritional status, growth, and tolerance. However, larger randomized trials with short- and longer-term efficacy and safety testing have started to produce an evidence base for

nutritional practice. Such studies are most advanced in preterm infants.

This chapter covers the following topics:

1. the important differences in nutrient requirements in preterm infants compared with those in infants born at term and
2. the practicalities of meeting these requirements during the early postpartum period and following discharge.

The discussion focuses on nutrition in relation to the short- and longer-term health and development of preterm infants. It does not attempt to provide a comprehensive review of nutrient requirements for preterm infants. For further information on specific nutrients the reader is referred to the recent review by Tsang et al. [1].

Major differences in nutritional requirements between preterm and term infants

Several approaches have been used to estimate the nutritional requirements of preterm infants, including (1) measuring the composition of "reference fetuses" at different stages of gestation to estimate fetal accretion rates for various nutrients, (2) nutritional balance studies in preterm infants, (3) relating nutrient intake to short-term growth, and (4) relating early nutrient intake to functional outcomes, both short term (e.g. infection, necrotizing enterocolitis [NEC]) and longer term. With increasing evidence that early diet has long-term consequences (as discussed subsequently), there is greater recognition of the need for feeding recommendations to be based, where possible, on health outcomes.

Protein

Results from a number of studies show that protein gain increases linearly with intakes between approximately 2 and 4 g/kg/24 hours [2]. Thus, to achieve nitrogen accretion at the same rate as seen in utero during the third trimester, the preterm infant requires substantially greater intakes of protein than would be obtained by a term infant fed on breast milk providing 1 to 2 g/kg/day.

There is evidence that both short- and long-term outcomes are improved by meeting the increased protein requirements of preterm infants. A recent systematic review [3] identified five randomized clinical trials (RCTs) comparing different protein intakes in preterm infants and reported improved weight gain and higher nitrogen accretion in infants receiving formulas with higher protein content ($\geq$ 3 g/kg/day but < 4 g/kg/day). None of the studies examined cognitive outcome. However, a study in 495 extremely low birth weight infants (ELBW)[4] suggested that in-hospital growth velocity had a significant impact on neurodevelopment and growth outcomes at 18 to 22 months postterm. Furthermore, preterm infants randomized to receive a formula containing 2 g/100 ml protein showed better short-term growth than those fed a standard formula containing 1.45 g/100 ml and also had significantly better neurodevelopment at 18 months and 7.5 to 8 years [5]. The beneficial effects were greater for boys than girls.

It is important to consider energy intake together with protein intake because, if energy intake is low, high protein intakes cannot be utilized, and the infant's metabolic machinery is stressed. The ratio of energy to protein also determines the relative proportions of fat and lean tissue, and the composition of tissue gained in preterm infants varies according to their diet. At present, it is not known whether it is preferable for a preterm infant to have a weight gain with 15% fat as in the fetus or 40% fat as in the term infant. The consequences of the altered fat distribution reported in preterm infants at term-equivalent compared with that of term infants at birth are also unclear [6]. However, in a randomized trial in preterm infants, despite major differences in growth rates between diet groups during the neonatal period, there were no differences in growth or body fatness [7] between groups at 8 to 12 years.

Despite recognition of the importance of an adequate protein intake for growth and outcome, preterm infants frequently demonstrate growth faltering during the neonatal period. Typically, a nutrient deficit accumulates during the early postnatal period when the infant is sick, and there is a delay in establishing enteral feeding. However, many infants fail to show catch-up growth and in the smallest, sickest infants, in whom fluid restriction may be imposed for medical reasons, the deficit often increases progressively. A recent study of nutrient intakes in hospitalized preterm infants found cumulative energy and protein deficits of 406 kcal/kg and 14 g/kg at 1 week and 813 kcal/kg and 23 g/kg at 6 weeks of age in infants less than 31 weeks gestation [8]. Recognizing this problem, recent guidelines have proposed higher enteral protein intakes of 3.8–4.4 g/kg/day in ELBW (< 1 kg) infants, with a protein:energy ratio of 2.5 to 3.4 g/100 kcal, and 3.4 to 4.2 g/kg/day in very low birth weight (VLBW; < 1.5 kg) infants, with a protein:energy ratio of 2.6 to 3.8 during the "stable growing" phase [9], to prevent growth faltering and to facilitate catch-up growth. It is important to monitor the *actual* protein intake received by the infant, not just the *prescribed* intake, because fluid restriction and perceived feed intolerance often lead to a marked difference between the two. Nutritional restriction for medical reasons must in all cases be weighed against the long-term consequences of suboptimal nutrition.

Amino acids

Certain amino acids may be particularly important in preterm infants. For example, a randomized trial of taurine supplementation in formula-fed preterm infants [10] showed some evidence of more rapid auditory maturation in the supplemented group at the equivalent of term. More recently, Wharton et al. [11] reported that preterm infants with the highest plasma taurine concentrations during the neonatal period have higher Bayley mental development index at 18 months and higher scores on the Wechsler Intelligence Scale for Children—Revised arithmetic subtest at age 7. Plasma arginine concentrations have been found to be inversely related to the severity of respiratory distress syndrome, and low concentrations have been reported in infants who develop NEC. A randomized trial of arginine supplementation versus placebo in preterm infants found a significantly reduced incidence of NEC in supplemented infants [12], although a recent Cochrane review [13] reported that follow-up of infants from this trial showed no difference in neurodevelopmental disability between groups.

Energy

Most measurements of energy expenditure have, for practical reasons, been performed on stable, growing preterm infants. There are no definite data suggesting an increased energy requirement in sick infants, and, in practice, the main challenge is ensuring that the desired nutrient intake is actually received by the infant in the face of fluid restriction due to the underlying illness and poor feed tolerance. Current recommended intakes are 110 to 130 kcal/kg/day for healthy, growing preterm infants [14], assuming a target weight gain of 16–20 g/kg/day.

Fat

Fat provides about half the energy for infants fed human milk. Preterm infants have lower fat absorption than term infants, largely because of reduced intestinal lipase activity. Although fat absorption from fresh breast milk may be as high as 90%, the range is large, and the figure is considerably lower from formula feeds or from pasteurized human milk in which the lipases have been denatured.

The type of fat is also important. Most modern formulas contain a fat blend designed to mimic the pattern of fatty acid saturation and chain lengths found in breast milk. When compared with breast milk, these mixtures have a reduced content of fatty acids esterified to glycerol in the 2 position and an increase in those esterified in the 1 and 3 positions. The latter undergo hydrolysis in the gut, releasing palmitic acid, which is poorly absorbed and tends to form calcium soaps. These soaps may be partly responsible for the harder stools seen in formula-fed infants and occasionally result in bowel obstruction, as well as influencing calcium absorption. Studies using a modified fat blend (Betapol) containing a higher proportion of fatty acids esterified in the 2 position to mimic that found in human milk show increased calcium absorption and fat absorption in term and preterm infants [15].

The role of n-3 and n-6 long-chain polyunsaturated fatty acids (LCPUFA) in preterm nutrition has been extensively investigated in recent years. These LCPUFA are synthesized from precursor essential fatty acids (EFA) and found in high concentrations in the central nervous system. In addition, LCPUFAs are highly bioactive, acting as precursors for eicosanoids and prostaglandins and affecting the expression and activity of a number of genes involved in metabolism. Rapid accumulation of LCPUFA, particularly docosahexaenoic acid, in the brain occurs from the third trimester to 18 months postpartum. Human milk contains both precursor EFA and adequate LCPUFA for structural lipid accretion. However, infant formulas traditionally contained only the parent EFA. Whether the addition of LCPUFA to preterm formulas results in improved clinical outcome remains controversial and has been the subject of numerous studies. One systematic review [16] concluded that supplementation results in more rapid visual maturation that is transient, whereas a Cochrane systematic review [17] concluded that there was no convincing evidence of cognitive benefit associated with supplementation. Two more recent studies reported some evidence for a beneficial effect of LCPUFA supplementation on neurodevelopment [18, 19], but no study has yet reported follow-up data beyond 2 years, and all studies in infants use tests of global cognitive function. LCPUFA supplementation may result in more subtle effects on areas of development that may be detected only by using more specific tests at a later age. Furthermore, given the bioactive nature of LCPUFA, it is plausible that supplementation may have long-term effects on other outcomes, as suggested recently for body composition [20] or cardiovascular risk factors [21].

Another important consideration is whether the addition of selected LCPUFA is safe. Various strategies have been used to supplement formula with LCPUFA, and they have not been without problems. There is a fine balance between the relative amounts of linoleic and linolenic acids and their longer-chain products, and it seems probable that the inconsistent findings in randomized trials may relate more to the different strategies and doses used to supplement the formula rather than to the actual LCPUFA themselves [22]. These issues require further investigation.

Calcium and phosphorus

The calcium and phosphorous requirements of the preterm infant have received considerable attention, because of the high incidence of metabolic bone disease (MBD) in this population. The majority of skeletal mineral is acquired during the last trimester, with intrauterine accretion rates of 140 and 75 mg/kg/day for calcium and phosphorus, respectively. Human milk fed at 200 ml/kg/day provides at the most 60 and 30 mg/kg/day, making the in utero rate of skeletal mineralization impossible. Calcium absorption from the gut further limits accretion, being 50% to 70% from human milk and as low as 20% from formula milk. Phosphate absorption is better – approximately 90% to 95% from both human milk and formula. However, when in short supply, it is used preferentially for tissue synthesis rather than bone mineralization. It is now recognized that the cause of MBD in preterm infants is an inadequate supply of mineral, particularly phosphorus, rather than a deficiency of vitamin D. Although MBD is usually asymptomatic, full-blown rickets and fractures may occur in severe cases.

Preterm infants fed human milk with its low mineral content are at greatest risk of developing MBD unless they receive phosphorous supplements. Those receiving modern preterm infant formulas should not require supplements. Current recommendations suggest an enteral mineral intake of between 120 and 200 mg/kg/day of calcium and 70 and 120 mg/kg/day phosphorus, with a calcium:phosphorus ratio of 1.7:2.0, and a 25-OH vitamin D intake of 200 to 1000 IU/day [23]. Although many preterm infants weighing less than 1.5 kg show evidence of reduced bone mineralization during the neonatal period, most are asymptomatic and appear to show catch-up in mineralization during the first few years of life [24]. An important question is whether early MBD has any long-term consequences. There is some evidence suggesting that even silent early bone disease retards linear growth up to 10 years later [25]. However, follow-up of preterm infants into early adult life suggests that those who received unsupplemented human milk (with very low early mineral intakes) have larger bones and a higher bone mass than those who received infant formulas (Fewtrell, unpublished). The significance of this finding for bone health and osteoporosis risk in later life is uncertain.

Iron

Preterm infants normally have adequate iron stores for the first 6 to 8 weeks of postnatal life, although they may be depleted more rapidly by frequent blood sampling. Beyond this, an iron intake of 2 to 3 mg/kg/day from all sources is recommended to prevent iron deficiency anemia, continuing until 12 months or until full mixed feeding provides an adequate iron intake. Infants receiving regular blood transfusions get substantial quantities of iron and do not need supplements until these are discontinued. A trial of high (20.7 mg/l) versus normal (13.4 mg/l) iron formulas in preterm infants found no difference in weight gain nor development at 12 months postterm [26]. However, a recent trial in VLBW infants receiving early versus late (14 days vs. 61 days) enteral iron supplementation showed a trend toward a beneficial effect of early supplementation on long-term neurocognitive and psychomotor development at age 5 years [27].

Zinc

Zinc plays a critical role in cell replication and growth and accumulates in the fetus during the last trimester at around 250 μg/kg/day. Dietary zinc together with release of zinc from body stores usually provides an adequate supply for the first few weeks of life, although zinc deficiency has been described as a late consequence of preterm birth (2–4 months). The amount of zinc provided by 200 ml/kg/day of human milk falls from 1650 μg on the first day of lactation to 160 μg after 4 months. Therefore, human milk collected during the early (but not later) months of lactation theoretically provides enough zinc to meet in utero accretion rates. A randomized study in preterm infants fed either a zinc-supplemented or placebo-supplemented term formula from the time at which they reached 1.8 kg for 6 months showed higher plasma zinc levels, significantly greater linear growth velocity, and higher motor development scores in the supplemented group [28]. The value of zinc supplementation for the long-term development and growth of preterm infants is thus an area requiring further investigation.

Vitamins

Preterm infants may have special requirements for some vitamins because of the following factors:

1. They are born with low body stores, especially of the fat-soluble vitamins, which normally accumulate during the third trimester.
2. They have reduced absorptive capacities for some vitamins (e.g. vitamin E).
3. They may benefit from "pharmacological" doses of some vitamins. For example, meta-analysis of data [29] from six trials of intramuscular vitamin A supplementation identified beneficial effects in terms of reducing death or oxygen requirement at 36 weeks gestation and 1 month of age and a trend

toward reduced incidence of retinopathy of prematurity. There is also some evidence from a meta-analysis of 26 RCTs that oral vitamin E might reduce the incidence of severe retinopathy and intraventricular hemorrhage. However, high-dose vitamin E (serum tocopherol > 3.5 mg/dl) was associated with an increased risk of sepsis [30].

Achieving optimal nutrition in preterm infants

Despite greater appreciation of the importance of adequate nutrition for outcome in preterm infants and the existence of specific nutritional recommendations, it is widely recognized that these infants often exhibit suboptimal growth, which may persist for some time after hospital discharge and which may have adverse consequences for cognitive outcome [4]. One practical problem for preterm infants following delivery is the initial inability to tolerate enteral feeds in sufficient amounts to ensure an adequate nutritional intake. In this situation, nutrition should be provided parenterally, starting with amino acid and dextrose solutions during the first day and rapidly building up to full nutrient requirements, including lipids. Parenteral nutrition should not be stopped until full enteral feeds are convincingly tolerated. Minimal enteral feeding – the practice of introducing small, nonnutritional quantities of milk to promote gut maturity – can proceed alongside parenteral nutrition and results in a reduction in time taken to tolerate full enteral feeds and a shorter total hospital stay [31].

The following options are available for enteral feeding in preterm infants:

- Human milk

    - Mother's own: "preterm milk" (MBM)
    - Banked donor milk (DBM)
    - Fortified human milk

- Preterm infant formula (PTF)
- Term infant formula (TF)

Human milk has significant advantages for preterm infants in both the short term (better feed tolerance, reduced risk of infection and NEC) and the longer term. Preterm infants fed MBM have higher developmental scores at 18 months and higher IQs at 7.5 to 8 years than those fed on other diets, even after adjusting for confounding factors [32]. Adolescents

born preterm and randomized to human milk during the neonatal period had significantly lower blood pressure and a more favorable lipid profile than those who received PTF, with a dose-response effect between these outcome measures and the proportion of human milk in the neonatal diet [33, 34]. The effect sizes observed in these studies were of a magnitude potentially important in public health terms in reducing the risk of cardiovascular disease. Interestingly, children who received human milk also had evidence of lower insulin resistance and better arterial distensibility (an early marker of vascular disease) than children from the PTF group (who had similar vascular function to children born at term) [35]. These effects appeared to be mediated by growth predominantly during the first 2 weeks of postnatal life and are consistent with the hypothesis that promoting growth early in the neonatal period may not be optimal for certain aspects of longer-term cardiovascular health [35].

Given these health benefits, it is important that mothers are strongly encouraged to provide their own breast milk for their infant. However, because preterm infants are generally unable to breast-feed effectively before 34 weeks, the mother needs to express her milk (sometimes for a prolonged period), which can then be fed to the infant through a nasogastric tube, cup, or bottle. This process makes great demands on the mother, and the importance of adequate support and advice cannot be overstated.

Despite the proven health benefits of human milk, in nutritional terms it does not meet the needs of preterm infants for several nutrients, including protein, energy, and minerals. To achieve adequate growth, avoid MBD, and, potentially, maximize cognitive outcome, human milk can be fortified with a human milk fortifier (HMF), derived from cow's milk, which is mixed with the mother's own breast milk before it is given to the infant. HMFs have been shown to improve short-term weight gain, linear and head growth, nitrogen retention, and blood urea levels [36]. However, long-term benefits have not been established, and the addition of an HMF may interfere with some of the anti-infective properties of human milk. Although HMFs continue to evolve, the addition of a fixed amount of fortifier to breast milk of variable nutritional content means that the nutritional intake of the infant remains unknown, with the possibility that the intake of some infants will remain suboptimal, whereas in others, it could exceed the upper recommended limit for certain nutrients. A small RCT

[37] showed that "adjustable" fortification of human milk (based on the infant's blood urea concentration) resulted in greater weight and head circumference gains, which were significantly correlated with protein intake, compared with "standard" fortification. The development of a "humanized" milk fortifier, produced from pooled DBM processed to ensure the highest safety standards, represents a potential advance because this would avoid exposure to cow's milk protein. However, the issue of uncertain nutrient intake would remain. Clinical trials of this new fortifier are under way.

When MBM is unavailable or is insufficient to meet the infant's full enteral requirements, the options are to supplement with DBM or PTF. DBM is derived from unrelated women who are breast-feeding either a preterm or term infant and who have "spare" milk. Donors are screened in the same way as blood donors, and milk is pasteurized to remove the risk of transmitting infection. The process of collection, freezing, thawing, and heat treatment [38] can damage antimicrobial factors in milk such as lysozyme, lactoferrin, immunoglobulins, and denatured milk lipase; milk cells seldom survive the banking process. For this reason, it cannot be automatically assumed that the benefits shown for MBM will necessarily apply to DBM.

The milk of mothers who have delivered preterm infants has a different composition from that of mothers delivered at term [39], with a higher concentration of total nitrogen, protein nitrogen, sodium, chloride, magnesium and iron, and copper and zinc, and a raised immunoglobulin A content in early lactation. The differences may relate to the low volume often produced by preterm donors. This milk is thus more suitable than term donor milk for feeding preterm infants, particularly in view of its higher concentration of protein. However, protein intakes from preterm human milk are variable and, by the second month, often fall to values at which theoretical needs would be met only at very high volume intakes.

A recent systematic review [40] that compared outcome in preterm infants fed DBM or formula identified only seven studies, five of them RCTs. Meta-analysis of data from three trials suggested that infants fed DBM had a significantly reduced risk of developing NEC (risk ratio 0.2), although feeding DBM was also associated with slower neonatal growth. However, all of the studies considered were 20 to 30 years old and from an era when DBM was fed without fortifi-

cation or mineral supplements, often as the sole diet. It is not clear whether similar effects would be seen when DBM is used in a more "modern" context – as a supplement to MBM and supplemented with minerals and/or HMF. Schanler et al. [41] performed an RCT examining the use of fortified DBM or PTF as a supplement to MBM and was unable to establish any short-term benefit for DBM over PTF. However, the study was only powered to detect a difference of 25% in the rate of NEC between DBM and PTF groups; a larger trial is required to address this issue specifically. DBM is expensive and often in short supply. There is a generally accepted need for more research to establish whether DBM as used in modern neonatal units is beneficial and safe, to identify groups of infants who benefit most, and to examine cost-benefit issues.

Preterm infant formulas are designed specifically to meet the increased nutrient requirements of this group. They promote more rapid growth [42], result in earlier discharge, and reduce the incidence of hyponatremia and MBD when compared to unsupplemented human milk. In addition, in a large RCT, infants randomized to receive PTF during the neonatal period had significantly better developmental scores at 18 months and 7.5 to 8 years than those randomized to a standard "term" formula [5, 43]. The advantages of PTF over TF were greatest in small-for-gestational-age and male infants. However, PTF also has some disadvantages; in the short term, it is less well tolerated than human milk with an increase in vomiting, abdominal distention, and risk of NEC.

For many years, standard TFs were used as an alternative to human milk for preterm infants. However, they contain inadequate nutrients to meet the requirements of the preterm infant. These formulas have little place in the nutritional management of preterm infants below 2 kg in body weight.

Postdischarge nutrition in preterm infants

The nutrition of preterm infants after they leave the neonatal unit has historically been relatively neglected. At this rather arbitrary time point, breast-milk fortifiers are stopped, or the infant is changed to a TF designed to meet the nutrient requirements of a healthy full-term infant, despite the fact that many infants are still preterm and growth retarded at the time. Many infants born appropriate for gestational age become growth retarded during their neonatal course, and data suggest that these early deficits persist to some degree into infancy and childhood [24]. However, although children born preterm remain, on average, shorter and lighter than children born at term, there is no evidence that nutrition during the period of hospitalization has any long-term effects on growth [44]. It is unclear whether nutrition during the period after hospital discharge ("postterm") influences longer-term growth. The small size of preterm infants at discharge is likely to be associated with deficits of a variety of nutrients, including calcium and phosphorus, zinc, and iron. Such deficits will inevitably increase in infants fed TF or unsupplemented breast milk after discharge.

Four dietary options are available for use in preterm infants after hospital discharge:

- human milk,
- term infant formula,
- preterm infant formula, and
- nutrient-enriched postdischarge formula (PDF).

Lucas et al. [45] reported extremely high mean daily milk intakes in preterm infants fed TF after discharge, reaching 230 ml/kg before 4 weeks postterm and remaining over 150 ml/kg/day beyond 6 months. Thus, given the opportunity, preterm infants will clearly consume a significantly greater quantity of nutrients than would be provided by TF fed at 150 ml/kg/day as recommended for term infants. One solution is to continue the use of PTF beyond discharge. However, theoretical concerns that infants fed on demand might consume high volumes of PTF with potentially toxic intakes of certain nutrients, such as vitamin D, led to the development of special PDFs. These contain (1) higher protein content to promote catch-up growth, accompanied by a modest increase in energy to allow utilization of the additional protein (a substantial increase in energy content might promote excess fat deposition and lead to the infant's downregulating formula intake), and (2) additional calcium, phosphorus, zinc, trace elements, and vitamins to support bone mineralization and the projected increase in growth rates.

Five RCTs reported increased weight and/or length in infants receiving PDF or PTF after discharge compared to TF [44]. However, a more recent study [46] reported slower growth in infants fed PDF compared with those randomized to TF. There are currently no follow-up data on growth and development in later childhood.

Breast-feeding postdischarge

It is unclear whether unsupplemented breast milk meets the nutritional requirements of preterm infants after discharge. Although the proportion of mothers exclusively breast-feeding their infant after discharge is still relatively small, a greater proportion of infants receive some breast milk for the first few weeks after discharge. A number of studies, inevitably nonrandomized and generally small, reported slower growth rates and lower bone mass in human milk-fed infants in the short term. Lucas et al. [47] studied 65 preterm infants who were breast-fed for at least 6 weeks after discharge. Although similar in size to formula-fed infants at discharge, by 6 weeks postterm, breast-fed infants were significantly lighter and shorter than formula-fed infants (on average 513 g lighter and 1.6 cm shorter than infants fed PDF). Slower growth persisted up to 9 months postterm, by which time all the breast-fed infants were receiving TF and solids, although there were no significant differences in head growth between diet groups. Collectively, these data suggest that preterm infants who are breast-fed after discharge grow more slowly and have lower bone mass in the short term than formula-fed infants. It is currently unclear whether this has longer-term consequences.

Introduction of solid foods

There are few data to guide either the optimal age for introducing solid foods or the optimal type of solid foods for preterm infants. The introduction of solids is likely to result in a reduction in milk intake. If the quality of solid food is poor, this may result in a reduction in overall nutrient density that could compromise growth and nutrient status. In a recent study, preterm infants were randomized either to "current" weaning practice or to a "new solid food strategy," which recommended early weaning (from 13 weeks chronological age) and the use of foods with a higher energy, protein, iron, and zinc content. The intervention group achieved increased protein and energy intake and better iron status by 6 months postterm and had improved linear growth velocity at 12 months [48].

Early nutrition and later health in preterm infants: an overview

Recent evidence suggests that human milk has an important place in neonatal intensive care. Human milk is better tolerated than formula, and enteral feeds can be established faster, reducing the requirement for parenteral nutrition with its known hazards. The use of breast milk is associated with a reduction in the incidence of NEC and systemic infection and is associated with improved cognitive outcome, lower blood pressure, and more favorable plasma lipid profile during childhood and adolescence. The slower initial growth rate seen in infants receiving human milk may be beneficial for later insulin resistance and arterial distensibility. However, in a preterm population, the risks and benefits of promoting growth must be balanced; the adverse consequences of poor early growth for short-term survival and for later cognitive development outweigh any slight increase in later cardiovascular risk associated with more rapid growth during very early postnatal life, and it is therefore essential to promote growth in these infants.

We recommend the use of breast milk, preferably the mother's own, but donor milk if it is not available, to establish enteral feeds. When mothers do not provide breast milk, PTF should be used. It may also be used as a supplement when mothers do not produce enough breast milk to meet the infant's requirements. Breast milk should be supplemented with phosphorus as a minimum, and a multinutrient fortifier should be added if growth is unsatisfactory on the maximum tolerated volume of breast milk. However, preterm infants are not a homogeneous population, and with the survival of ELBW babies, any single diet is now unlikely to be optimal from birth to discharge. Further work is required to explore how diets can be tailored to individual patients' needs.

After discharge (post-term), it is important to provide adequate nutrition to facilitate catch-up growth and reverse nutrient deficits that accumulate postnatally. This can be achieved using a postdischarge formula. Available data suggest that preterm infants who are breast-fed after discharge might benefit from additional nutrients, but longer-term outcome data are required to investigate the consequences of the slower

growth and bone mineralization seen in these infants. In practice, it is difficult to envisage how nutritional supplementation could easily be given to a fully breast-fed infant without interfering with the process of lactation. Nevertheless, because the majority of preterm breast-fed infants (particularly the smallest, who are likely to be most at risk of growth problems) receive at least some formula milk, it would make sense for this to be PDF rather than TF. Another solution is to focus more attention on the age of introduction of solid food, ensuring that the diet is of a high nutrient density.

Summary points

- Early nutrition affects both the short-term and longer-term health and development of preterm infants.
- There are major differences in the nutritional needs of preterm infants compared with those of infants born at term, determined by the degree of prematurity, events in utero that may have compromised fetal nutrition, the severity of neonatal illness, and its treatment.
- Early growth failure in preterm infants has adverse consequences for short-term outcomes and for longer-term neurodevelopment and should be prevented.
- Human milk has many health benefits for preterm infants including a lower risk of infection and NEC, improved cognitive outcome, and reduced risk factors for cardiovascular disease. However, in nutritional terms it does not meet the requirements of preterm infants for several nutrients. It therefore requires supplementation with phosphorus as a minimum and generally with a multinutrient fortifier to ensure adequate growth.

References

1. Tsang RC, Uauy R, Koletzko B, and Zlotkin SH, Nutrition of the Preterm Infant: Scientific Basis and Practical Guidelines (Cincinnati, OH: Digital Educational Publishing, 2005).

2. Micheli J-L, and Schutz Y, Protein. In ed., Tsang RC, Lucas A, Uauy R, and Zlotkin SH, Nutrition of the Preterm Infant: Scientific Basis and Practical Guidelines (New York: Caduceus Medical Publishers 1993), pp. 29–46.

3. Premji SS, Fenton TR, and Sauve RS, Higher versus lower protein intake in formula-fed low birth weight infants. *Cochrane Database Syst Rev* (2006), 1:CD003959.

4. Ehrenkranz RA, Dusick AM, Vohr BR, Wright LL, Wrage LA, and Poole WK, Growth in the neonatal intensive care unit influences neurodevelopmental and growth outcomes of extremely low birth weight infants. *Pediatrics* (2006), 117:1253–61.

5. Lucas A, Morley R, and Cole TJ, Randomised trial of early diet in preterm babies and later intelligence quotient. *BMJ* (1998), 317:1481–7.

6. Uthaya S, Thomas EL, Hamilton G, Dore CJ, Bell J, and Modi N, Altered adiposity after extremely preterm birth. *Pediatr Res* (2005), 57:211–15.

7. Fewtrell MS, Lucas A, Cole TJ, and Wells JC, Prematurity and reduced body fatness at 8–12 y of age. *Am J Clin Nutr* (2004), 80:436–40.

8. Embleton NE, Pang N, and Cooke RJ, Postnatal malnutrition and growth retardation: an inevitable consequence of current recommendations in preterm infants? *Pediatrics* (2001), 107:270–3.

9. Rigo J, Protein, Amino acid and other nitrogen compounds. In: ed. Tsang RC, Uauy R, Koletzko B, and Zlotkin SH, Nutrition of the Preterm Infant: Scientific Basis and Practical Guidelines (Cincinnati, OH: Digital Educational Publishing, 2005), pp. 45–80.

10. Tyson JE, Lasky R, Flood D, Mize C, Picone T, and Paule CL, Randomized trial of taurine supplementation for infants less than or equal to 1,300-gram birth weight: effect on auditory brainstem-evoked responses. *Pediatrics* (1989), 83:406–15.

11. Wharton BA, Morley R, Isaacs EB, Cole TJ, and Lucas A, Low plasma taurine and later neurodevelopment. *Arch Dis Child Fetal Neonatal Ed* (2004), 89:F497–8.

12. Amin HJ, Zamora SA, McMillan DD, Fick GH, Butzner JD, Parsons HG, and Scott RB, Arginine supplementation prevents necrotizing enterocolitis in the premature infant. *J Pediatr* (2002), 140:425–31.

13. Shah P and Shah V, Arginine supplementation for prevention of necrotising enterocolitis in preterm infants. *Cochrane Database Syst Rev* (2007), 3:CD004339.

14. Leitch CA and Denne SC, Energy. In: ed. Tsang RC, Uauy R, Koletzko B, Zlotkin SH, Nutrition of the Preterm Infant: Scientific Basis and Practical Guidelines (Cincinnati, OH: Digital Educational Publishing, 2005), pp. 23–44.

15. Carnielli VP, Luijendijk IH, Van Goudoever JB, Sulkers EJ, Boerlage AA, Degenhart HJ, and Sauer PJ, Structural position and amount of palmitic acid in infant formulas: effects on fat, fatty acid, and mineral balance. *J Pediatr Gastroenterol Nutr* (1996), 23:553–60.

16. SanGiovanni JP, Parra-Cabrera S, Colditz GA, Berkey CS, and Dwyer JT, Meta-analysis of dietary essential fatty acids and long-chain polyunsaturated fatty acids as they relate to visual resolution acuity in healthy preterm infants. *Pediatrics* (2000), 105:1292–8.

17. Simmer K and Patole S, Longchain polyunsaturated fatty acid supplementation in preterm infants. *Cochrane Database Syst Rev* (2004), 1:CD000375.

18. Fewtrell MS, Abbott RA, Kennedy K, Singhal A, Morley R, Caine E, et al., Randomized, double-blind trial of long-chain polyunsaturated fatty acid supplementation with fish oil and borage oil in preterm infants. *J Pediatr* (2004), 144:471–9.

19. Clandinin MT, Van Aerde JE, Merkel KL, Harris CL, Springer MA, Hansen JW, et al., Growth and development of preterm infants fed infant formulas containing docosahexaenoic acid and arachidonic acid. *J Pediatr* (2005), 146:461–8.

20. Groh-Wargo S, Jacobs J, Auestad N, O'Connor DL, Moore JJ, and Lerner E, Body composition in preterm infants who are fed long-chain polyunsaturated fatty acids: a prospective, randomized, controlled trial. *Pediatr Res* (2005), 57:712–18.

21. Forsyth JS, Willatts P, Agostoni C, Bissenden J, Casaer P, and Boehm G, Long chain polyunsaturated fatty acid supplementation in infant formula and blood pressure in later childhood: follow up of a randomised controlled trial. *BMJ* (2003), 326:953.

22. Fewtrell MS, Long-chain polyunsaturated fatty acids in early life: effects on multiple health outcomes. A critical review of current status, gaps and knowledge. *Nestle Nutr Workshop Ser Pediatr Program* (2006), 57:203–14.

23. Atkinson SA and Tsang RC, Calcium, magnesium, phosphorus and vitamin D. In ed. Tsang RC,

Uauy R, Koletzko B, and Zlotkin SH, Nutrition of the Preterm Infant: Scientific Basis and Practical Guidelines (Cincinnati, OH: Digital Educational Publishing, 2005), pp. 245–76.

24. Fewtrell MS, Prentice A, Jones SC, Bishop NJ, Stirling D, Buffenstein R, et al. Bone mineralization and turnover in preterm infants at 8–12 years of age: the effect of early diet. *J Bone Miner Res* (1999), **14**:810–20.

25. Fewtrell MS, Cole TJ, Bishop NJ, and Lucas A, Neonatal factors predicting childhood height in preterm infants: evidence for a persisting effect of early metabolic bone disease? *J Pediatr* (2000), **137**:668–73.

26. Friel JK, Andrews WL, Aziz K, Kwa PG, Lepage G, and L'Abbe MR, A randomized trial of two levels of iron supplementation and developmental outcome in low birth weight infants. *J Pediatr* (2001), **139**:254–60.

27. Steinmacher J, Pohlandt F, Bode H, Sander S, Kron M, and Franz AR, Randomized trial of early versus late enteral iron supplementation in infants with a birth weight of less than 1301 grams: neurocognitive development at 5.3 years' corrected age. *Pediatrics* (2007), **120**:538–46.

28. Friel JK, Andrews WL, Matthew JD, Long DR, Cornel AM, Cox M, et al., Zinc supplementation in very-low-birth-weight infants. *J Pediatr Gastroenterol Nutr* (1993), **17**:97–104.

29. Darlow B and Graham P, Vitamin A supplementation to prevent mortality and short and long-term morbidity in very low birthweight infants. *Cochrane Database Syst Rev* (2007), **4**:CD000501.

30. Brion LP, Bell EF, and Raghuveer TS, Vitamin E supplementation for prevention of morbidity and mortality in preterm infants. *Cochrane Database Syst Rev* (2003), **3/4**:CD003665.

31. Tyson JE and Kennedy KA, Trophic feedings for parenterally fed infants. *Cochrane Database Syst Rev* (2005), **3**:CD000504.

32. Lucas A, Morley R, Cole TJ, Lister G, and Leeson-Payne C, Breast milk and subsequent intelligence quotient in children born preterm. *Lancet* (1992), **339**:261–4.

33. Singhal A, Cole TJ, and Lucas A, Early nutrition in preterm infants and later blood pressure: two cohorts after randomised trials. *Lancet* (2001), **357**:413–19.

34. Singhal A, Cole TJ, Fewtrell M, and Lucas A, Breastmilk feeding and lipoprotein profile in adolescents born preterm: follow-up of a prospective randomised study. *Lancet* (2004), **363**:1571–8.

35. Singhal A and Lucas A, Early origins of cardiovascular disease: is there a unifying hypothesis? *Lancet* (2004), **363**:1642–5.

36. Kuschel CA and Harding JE, Multicomponent fortified human milk for promoting growth in preterm infants. *Cochrane Database Syst Rev* (2004), **1/2**:CD000343.

37. Arslanoglu S, Moro GE, and Ziegler EE, Adjustable fortification of human milk fed to preterm infants: does it make a difference? *J Perinatol* (2006), **26**:614–21.

38. Garza C, Johnson CA, Harrist R, and Nichols BL, Effects of methods of collection and storage on nutrients in human milk. *Early Hum Dev* (1982), **6**:295–303.

39. Atkinson SA, The effects of gestational stage at delivery on human milk composition. In ed. Jensen RG, *Handbook of Milk Composition* (San Diego, CA: Academic Press, 1995), pp. 222–37.

40. Boyd CA, Quigley MA, and Brocklehurst P, Donor breast milk versus infant formula for preterm infants: systematic review and meta-analysis. *Arch Dis Child Fetal Neonatal Ed* (2007), **92**:F169–75.

41. Schanler RJ, Lau C, Hurst NM, and Smith EO, Randomized trial of donor human milk versus preterm formula as substitutes for mothers' own milk in the feeding of extremely premature infants. *Pediatrics* (2005), **116**:400–6.

42. Lucas A, Gore SM, Cole TJ, Bamford MF, Dossetor JF, Barr I, et al., Multicentre trial on feeding low birthweight infants: effects of diet on early growth. *Arch Dis Child* (1984), **59**:722–30.

43. Lucas A, Morley R, Cole TJ, Gore SM, Lucas PJ, Crowle P, et al., Early diet in preterm babies and developmental status at 18 months. *Lancet* (1990), **335**:1477–81.

44. Fewtrell MS, Growth and nutrition after discharge. *Semin Neonatol* (2003), **8**:169–76.

45. Lucas A, King F, and Bishop NB, Postdischarge formula consumption in infants born preterm. *Arch Dis Child* (1992), **67**:691–2.

46. Koo WW and Hockman EM, Posthospital discharge feeding for preterm infants: effects of standard compared with enriched milk formula on growth, bone mass, and body composition. *Am J Clin Nutr* (2006), **84**:1357–64.

47. Lucas A, Fewtrell MS, Morley R, Singhal A, Abbott RA, Isaacs E, et al., Randomized trial of nutrient-enriched formula versus standard formula for postdischarge preterm infants. *Pediatrics* (2001), **108**:703–11.

48. Marriott LD, Foote KD, Bishop JA, Kimber AC, and Morgan JB, Weaning preterm infants: a randomised controlled trial. *Arch Dis Child Fetal Neonatal Ed* (2003), **88**:F302–7.

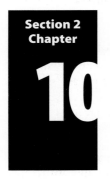
Influences of timing and duration of formula feeding on infant growth

William C. Heird

Introduction

All national and international groups responsible for making nutritional recommendations for infants endorse exclusive breast-feeding for the first several months of life [1–3]. Some state "for 6 months," others state "for about 6 months," and still others state "for 4 to 6 months." Continued breast-feeding for as long as 2 years or more along with timely introduction of appropriate complementary foods is also endorsed. However, these bodies recognize that many infants, for a variety of reasons, either are not breast-fed or are not breast-fed for the recommended time. For these infants, the only acceptable alternative is thought to be a modern infant formula. Thus, in the United States, where about 75% of infants are breast-fed at hospital discharge but only about 30% are still breast-fed at 4 months of age, at least 25% of all infants are fed formula (or another liquid) for the first year of life and 75% or more are fed formula (or another liquid) after 4 months of age. Breast-feeding is more common in some other developed countries and particularly in developing countries. Nonetheless, many infants are formula-fed for a large part of the first year of life, and those who are not breast-fed or formula-fed receive a variety of liquids that contribute to higher rates of malnutrition, morbidity, and mortality [4].

Although infants fed modern formulas do not experience many of the advantages afforded by human milk (e.g. fewer common infections), they do quite well. As stated by Fomon [5], "in industrialized countries, any woman with the least inclination toward breast-feeding should be encouraged to do so and all assistance possible should be provided by physicians, nurses, nutritionists and other health workers. At the same time there is little justification for attempts to coerce women to breastfeed. No woman in an industrialized country should be made to feel guilty because she elects not to breastfeed her infant." As described subsequently, this statement would not have been true as recently as about 60 years ago.

To provide a historical perspective into the evolution of modern infant formulas, this chapter begins with a brief history of formula feeding. This is followed by discussions of the types and composition of modern infant formulas available, the regulation of infant formula composition and marketing, the growth of formula-fed versus breast-fed infants, and the appropriate introduction of complementary foods for both breast-fed and formula-fed infants.

History of infant formulas

Despite attempts over several centuries to feed infants who are not breast-fed, modern infant formulas are a relatively recent phenomenon. The patenting of a method for condensing cow's milk by Borden in the late 1800s is usually cited as the major factor in development of modern infant formulas. However, other accomplishments were necessary before major progress was made. The introduction of glass bottles and rubber nipples in the mid- to late 1800s made it easier to keep feeding utensils clean. In addition, commercial-scale pasteurization was available by the late 1800s, and sanitary, closed-top metal containers that allowed safe long-term storage of formula components and complete formulas were introduced in the early 1900s. Another crucial factor was knowledge of the composition of human and animal milks and, hence, how to modify animal milks to more closely mimic the composition of human milk. Finally, by the early 1920s, the general level of sanitation had improved and home refrigerators were available.

With more widespread use of formulas, it was realized that scurvy and rickets were more common in formula-fed than in breast-fed infants. These vitamin-deficiency diseases were initially attributed directly to the use of the artificial formulas or failure to breast-feed, but eventually it was recognized that the problem was not formula per se but that the vitamins were destroyed by heat processing.

The advances in formula composition and manufacture between the late 1800s and early 1900s were so dramatic that by the early 1900s, formula feeding was no longer considered hazardous, and pediatricians around the world began recommending a variety of artificial feedings for infants who could not be breast-fed. This, of course, led to the development and marketing of a number of complete formulas. One of these, a synthetic milk-adapted (SMA) product, was the forerunner of a formula that is still available.

Despite availability of complete formulas that required only mixing with water before being fed to the infant, formulas made at home from evaporated milk, sugar, and water remained popular until the late 1950s, by which time they had largely been replaced by "complete" formulas. Initially, only powdered and concentrated liquid products were available, but ready-to-feed formulas were soon introduced. The convenience of ready-to-feed formulas made them quite popular, but recently, powdered formula has regained popularity, probably because of its lower price and its convenience for feeding away from home.

Although some of the changes in formula composition and manufacture since the late 1960s are important, changes during this time pale in comparison to previous advances. Perhaps the most important of the more recent changes is the availability and use of iron-fortified formulas, which are credited with markedly reducing iron-deficiency anemia throughout the world. In addition, a number of human milk components have been added to formulas over the past few decades [11]. These include taurine, carnitine, nucleotides, and, more recently, the long-chain polyunsaturated fatty acids docosahexaenoic acid (DHA) and arachidonic acid (AA). Currently, some formulas contain prebiotics and/or probiotics that are thought to support the growth of beneficial bacteria and inhibit the growth of pathogenic bacteria.

Composition of current infant formulas

A number of formulas are now available for feeding the normal term infant. There are also special formulas for feeding preterm infants as well as formulas for feeding infants with inborn errors of metabolism (e.g. phenylketonuria) and diseases associated with gastrointestinal intolerance. Modern infant formulas differ considerably from evaporated milk formulas. They contain less protein, their carbohydrate content has been modified to include more lactose (unless intended for infants with lactose intolerance), and butter fat has been largely replaced by mixtures of vegetable oils that are better absorbed than butter fat. As described in the following section, all must support normal growth for the first 4 to 6 months of life when fed as the sole source of nutrition.

Although the composition of infant formulas has evolved over many years, research to improve acceptability and nutritional quality continues. In general, human milk serves as a model for the composition of infant formulas, but it has been impossible to duplicate the exact composition of human milk, which, in addition to nutrients, contains hormones, growth factors, immunologically active agents, enzymes, cells, and other factors [12]. In addition, the bioavailability of some nutrients in human milk is greater than in formula; thus, current efforts focus on duplicating the biological effects of human milk rather than its precise content.

The most commonly used infant formulas are standard cow's milk–based formulas, but for the past quarter century, approximately 25% of all formulas sold in the United States have been soy-based. However, these formulas are much less popular in most other countries. A variety of hydrolyzed protein formulas with peptides of different lengths are also available, as are formulas containing only amino acids. Each of these is now discussed briefly.

Cow's milk–based formulas

A standard cow's milk–based formula is the feeding of choice for normal term infants who are not breast-fed or are not breast-fed for the recommended 12 months. The nutrient composition of some of the most popular cow's milk–based formulas is shown in Table 10.1. The compositions do not differ appreciably. The protein content of these formulas is either unmodified cow's milk protein or whey-predominant cow's milk protein, a mixture of cow's milk and demineralized whey proteins. The earliest such formulas had a ratio of 60% whey proteins and 40% caseins, mimicking the percentage of these two proteins in human milk. Although it is now recognized that the composition of human milk and bovine whey proteins and caseins differs considerably, such formulas remain popular. More recently, formulas with other mixtures of caseins and whey proteins (e.g. 48% whey proteins, 52% caseins) have become available. The plasma amino acid

Table 10.1 Nutrient content (per liter) of representative cow's milk–based infant formulas

	Enfamil® Lipil®* (Mead Johnson, Evansville, IN)	NAN® (Nestle, Glendale, CA)	Similac®* (Abbott, Columbus, OH)
Energy, kcal	680	676	676
Protein, g	14.5	15	14
Casein, % of total protein	40	40	52
Whey, % of total protein	60	60	48
Fat, g	36	35	36.5
Polyunsaturated, %	20	22	24
Monounsaturated, %	37	33	39
Saturated, %	43	45	37
Oils	Palm olein, high-oleic sunflower, soy, coconut, DHA, AA	Palm olein, soy, coconut, high-oleic sunflower, safflower, DHA, AA	High-oleic safflower, coconut, soy, DHA, AA
Carbohydrate, g	73	76	73
	Lactose	Lactose, corn syrup	Lactose
Minerals			
Calcium, mg	530	510	527
Phosphorus, mg	360	286	284
Magnesium, mg	54	48	41
Iron, mg	12.2	10.2	12.2
Zinc, mg	6.8	5.4	5.1
Manganese, μg	100	48	34
Copper, μg	510	544	608
Iodine, μg	68	82	41
Sodium, mEq	8.0	7.1	7.1
Potassium, mEq	18.7	17.4	18.1
Chloride, mEq	12.1	12.5	12.4
Vitamins			
A, IU	2000	2027	2027
D, IU	410	405	405
E, IU	13.5	13.6	10.1
K, μg	54	54	54
Thiamine (B_1), μg	540	405	676
Riboflavin (B_2), μg	950	952	1014
Pyridoxine, μg	410	510	405
B_{12}, μg	2.0	1.7	1.7
Niacin, mg	6.8	5.1	7.1
Folic acid, μg	108	102	101
Pantothenic acid, mg	3.4	3.1	3.0
Biotin, μg	20	14.9	29.7

patterns of infants fed formulas with modified and unmodified cow's milk protein differ somewhat, but there is no convincing evidence that one mixture is more or less efficacious than another [13].

Fat provides 40% to 50% of the energy content of cow's milk–based formulas. This is usually a mixture of vegetable oils, but some, primarily those intended for the European market, also contain a small amount of butterfat. As shown in Table 10.1, the fat blends of the common cow's milk–based formulas differ somewhat, but all provide a mixture of saturated, monosaturated, and unsaturated fatty acids, mimicking the balance of these fatty acids in human milk or the response of the breast-fed infant. More recently, small amounts of the long-chain polyunsaturated fatty acids DHA and AA have been added to mimic the contents of these fatty acids in human milk [14]. The source of these fatty acids in most formulas is a mixture of single cell oils, but fish oils and egg yolk phospholipid are also available and are used in some formulas manufactured outside the United States.

There are some differences in fat absorption and mineral absorption as well as the plasma lipid profile among infants fed the various combinations of oils. However, these are not marked. All current infant formulas are well tolerated, and all result in fat and mineral absorption that differ minimally from fat and mineral absorption of breast-fed infants.

Although some cow's milk–based formulas contain other sugars, lactose is the major carbohydrate of most, and it is well tolerated by most infants. Some formulas also contain small amounts of starch or other complex carbohydrates for technical reasons.

Soy-based formulas

Modern soy-based formulas, like modern cow's milk–based formulas, support growth similar to that of breast-fed infants. The nutrient contents of some common soy-based formulas are shown in Table 10.2. Again, the compositions of the various formulas differ minimally. Although native soy protein is deficient in methionine, the soy-based formulas are supplemented with methionine, which makes the nutritional quality of this protein equal to that of cow's milk–based protein [15]. Nevertheless, soy-based formulas contain about 25% more protein than cow's milk–based formulas, presumably because of the assumption that the nutrient quality of soy protein (fortified with methionine) is less than that of human milk or cow's milk.

Soy-based formulas contain no lactose, making them appropriate for infants with lactose intolerance. Other indications include documented immunoglobulin E–mediated allergy to cow's milk protein, documented transient or congenital lactase deficiency, galactosemia, or simply the desire of the parents to have their infant receive a vegetarian diet [16]. Soy-based formulas, like cow's milk–based formulas, can also be used for infants whose nutritional needs are not met by human milk.

The same vegetable oils used in cow's milk–based formulas are used in soy-based formulas. The mineral and vitamin content of soy-based formulas, like the content of protein, is higher than the contents of these nutrients in human milk or cow's milk–based formulas. This is thought to compensate for presumed lower mineral availability, secondary, in part, to substances in soybeans such as phytate.

Protein hydrolysate formulas

These formulas were developed for infants who could not digest or were intolerant to both cow's milk and soy protein. The protein is hydrolyzed to amino acids and peptides that are incapable of causing, or unlikely to cause, an immunological response in most infants. Such formulas are indicated for infants who are intolerant of both cow's milk and soy protein and for those with significant malabsorption secondary to gastrointestinal or hepatobiliary disease. They also are used for infants with a strong family history of food sensitivities, but it is not clear that use of these formulas prevent symptoms of food intolerances [17]. Although nutritionally efficacious, these formulas have an unpleasant taste, are expensive, and have a high osmolality.

Formulas based on hydrolysates of cow's milk, casein, and whey are available. The proteins are heat treated and systematically hydrolyzed, resulting in a hydrolysate of free amino acids and peptides of varying length. The hydrolysate is then supplemented with the amino acids destroyed in the hydrolysis process. The available formulas contain different amounts of peptides of varying chain lengths. More extensive hydrolysis results in less allergenicity but higher cost. Unfortunately, the allergenicity can be determined only by clinical trial.

Most hydrolyzed formulas are lactose free. They may contain sucrose, corn syrup solids, tapioca starch, corn starch, or other starches in various amounts. Many hydrolysate formulas contain medium-chain

95

Table 10.2 Nutrient content (per liter) of representative soy-based infant formulas

	Prosobee® (Mead Johnson, Evansville, IN)	Good Start® Essentials Soy (Nestle, Glendale, CA)	Isomil® (Abbott, Columbus, OH)
C (ascorbic acid), mg	81	61	61
Choline, mg	81	82	108
Inositol, mg	41	122	32
Energy, kcal	680	676	676
Protein, g	16.9	19	16.6
Source	Soy protein isolate	100% soy protein isolate	Soy protein isolate, L-methionine
Fat, g	36	34	37
Polyunsaturated, %	19	22	
Monounsaturated %	38	33	
Saturated, %	40	45	
Oils	Palm olein, soy, coconut, high oleic sunflower	Palm olein, soy, coconut, high oleic safflower	High-oleic safflower, coconut, soy
Carbohydrate, g	72 Corn syrup solids	74 Corn maltodextrin, sucrose	69.6 Corn syrup solids, sucrose
Minerals			
Calcium, mg	710	704	709
Phosphorus, mg	560	423	507
Magnesium, mg	74	74	50.7
Iron, mg	12.2	12.1	12.2
Zinc, mg	8.1	6	5.1
Manganese, μg	169	228	169
Copper, μg	510	805	507
Iodine, μg	101	101	101
Sodium, mEq	10.4	10.2	12.9
Potassium, mEq	21	20	18.7
Chloride, mEq	15.2	13.5	11.8
Vitamins			
A, IU	2000	2012	2027
D, IU	410	402	405
E, IU	13.5	20.1	10.1
K, μg	54	54	74
Thiamine (B_1), μg	540	402	405
Riboflavin (B_2), μg	610	631	608
Pyridoxine, μg	410	402	405
B_{12}, μg	2	2.1	3.0
Niacin, mg	6.8	8.72	9.1
Folic acid, μg	108	107	101
Pantothenic acid, mg	3.4	3.2	5.1
Biotin, μg	20	52	30.4
C (ascorbic acid), mg	81	107	61
Choline, mg	81	80	54
Inositol, mg	41	121	33.8

triglycerides to facilitate fat absorption, but they also contain enough polyunsaturated vegetable oils to supply essential fatty acids.

Amino acid–based formulas

Formulas containing only amino acids are intended for use in infants with extreme protein hypersensitivity, that is, those with persistent symptoms when fed an extensively hydrolyzed protein formula. These formulas are much more expensive than cow's milk– or soy-based formulas and are also more expensive than hydrolyzed formulas.

Follow-up formulas

Follow-up, or follow-on, formulas are intended for infants over 6 months of age. In general, they contain more protein and more of some minerals than regular infant formulas. Part of the rationale for such a formula is to compensate for a possibly low protein intake and, particularly, a low iron intake after complementary feedings begin to displace human milk or formula intake. Although nutritionally adequate, these formulas offer no advantage for infants whose diets contain adequate iron and other nutrients from a combination of formula, complementary foods, and supplements. Such formulas are popular in Europe and other parts of the world but are rarely used in the United States. Moreover, advisory committees in Europe no longer endorse use of these formulas [18], and they have never been endorsed by U.S. advisory committees.

Whole and reduced-fat cow's milk is often used in lieu of formula, in part because of its lower cost. Thus, availability of a simpler, less expensive formula for use after 6 months of age would be a welcome addition. Availability of such a formula should delay introduction of cow's milk, which has a high renal solute load and may contribute to fecal iron loss and anemia.

Regulation of infant formulas [19, 21]

Infant formula is regulated as a food intended solely for infants, that is, it simulates human milk or is suitable as a complete or partial substitute for human milk. In the United States, marketing of infant formula is regulated by the federal Food, Drug, and Cosmetic Act and subsequent regulations of the Food and Drug Administration (FDA). Similar regulations are in place in most other countries, but the details of these regulations differ somewhat from country to country. Only the U.S.

regulations, with which the author is most familiar, are discussed.

The regulations provide specific controls for the nutrient composition, production, and marketing of infant formulas. Current specifications for the nutrient composition of formulas marketed in the United States as well as other recent recommendations are shown in Table 10.3 [18, 21, 22]. Like the nutrient contents of available infant formulas, the recommendations of the various groups differ minimally.

The purpose of the infant formula provisions of the regulatory acts is to protect the health of infants fed the infant formula product. These were strengthened in the mid 1980s in response to a series of events in the late 1970s. An infant formula manufacturer in the United States changed its monitoring practices to exclude chloride, the concentration of which, historically, had been predictable from the sodium concentration. However, the source of another ingredient was changed, negating the historical predictability of chloride content from sodium content. As a result, chloride-deficient formulas were released, and infants fed these formulas developed chloride deficiency with hypochloremic metabolic alkalosis [23].

This incident precipitated passage of the Infant Formula Act of 1980, which amended the Food, Drug, and Cosmetic Act to ensure the adequacy of the nutrient composition of infant formulas. Subsequently, the statutory requirements for infant formula under the act were revised, giving the FDA even broader regulatory authority, including the requirements for the nutrient content of infant formula, quality control procedures, record keeping, and procedures for "recalling" unsafe infant formula from the marketplace.

Currently, infant formula manufacturers must submit information, including information on processing, to the FDA before any new formula or any formula manufactured by a previously unknown manufacturer is marketed. The FDA has responsibility under the act to review the new infant formula submission to enhance the likelihood that the product produced will be safe. If the information in the submission meets the requirements of the act, the FDA will not object to marketing of the formula. Interestingly, the FDA is not authorized to "approve" infant formulas before they are marketed, but it has compliance authority if an infant formula is marketed over its objections.

An infant formula submission must include a quantitative formulation and listing of all ingredients in the formula, including amounts. Only ingredients

Table 10.3 Recommendations for the nutrient content of infant formulas (amount/100 kcal unless otherwise noted)

	FDA[21]		LSRO[22]		ESPGHAN[18]	
	Minimum	Maximum	Minimum	Maximum	Minimum	Maximum
Energy (kcal/dl)	—	—	63	71	60	70
Total fat (g)	3.3	6.0	4.4	6.4	4.4	6.0
% energy	40	54	40	57.2	40	54
LA (% FA) **	2.7	—	8	35	75	27
ALA (% FA) ***	—	—	1.75	4	2.5	—
LA/ALA	—	—	6:1	16:1	5:1	15:1
Protein (g)	1.8	4.5	1.7	3.4	1.8 (soy, 2.25)	3.0
Carbohydrates (g)	—	—	9.0	13	9.0	14
Carnitine (mg)	—	—	1.2	2.0	1.2	—
Taurine (mg)	—	—	0	12	0	12
Nucleotides (mg)	—	—	0	16	0	5
Choline (mg)	7.0	—	7	30	7.0	50
Inositol (mg)	4.0	—	4	40	4	40
Calcium (mg)	80	—	50	140	50	140
Phosphorus (mg)	30	—	20	70	25 (milk) 30 (soy)	90 (milk) 100 (soy)
Magnesium (mg)	6.0	—	4.0	17	5	15
Iron (mg)	0.15	3.0	0.2	1.65	0.3	2.0
Zinc (mg)	0.5	—	0.4	1	0.5	1.5
Manganese (μg)	5.0	—	1.0	100	1	50
Copper (μg)	60	—	60	160	35	80
Iodine (μg)	5.0	—	8	35	10	50
Sodium (mg)	20	60	25	50	20	60
Potassium (mg)	80	200	60	160	60	160
Chloride (mg)	55	150	50	160	50	160
Selenium (μg)	—	—	1.5	5.0	1	9
Fluoride (μg)	—	—	0	60	—	60
Vitamin A (IU)	250	750	200	500	200	600
Vitamin D (IU)	40	100	40	100	40	100
Vitamin E (mg/αTE/g PUFA)	0.7	—	0.5	5.0	0.5	5.0
Vitamin K (μg)	4.0	—	1.0	25	4	25
Thiamine; vit B_1, (μg)	40	—	30	200	60	300
Riboflavin; vit B_2, (μg)	60	—	80	300	80	400
Niacin; vit B_3, (μg)	250	—	550	2000	300	1500
Pyridoxine; vit B_6 (μg)	35	—	30	130	35	175
Vitamin B_{12} (μg)	0.15	—	0.08	0.7	0.1	0.5
Folic acid (μg)	40	—	11	40	10	50
Pantothenic acid (μg)	300	—	300	1200	400	2000
Biotin (μg)	1.5	—	1.0	15	1.5	7.5
Vitamin C (mg)	8.0	—	6	15	10	30

ALA = α-linolenic acid; ESPGHAN = European Society of Pediatric Gastroenterology, Hepatology and Nutrition. Report of International Expert Group (IEG) for Codex Committee on Nutrition and Foods for Special Dietary Uses (CCNFSDU); FDA = U.S. Food and Drug Administration; LA = linoleic acid; LSRO = Life Sciences Research Organization for U.S. FDA.

Table 10.4 Median weight (kg)/age and length (cm)/age of male and female children constituting the populations of the World Health Organization (WHO; predominantly breast-fed) and Centers for Disease Control and Prevention (CDC; predominantly formula-fed) Growth Standard/Reference studies [24, 25]

Age (m)	Weight for age				Length for age			
	Male		Female		Male		Female	
	WHO	CDC	WHO	CDC	WHO	CDC	WHO	CDC
0	3.3	3.5	3.2	3.4	49.9	52.7	49.1	51.7
1	4.5	4.9	4.2	4.5	54.7	56.6	53.7	55.3
2	5.6	5.7	5.1	5.2	58.4	59.6	57.1	58.1
3	6.4	6.4	5.8	5.9	61.4	62.1	59.8	60.5
4	7.0	7.0	6.4	6.4	63.9	64.2	62.1	62.5
5	7.5	7.6	6.9	7.0	65.9	66.1	64.0	64.4
6	7.9	8.2	7.3	7.5	67.6	67.9	65.7	66.1
12	9.6	10.5	8.9	9.7	75.7	76.1	74.0	74.4
24	12.2	12.7	11.5	12.1	87.1	86.9	85.7	85.4
36	14.3	14.4	13.9	13.9	96.1	95.3	95.1	94.2
48	16.3	16.3	16.1	15.9	103.3	102.5	102.7	101.3
60	18.3	18.5	18.2	18.0	110.0	109.2	109.4	108.0

that have been shown to be safe and suitable under the applicable food safety provisions of the act may be used in infant formulas. The manufacturer also must provide assurance that the formula meets the nutrient content and quantity specifications as well as the nutrient quality standards of the act and demonstrate that all required nutrients are present and available at the specified levels throughout the shelf life of the product. Finally, the manufacturer must demonstrate that the formula contains no contaminant and that the concentrations of required nutrients do not exceed the maximum level allowed.

In some cases, exemptions from the nutrient specifications are permitted. These allow availability of formulas for feeding infants with special medical and dietary needs, for example, formulas for children with inborn errors of metabolism and formulas for low birth weight infants whose nutrient requirements are thought to differ from those of term infants.

Infant formulas, as the sole source of nutrition, must contain all nutrients required to support normal growth and development. Ordinarily, manufacturers submit documentation that the formula, when fed as the sole source of nutrients, supports normal growth and development for approximately 60 days. The clinical studies are generally conducted in accordance with specific recommendations for infant pop-ulations and general recommendations for rigorous clinical trial design, conduct, and analysis.

The labels of infant formulas must include instructions for use, including pictorial instructions; a statement warning against improper preparation or use; a statement cautioning that the infant formula should be used only as directed by a physician; and a "use by" date that ensures the formula will deliver no less than the quantity of nutrients stated on the product label at that date. To comply with the World Health Organization (WHO) Code for Marketing Infant Formulas [24], the label also must state that breast-feeding is the preferred method of feeding infants. Many infant formula labels also contain claims. These must be truthful and not misleading; however, there is no requirement that label claims be approved by the FDA.

Growth of formula-fed infants

Most reports from industrialized countries indicate that weight and length gains of formula-fed infants are greater than those of breast-fed infants. However, rates of gain during the first few weeks to months of life generally are about the same in breast-fed and formula-fed infants or are somewhat greater in breast-fed infants. Examples of early growth are illustrated in Table 10.4, which shows the median weight and length (height)

99

Table 10.5 Weight and length gains of breast-fed and formula-fed infants

	Length gain (mm/d ± SD)			
	Males		Females	
Interval	Breast-fed	Formula-fed	Breast-fed	Formula-fed
8–56 d	1.22 ± 0.16	1.28 ± 0.17	1.15 ± 0.17	1.2 ± 0.14
8–112 d	1.07 ± 0.18	1.13 ± 0.11	1.01 ± 0.11	1.04 ± 0.09

	Weight gain (g/d)			
	Males		Females	
Interval	Breast-fed	Formula-fed	Breast-fed	Formula-fed
8–56 d	37.1 ± 8.7	38.3 ± 7.0	31.7 ± 7.9	32.1 ± 6.5
8–112 d	29.8 ± 5.8	32.2 ± 5.6	26.2 ± 5.6	27.5 ± 4.9

for age at various ages of both males and females participating in the recent WHO Multicenter Growth Reference Study [25], as well as the same data from infants comprising the current WHO/Centers for Disease Control and Prevention growth references [26]. The former group was primarily breast-fed, and the latter was primarily formula-fed. Table 10.5 shows the median daily rates of increase in weight and length of more than 300 breast-fed and formula-fed infants studied during the 1980s at the University of Iowa [27].

Although the rates of gain in weight and length of formula-fed and breast-fed infants, overall, are not dramatically different, the small differences have given rise, on one hand, to arguments that the breast-fed infants' lower rates of gain indicate that breast-feeding may be less than optimal and, on the other, to arguments that formula feeding is excessive and contributes to subsequent development of obesity.

The differences or lack of differences described here concerns infants in industrialized countries. In less industrialized countries, a number of factors interact to increase the variability of weight and length gains. In these countries, formula feeding is often dangerous because of overdilution of the formula, an unsafe water supply, lack of refrigeration, and other factors that are less common than in industrialized countries.

Most exclusively breast-fed infants need additional nutrients by 6 months of age, and some need them earlier. Deciding when to start complementary foods requires balancing the physiological and developmental readiness of the infant and the nutrient require-

ments for growth and development, as well as other health considerations. Thus, it is difficult to specify an age for introduction of complementary foods that is appropriate for all infants.

Complementary feeding

An attempt to formulate guidelines for complementary feeding was made recently by a group convened by the American Dietetic Association and Gerber Products Company to formulate feeding recommendations for 6- to 24-month-old infants and toddlers [28]. This group assumed that the nutrient needs of these children were equal to the Dietary Reference Intakes (DRIs) issued by the Food and Nutrition Board–Institute of Medicine/Health Canada [29–34]. Thus, recommendations concerning the amounts of nutrients needed by breast-fed infants from complementary foods were estimated as the difference between the content of each nutrient in the average intake of human milk and the DRI for that nutrient. Examples of this exercise for 6- to 8-month-old infants are shown in Table 10.6. This process is similar to that used to estimate the complementary food needed by children in developing countries [35].

Because the average intake of infant formula supplies the amount of each nutrient needed for normal growth through the first 12 months of life, formula-fed infants do not require complementary foods to support normal growth. This is illustrated in Table 10.7, which was compiled in the same way as Table 10.6 but substituting the amounts of each nutrient in 708 ml of a common cow's milk–based formula. Although formula-fed infants do not need complementary foods to support normal growth, these foods are essential for development of oromotor skills and the development of familiarity with different flavors and textures. It is clear from Tables 10.6 and 10.7 that complementary foods that meet the nutrient needs of breast-fed infants are likely also to be adequate for formula-fed infants receiving appropriate volumes of formula.

These exercises indicate that less than 50% of the recommended daily allowance for iron and zinc and less than 50% of the adequate intake (i.e. the amount received by normally growing breast-fed infants) for manganese, fluoride, vitamin D, vitamin B_6, niacin, vitamin E, magnesium, phosphorus, biotin, and thiamin are met by the average intake of human milk from 6 to 8 months of age (708 ml). Thus, the complementary foods chosen should be good sources of these nutrients.

Table 10.6 Calculation of nutrients needed from complementary foods by 6- to 8-month-old breast-fed children

Nutrient	DRI (6–8 mo)	Intake from 708 ml breast milk	Intake – DRI	% DRI needed
Energy	649 kcal/d	486 kcal/d	163 kcal/d	25%
Protein	9.9 g/d	7.4 g/d	−2.5 g/d	25%
Fat	30 g/d	22.5 g/d	−7.5 g/d	25%
Vit A	500 µg/d	354 µg/d	−146 µg/d	29%
Vit C	50 mg/d	28.3 mg/d	−22 mg/d	44%
Vit D	5 µg/d	0.39 µg/d	−4.6 µg/d	92%
Vit E	5 mg/d	1.6 mg/d	−3.4 mg/d	68%
Vit K	2.5 µg/d	1.5 µg/d	−1.0 µg/d	40%
Thiamine	0.3 mg/d	0.15 mg/d	−0.15 mg/d	50%
Riboflavin	0.4 mg/d	0.25 mg/d	−0.15 mg/d	60%
Niacin	4 mg/d	1.1 mg/d	−2.9 mg/d	72.5%
Vit B_6	300 µg/d	66 µg/d	−234 µg/d	78%
Folate	80 µg/d	60 µg/d	−20 µg/d	25%
Vit B_{12}	0.5 µg/d	0.7 µg/d	0.2 µg/d	0%
Pantothenic acid	1.8 mg/d	1.3 mg/d	−0.5 mg/d	28%
Biotin	6 µg/d	2.8 µg/d	−3.2 µg/d	53%
Calcium	270 mg/d	198 mg/d	−72 mg/d	27%
Chromium	5.5 µg/d	35.4 µg/d	30 µg/d	0%
Copper	220 µg/d	180 µg/d	−40 µg/d	18%
Chloride	570 mg/d	297 mg/d	−273 mg/d	48%
Fluoride	500 µg/d	11.3 µg/d	−489 µg/d	98%
Iodine	130 µg/d	78 µg/d	−52 µg/d	40%
Iron	11 mg/d (RDA)	0.21 mg/d	−10.8 mg/d	98%
Magnesium	75 mg/d	25 mg/d	−50 mg/d	67%
Manganese	600 µg/d	4.3 µg/d	−596 µg/d	99%
Phosphorus	275 mg/d	99 mg/d	−176 mg/d	64%
Potassium	700 mg/d	372 mg/d	−328 mg/d	47%
Selenium	20 µg/d	14.2 µg/d	−5.8 µg/d	39%
Sodium	370 mg/d	127 mg/d	−243 mg/d	66%
Zinc	3 mg/d	0.85 mg/d	−2.15 mg/d	72%

DRI = Dietary Reference Intake; RDA = recommended daily allowance.

Because iron deficiency can result in cognitive and motor deficits, some of which may not be reversible [36], prevention of iron deficiency is particularly important. By about 6 months of age, most term breast-fed infants require an additional source of dietary iron to meet their iron requirement. Good sources include meats, especially red meats, and iron-fortified infant cereals. A serving of 30 g of infant cereal provides the daily iron requirement, and feeding the cereal with vitamin C–rich foods (such as strained fruits) helps ensure that the iron from the cereal will be absorbed. Formula-fed infants should receive only iron-fortified formula, which also should be used for supplementing breast-fed infants.

Table 10.7 Calculation of nutrients needed from complementary foods by 6- to 8-month-old formula-fed children

Nutrient	DRI (7–12 mo)	Formula intake (708 ml)	Intake – DRI	% DRI
Energy	649 kcal/d	474 kcal/d	−175 kcal/d	27%
Protein	9.9 g/d	10 g/d	—	—
Fat	30 g/d	25.5 g/d	−4.5 g/d	15%
Vit A	500 μg/d	1423 μg/d	923 μg/d	0%
Vit C	50 mg/d	43 mg/d	−7 mg/d	14%
Vit D	5 μg/d	7.1 μg/d	2.1 μg/d	0%
Vit E	5 mg/d	7 mg/d	2 mg/d	0%
Vit K	2.5 μg/d	38 μg/d	36.5 μg/d	0%
Thiamine	0.3 mg/d	0.47 mg/d	0.17 mg/d	0%
Riboflavin	0.4 mg/d	0.7 mg/d	0.3 mg/d	0%
Niacin	4 mg/d	4.9 mg/d	0.9 mg/d	0%
Vit B_6	300 μg/d	285 μg/d	−15 μg/d	5%
Folate	80 μg/d	71 μg/d	−9 μg/d	11%
Vit B_{12}	0.5 μg/d	1.2 μg/d	0.7 μg/d	0%
Pantothenic acid	1.8 mg/d	2.35 mg/d	0.55 mg/d	0%
Biotin	6 μg/d	21 μg/d	15 μg/d	0%
Calcium	270 mg/d	370 mg/d	100 mg/d	0%
Chromium	5.5 μg/d	26 μg/d	210 μg/d	0%
Copper	220 mg/d	430 mg/d	0.21 mg/d	0%
Chloride	570 mg/d	304 mg/d	−266 mg/d−	47%
Fluoride	500 μg/d	—	—	—
Iodine	130 μg/d	29 μg/d	−100 μg/d	77%
Iron	11 mg/d	8.5 mg/d	−2.5 mg/d	23%
Magnesium	75 mg/d	29 mg/d	−46 mg/d	61%
Manganese	600 μg/d	24 μg/d	−576 μg/d	96%
Phosphorus	275 mg/d	199 mg/d	−76 mg/d	28%
Potassium	700 mg/d	516 mg/d	−154 mg/d	22%
Selenium	20 μg/d	114 μg/d	94 μg/d	65%
Sodium	370 mg/d	130 mg/d	−240 mg/d	−2%
Zinc (mg)	3 mg/d	3.6 mg/d	0.6 mg/d	—

DRI = Dietary Reference Intake.

Both human milk and currently available infant formulas provide generous amounts of the essential fatty acids, linoleic acid, and α-linolenic acid. However, cow's milk, especially skim and low fat milk, has very low levels of these fatty acids, and low linoleic acid intake has been documented in infants and toddlers fed cow's milk [37]. The extent to which these low intakes are associated with signs and symptoms of deficiency (poor growth, scaly skin lesions, impaired wound healing, impaired visual acuity) is not clear, but to help ensure adequate intakes, cow's milk should not be introduced until after 1 year of age, and only whole milk should be fed until at least 2 years of age.

There has been considerable concern that infants receiving adequate amounts of linoleic and α-linolenic acids may also need a dietary source of the long-chain polyunsaturated products of these fatty acids, for example, AA and DHA, particularly the latter. Because human milk contains these fatty acids and formulas supplemented with them are available, intakes by breast-fed infants and infants fed supplemented formula are probably adequate through approximately 1 year of age [38, 39]. It is not clear whether toddlers will benefit from supplements of these long-chain fatty acids. Nonetheless, DHA-supplemented complementary foods are now available.

There is no convincing evidence that the order of introduction of foods other than those rich in iron is important. However, only one new food should be introduced at a time, and others should not be introduced for 3 to 4 days to allow time for detection of any difficulty with the newly introduced food.

Current recommendations for infants with a strong family history of food allergy (i.e. those whose parents or siblings have or had significant allergic reactions) are that they should be breast-fed for as long as possible and should not receive complementary foods until 6 months of age. Until recently, it was recommended that introduction of the major food allergens be delayed until after the first year of age and that introduction of foods associated with "lifelong" sensitization (peanuts, tree nuts, fish, and shellfish) be delayed even longer. However, recent recommendations do not stress such caution.

The parents' approach to child feeding is central to the child's early feeding experience. The appropriate approach is often described as a division of responsibility between parent(s) and child. The parents' responsibility is to set the environment and provide appropriate healthy foods, and the child's responsibility is to decide whether to eat and, if so, how much [40]. In this regard, it is important to note that some foods must be presented several times before they are finally accepted by the child. It also is important to avoid major encounters with the child if he or she continues to refuse a specific food, particularly one that has no unique nutritional quality.

References

1. World Health Organization. Infant and Young Child Nutrition – Global Strategy for Infant and Young Child Feeding. Available at: http://www.who.int/gb/ebwha/pdf_files/WHA55/ea5515.pdf (accessed February 18, 2008).

2. American Academy of Pediatrics Committee on Nutrition. Breast-feeding. In: Pediatric Nutrition Handbook, 5th edn (Elk Grove Village, IL: American Academy Press, 2004), pp. 55–85.

3. Agostoni C, Decsi T, Fewtrell M, Goulet O, Kolacek S, Koletzko B, et al., for the ESPGHAN Committee on Nutrition. Complementary feeding: A commentary by the ESPGHAN Committee on Nutrition. *J Pediatr Gastroenterol Nutr* (2008), **46**: 99–110.

4. Marriott BM, Campbell L, Hirsch E, and Wilson D, Preliminary data from demographic and health surveys on infant feeding in 20 developing countries. *J Nutr* (2007), **137**:518S–23S.

5. Fomon SJ, Recommendations for feeding normal infants. In: ed. Fomon SJ, Nutrition of Normal Infants (St. Louis, Mosby-Year Book, 1993), pp. 455–8.

6. Cone TE Jr., History of American Pediatrics (Boston, MA: Little, Brown and Company, 1979).

7. Fomon SJ, History. In: ed. Fomon SJ, Nutrition of Normal Infants (St. Louis, MO: Mosby-Year Book, 1993), pp. 6–14.

8. Hansen JW, and Boettcher JA, Human milk substitutes. In ed. RC Tsang, SH Zlotkin, BL Nichols, and JW Hansen, Nutrition during Infancy, Principles and Practice, 2nd edn (Cincinnati, OH: Digital Educational Publishing, 1997), 441–66.

9. Wood AL, The history of artificial feeding of infants. *J Am Diet Assoc* (1955), **31**:474–82.

10. Stoker TW and Kleinman RE, Standard and specialized enteric feeding practices in nutrition. In eds. WA Walker and JB Watkins, Nutrition in Pediatrics, 2nd edn (Hamilton, Canada: BC Decker, 1997), pp. 727–33.

11. Heird WC, Progress in promoting breast-feeding, combating malnutrition, and composition and use of infant formula, 1981–2006. *J Nutr* (2007), **137**:499S–502S.

12. Koldovsky O, Search for role of milk-borne biologically active peptides for the suckling. *J Nutr* (1989), **119**:1543–51.

13. Järvenpää A-L, Rassin DK, Räihä DK, and Gaull GE, Milk protein quantity and quality in the term infant: I. Metabolic responses and effects on growth. *Pediatrics* (1982), **70**:214–20.

14. Heird WC and Lapillonne A, The role of essential fatty acids in development. *Annu Rev Nutr* (2005), **25**:549–71.

15. Fomon SJ, Ziegler EE, Filer LJ Jr., and Nelson SE, and Edwards BB, Methionine fortification of a soy protein formula fed to infants. *Am J Clin Nutr* (1979), **32**:2360–471.

16. American Academy of Pediatrics Committee on Nutrition, Soy protein-based formulas: recommendations for use in infant feeding. *Pediatrics* (1998), **101**:148–53.

17. Greer FR, Sicherer SH, Burks AW, and the Committee on Nutrition and Section on Allergy and Immunology, Effects of early nutritional interventions on the development of atopic disease in infants and children: the role of maternal dietary restriction, breast-feeding, timing of introduction of complementary foods, and hydrolyzed formulas. *Pediatrics* (2008), **121**:183–91.

18. Koletzko B, Baker S, Cleghorn G, Neto UF, Gopalan S, Hernell O, et al., Global standard for the composition of infant formula:

recommendations of an ESPGHAN Coordinated International Expert Group (medical position paper). *J Pediatr Gastroenterol Nutr* (2005), **41**: 584–99.

19. American Academy of Pediatrics Committee on Nutrition. Current legislation and regulations for infant formulas. In: ed. RE Kleinman, Pediatric Nutrition Handbook, 5th edn (Elk Grove Village IL: American Academy Press, 2004), pp. 99–101.

20. Fomon SJ. Regulations for nutrient content of infant formulas and follow-up formulas. In: Nutrition of Normal Infants (St. Louis, MO: Mosby-Year Book, 1993), pp. 434–9.

21. Code of Federal Regulations. Title 21, Parts 106 and 107. Washington, DC: US Government Printing Office.

22. Raiten DJ, Talbot JM, and Waters JH, for the Life Sciences Research Office (LSRO) of the American Society for Nutritional Sciences. Assessment of nutrient requirements for infant formulas. *J Nutr* (1998), **128** (No. 11S): 2059S–293S.

23. Grossman H, Duggan E, Mccamman S, Welchert E, and Hellerstein S, The dietary chloride deficiency syndrome. *Pediatrics* (1980), **66**:366–74.

24. World Health Organization, International code of marketing of breast-milk substitutes 1981). Available at: http://www.who.int/nutrition/publications/code_english.pdf (accessed February 18, 2008).

25. WHO Multicentre Growth Reference Study Group, WHO child growth standards based on length/height, weight and age. *Acta Paediatrica* (2006), Suppl **450**:76–85

26. Kuczmarski RJ, Ogden CL, Gummer-Strawn LM, et al., *CDC Growth Charts: United States. Advance Data from Vital and*

Health Statistics of the Center for Disease Control and Prevention/ National Center for Health Statistics. Number 314, December 4, 2000 (revised).

27. Fomon SJ and Nelson SE, Size and growth. In ed. Craven L, Nutrition of Normal Infants (St. Louis, MO: Mosby-Year Book, 1993), pp. 36–84.

28. Butte N, Cobb K, Dwyer J, Graney L, Heird W, Rickard K, American Dietetic Association, and Gerber Products Company, The Start Healthy Feeding Guidelines for Infants and Toddlers. *J Am Diet Assoc* (2004), **104**:442–54.

29. Institute of Medicine, Food and Nutrition Board, Dietary Reference Intakes: Energy, Carbohydrate, Fiber, Fat, Fatty Acids, Cholesterol, Protein, and Amino Acids (Washington, DC: National Academy Press, 2002).

30. Institute of Medicine, Food and Nutrition Board, Dietary Reference Intakes for Vitamin A, Vitamin K, Arsenic, Boron, Chromium, Copper, Iodine, Iron, Manganese, Molybedenum, Nickel, Silicon, Vanadium, and Zinc (Washington, DC: National Academy Press, 2001).

31. Institute of Medicine, Food and Nutrition Board, Dietary Reference Intakes for Vitamin C, Vitamin E, Selenium, and Carotenoids (Washington, DC: National Academy Press, 1997).

32. Institute of Medicine, Food and Nutrition Board, Dietary Reference Intakes for Thiamin, Riboflavin, Niacin, Vitamin B6, folate, Vitamin B12, Pantothenic Acid, Biotin, and Choline (Washington, DC: National Academy Press, 1998).

33. Institute of Medicine, Food and Nutrition Board, Dietary Reference Intakes for Calcium, Phosphorus, Magnesium, Vitamin D, and Fluoride (Washington, DC: National Academy Press, 1997).

34. Institute of Medicine, Food and Nutrition Board, Dietary Reference Intakes for Water, Potassium, Sodium, Chloride, and Sulfate (Washington, DC: National Academy Press, 2004).

35. Brown K, Dewey K, and Allen L, Complementary Feeding of Young Children in Developing Countries: A Review of Scientific Knowledge (Geneva: World Health Organization, 1998).

36. Lozoff B, Jimenez E, Hagen J, et al. Poorer behavioral and developmental outcome more than 10 years after treatment for iron deficiency in infancy. *Pediatrics* (2000), **105**: E51.

37. Ernst JA, Brady MS, Rickard KA. Food and nutrient intake of 6-to 12-month-old infants fed formula or cow milk: a summary of four national surveys. *J Pediatr* (1990), **117**: S86–S100.

38. Hoffman DR, Birch EE, Castañeda YS, Fawcett SL, Wheaton DH, Birch DG, and Uauy R, Visual function in breast-fed term infants weaned to formula with or without long-chain polyunsaturates at 4 to 6 months: a randomized clinical trial. *J Pediatr* (2003), **142**:669–77.

39. Hoffman DR, Theuer RC, Castañeda YS, Wheaton DH, Bosworth RG, O'Connor AR, et al., Maturation of visual acuity is accelerated in breast-fed term infants fed baby food containing DHA-enriched egg yolk. *J Nutr* (2004), **134**:2307–13.

40. Satter E, The feeding relationship. In ed. Kessler DB and Dawson P, Failure to Thrive and Pediatric Undernutrition: A Transdisciplinary Approach (Baltimore, MD: Paul H. Brookes, 1999), pp. 121–50.

Nutritional regulation and requirements for lactation and infant growth

Maternal and offspring benefits of breast-feeding

Alison C. Tse and Karin B. Michels

Introduction

Infant feeding practices have undergone changes during the past century, especially in the developed world. Commercially prepared infant formula first became available in the late 19th century, supplementing the range of choices available and eventually replacing cow's milk as a substitute for breast milk. In the first half of the 20th century, bottle-feeding was more popular among women of higher socioeconomic status (SES), in part as a result of marketing of breast-milk substitutes as equal, if not superior, to maternal milk [1]. Breast-feeding is currently more common among white (compared with black), older, more educated, and higher-income women in the United States [2] (Table 11.1). According to the U.S. Centers for Disease Control and Prevention (CDC), 11.3% of mothers exclusively breast-feed at 6 months and 20.9% of mothers breast-feed (either exclusively or partially) at 12 months [2]. Breast-feeding rates in the United States increased substantially during the 1970s and reached a peak in the early 1980s. Following a general trend of a decline from the early to late 1980s and a substantial increase into the new millennium, breast-feeding rates in the United States appear to be leveling off [3] (Fig. 11.1).

Breast milk is higher in lactose and lower in protein than cow's milk [1]. Although the protein in cow's milk is predominantly casein, the major protein in human milk is whey. In addition to containing more cholesterol than cow's milk, human milk differs greatly in the composition of fatty acids [4]. Compared with cow's milk, human milk contains fewer short-chain polyunsaturated and saturated fatty acids but substantially more long-chain polyunsaturated fatty acids (LCPU-FAs). Early formulas were high in protein and butterfat, but most currently available formulas are designed to more closely approximate breast milk's nutrient content [1, 5].

Although the benefits of breast-feeding for the child's health have long been suspected, benefits for maternal health have only recently been recognized. Reported child benefits include decreased risks of infections (including gastrointestinal and lower respiratory infections), lower risk of obesity, and better cognitive development. Breast-feeding has also been linked to decreased incidence of maternal breast cancer and increased postpartum weight loss. More recently reported maternal benefits include decreased risks of Type II diabetes (TIIDM) and cardiovascular disease (CVD). In 2000, the U.S. Department of Health Services reported breast-feeding rate goals of 75% for initiation, 50% at 6 months, and 25% at 12 months by 2010 [6].

In evaluating studies on the benefits of breast-feeding for maternal and child health, several methodological issues must be considered. Because it is not without ethical concern to randomize infants to breast-feeding or formula, most of the studies are observational, mostly of cohort and case-control design. A cohort study is composed of a group of individuals from a population who are defined according to their exposure levels at baseline and followed over time for the occurrence of outcomes of interest [7]. However, cohort studies are costly and time-consuming because of the large number of participants who must be followed for a long duration. Conversely, in a case-control study, individuals are defined by whether they have the disease of interest. Exposure histories are then compared between cases and controls who are representative of the population from which cases have arisen. Although case-control studies are less expensive and time-consuming, bias may be introduced if participants associate their case status with a lack of breast-feeding or if controls are not representative of the source population for cases.

An inherent limitation of observational studies on breast-feeding is that the choice to breast-feed may be dependent on demographic or lifestyle factors that also are related to health status. To minimize bias in

Table 11.1 Estimated percentage of U.S. infants born in 2004 who were ever breast-fed, exclusively breast-fed through age 6 months, and breast-fed through age 12 months, by selected sociodemographic characteristics in the National Immunization Survey [6]

Characteristics	Ever breast-feeding (%)	Exclusive breast-feeding through age 6 months[a] (%)	Breast-feeding at 12 months (%)
U.S. overall	73.8	11.3	20.9
Race/Ethnicity			
White, non-Hispanic	73.9	11.7	20.8
Hispanic	81.0	11.6	24.1
Black, non-Hispanic	56.2	7.5	11.9
Asian or Pacific Islander	81.7	15.8	29.1
American Indian or Alaska Native	77.5	11.4	24.3
Maternal age at birth (yr)			
< 20	55.8	6.1	8.6
20–29	69.8	8.4	16.7
≥ 30	77.9	13.8	24.9
Education			
< High school	67.7	9.1	18.5
High school	65.7	8.2	16.8
Some college	75.2	12.3	18.5
College graduate	85.3	15.4	28.2
Marital status			
Married	79.6	13.4	24.5
Unmarried	60.0	6.1	12.4
Income: poverty ratio			
< 100	65.9	8.3	18.6
100–184	70.8	8.9	16.6
185–349	75.1	11.8	21.3
≥ 350	81.5	14.0	23.6

[a] Exclusive breast-feeding is defined as only breast milk (no solids, water, or other liquids).

epidemiological studies, care must be taken to measure adequately and control for such confounding factors [7]. However, it is difficult to capture these differences completely, and residual or unmeasured confounding may persist. Second, differences between the assessment and definition of breast-feeding make comparisons across studies difficult. In most studies, breast-feeding is assessed as a dichotomous variable (i.e. ever vs. never) and/or as a lifetime duration in months. Few studies have attempted to assess the impact of exclusive breast-feeding, and a significant gap in the literature stems from a lack of differentiation between partial and exclusive breast-feeding in many studies. The World Health Organization (WHO) defines exclusive breast-feeding as follows: "The infant has only breast milk from his/her mother or a wet nurse, or expressed breast milk, and no other liquids or solids with the exception of drops or syrups consisting of vitamins, mineral supplements, or medicine" [8].

The purpose of this chapter is to evaluate critically some of the reported infant and maternal benefits of breast-feeding. For each topic, we start by briefly reviewing the relevant mechanisms and then focus on the epidemiological evidence, evaluating the

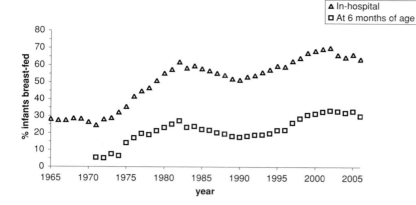

Figure 11.1 U.S. breast-feeding rates, 1965–2006, in the Ross Laboratories Mothers' Survey [3].

Benefits for child

Immune function

Breast milk contains several components that promote passive and active immunity [9]. These factors are either present in low levels or absent in formula. Immunoglobulins (IGs), including IgA antibodies, directed at microbes in the maternal environment, are transferred from the mother to the infant through breast milk. Lactoferrin, an iron-binding protein present at high levels in human milk, is relatively resistant to enzymatic degradation and is microbicidal and anti-inflammatory. Oligosaccharides present in breast milk may prevent colonization of mucous membranes by competing with microbes for receptors.

Perhaps the strongest evidence for an association between breast-feeding and gastrointestinal infections comes from the Promotion of Breast-feeding Intervention Trial (PROBIT), a randomized trial of 17 046 infants followed for 1 year in Belarus, an eastern European country [10]. Matched on several potential confounders, study hospitals and their corresponding clinics were assigned to a breast-feeding promotion intervention or no intervention. Adjusting for birth weight and number of children in the household, infants in the intervention group had a lower risk of gastrointestinal infection (odds ratio [OR] = 0.60, 95% CI [confidence interval] 0.40–0.91) but not hospitalization for gastrointestinal tract infection during the first year of life (OR = 0.92, 95% CI 0.62–

The text continues: methodological strengths and limitations. We do not address special issues such as HIV transmission via breast milk, which is beyond the scope of this chapter.

1.37). Adjusting for the same confounders and maternal smoking during pregnancy, no associations were found between assignment to breast-feeding intervention and two or more respiratory tract infections (OR = 0.87, 95% CI 0.62–1.37) or hospitalization for respiratory tract infection (OR = 0.85, 95% CI 0.57–1.27).

Observational data from well-defined cohorts in developed countries also support the hypothesis of a protective association between breast-feeding and infections. The association of breast-feeding with onset of otitis media was examined in a prospective cohort of 1013 infants in a health maintenance organization in Arizona [11]. After adjustment for sex, day-care attendance, presence of siblings at home, maternal smoking, and parental history of hay fever, infants who were breast-fed for 6 months or longer had decreased risks of both acute otitis media (OR = 0.61, 95% CI 0.40–0.92) and recurrent otitis media (OR = 0.39, 95% CI 0.21–0.73) during the first year of life when compared with non-breast-fed infants.

The associations of current and past breast-feeding with hospitalization for diarrheal and lower respiratory tract infections (LRTIs) were examined in a nationally representative cohort of 15 980 British infants born between 2000 and 2002 [12]. In the first 8 months of life, exclusively breast-fed infants (but not partially breast-fed infants) had a lower risk of developing diarrhea compared with infants who were not breast-fed, after adjustment for infant's age, maternal age, mode of delivery, and maternal education (OR for exclusively breast-fed = 0.37, 95% CI 0.18–0.78; OR for partially breast-fed = 0.63, 95% CI 0.32–1.25). Similarly, exclusively breast-fed infants (but not partially breast-fed infants) had a lower risk of LRTI, which was defined as chest infection or pneumonia, but not wheezing or asthma, after adjusting for the same confounders (OR for LRTI in exclusively breast-fed = 0.66, 95% CI 0.47–0.92; OR for partially breast-fed = 0.69, 95% CI 0.47–1.00). The protective effect of breast-feeding on both types of infections did not appear to persist following cessation of breast-feeding.

The relation between infant feeding practices and infections in the developing world deserves special attention because of the substantial proportion of neonatal deaths due to infections, which in part can be attributed to limited access to clean, nutritious alternatives to breast milk. In a recent meta-analysis of six studies conducted in Brazil, the Gambia, Ghana, Pakistan, the Philippines, and Senegal, infants who were not breast-fed had increased risks of death during the first 6 and 12 months of life due to diarrhea (6 months OR = 6.1, 95% CI 4.1–9.0; 12 months OR = 1.9, 95% CI 1.2–3.1) and acute respiratory infection (ARI; 6 months OR = 2.4, 95% CI 1.6–3.5; 12 months OR = 2.5, 95% CI 1.4–4.6) after adjustment for maternal education [13]. In a clustered randomized trial of a community-based promotion of exclusive breast-feeding in 1115 infants in Haryana, India, infants in the intervention group had a significantly lower 7-day diarrhea prevalence at 3 months (OR = 0.64, 95% CI 0.44–0.95) and 6 months (OR = 0.85, 95% CI 0.72–0.99) after adjusting for maternal working status [14].

Observational data from developed countries suggest that breast-feeding decreases the risks of gastrointestinal and LRTIs and otitis media [11, 12]. In developing countries, an association between breast-feeding and decreased risks of diarrheal and ARI mortality in the first year of life has been suggested. Given the high mortality in developing countries from infections early in life, these results may have substantial public health implications [13, 14]. Additionally, the high morbidity in developed countries due to infections early in life suggests that increasing breast-feeding rates may have a large public health impact [12].

Overweight and obesity

On the basis of early epidemiological reports on an inverse link between breast-feeding and childhood body mass, public health organizations such as the CDC and lay organizations such as La Leche League International, an organization that promotes breast-feeding through mother-to-mother support, have recommended breast-feeding to prevent pediatric obesity and overweight [15, 16]. Breast-fed infants have

lower rates of weight and fat mass gain compared with formula-fed infants during the first year of life, which may be explained by lower total energy and protein intakes in breast-fed infants compared with formula-fed infants [17]. Rapid growth during early childhood may have adverse implications for growth and body mass later in life [18]. Compared with breast-fed infants, formula-fed infants have higher serum concentrations of insulin-like growth factor 1 (IGF-1)[19] and higher plasma concentrations of insulin, which stimulates greater deposition of body fat and could lead to insulin resistance [20]. Formula-fed infants have lower serum concentrations of leptin, a hormone that regulates food intake and energy balance [21]. Breast-feeding may also foster maternal feeding styles that are less controlling and more responsive to infant cues of hunger and satiety, leading to the development of greater self-regulation of energy intake and ability to respond to internal appetite cues [22].

Observational studies on the association between breast-feeding and obesity are subject to confounding by SES. In many early studies, differences in SES between breast-fed and non-breast-fed children were not adequately accounted for. In a meta-analysis of 28 observational studies, the unadjusted summary estimate suggested that having been breast-fed was protective against obesity measured at varying time points later in life (range of mean age of evaluation of obesity = 0.5–33 years; OR = 0.87, 95% CI 0.85–0.89) [23]. The association did not differ by the age at which obesity was measured. However, the crude summary estimate for the association in six studies that assessed maternal smoking, SES, and parental body mass index (BMI; OR = 0.86, 95% CI 0.81–0.91) attenuated greatly when all three of these confounders were adjusted for (OR = 0.93, 95% CI 0.88–0.99).

Evidence from the largest study to date, the Nurses' Health Study II (NHS II), suggests that any inverse association between having been breast-fed and adiposity in childhood is not maintained into early or mid-adulthood [24]. The association between duration of breast-feeding and overweight and obesity across the life course was examined in a cohort of 35 500 U.S. female nurses for whom breast-feeding information was obtained from their mothers. Several indicators of SES and other confounders were controlled, limiting the extent of residual confounding. Compared with women who were breast-fed exclusively for less than 1 week, women who were exclusively breast-fed for 6 months or longer (but not shorter durations)

Table 11.2 Associations of exclusive breast-feeding duration in infancy with early life body shape and adult overweight and obesity in the Nurses' Health Study II [23]

	Body shape[a]		Obesity[b]		Overweight[b]	
	Age 5	Age 10	Age 18	Adulthood[c]	Age 18	Adulthood[c]
None or < 1 week	1	1	1	1	1	1
1 week–3 months	1.00 (0.86–1.16)	1.05 (0.92–1.20)	1.09 (0.87–1.37)	0.98 (0.89–1.08)	0.95 (0.83–1.09)	1.01 (0.93–1.10)
3–6 months	0.98 (0.81–1.19)	1.12 (0.95–1.31)	0.86 (0.63–1.17)	1.03 (0.92–1.16)	1.01 (0.82–1.18)	0.99 (0.90–1.10)
>9 months	0.81 (0.65–1.01)	0.93 (0.77–1.11)	1.01 (0.73–1.39)	0.94 (0.83–1.07)	1.12 (0.94–1.33)	0.98 (0.87–1.10)
p for trend	0.1	0.92	0.72	0.63	0.35	0.75

[a] OR for highest vs. lowest category, adjusted for age at return of questionnaire, year of birth, maternal pre-pregnancy weight, maternal pregnancy weight gain, birth weight, gestational age, maternal education, paternal education, maternal occupation, paternal occupation, and home ownership. NHS II participants were asked to recall their body shape at ages 5 and 10 using a nine-level figure drawing, which was validated previously.

[b] OR adjusted for the same as above and age at menarche, parity, age at first birth, physical activity, alcohol consumption, smoking, daily energy intake, menopausal status, income, and husband's education. Body mass index (BMI) was calculated as height in meters squared divided by weight in kilograms. Obesity was defined as a BMI greater than or equal to 30.

[c] At end of follow-up in 2001 (age range: 37–54 years). Overweight was defined as a BMI of greater than or equal to 25, but less than 30.

had a slightly decreased risk of high adiposity at age 5 after adjustment for maternal characteristics, participant characteristics, and several indicators of SES (Table 11.2). However, no reduction in risk of high adiposity at age 10 was seen in women who were exclusively breast-fed for any duration. Moreover, women who were exclusively breast-fed in infancy for any duration did not have reduced risks of overweight or obesity at age 18 or later in adulthood.

The association between having been breast-fed with obesity and overweight may be largely explained by lifestyle factors associated with socioeconomic gradients [23, 24]. Even if the association of breast-feeding with childhood and adolescent obesity is real, the effect size likely is small, and the role of exclusive versus partial breast-feeding needs to be clarified [23, 24]. The existing data suggest that breast-feeding may somewhat reduce the risk of child overweight and obesity, although differences in body mass do not appear to persist into adulthood [24].

Cognition

Compared with formula, breast milk is hypothesized to foster improved cognitive development through the superiority of its nutrients. Breast-fed infants have higher docosahexaenoic acid (DHA) concentrations in their cerebral tissues than bottle-fed infants [25]. Breast milk may support cognitive development by providing LCPUFAs, including DHA and arachidonic acid (AA), which are hypothesized to be crucial for

early brain development [26, 27]. Commercially prepared formulas supplemented with DHA and AHA levels comparable to those of human milk are now available [26].

In a meta-analysis of 11 observational studies, children who were breast-fed had cognitive function scores that were 5.32 points higher than those of non-breast-fed children at ages 6 months to 15 years (95% CI 4.51–6.13) in the unadjusted estimate [27]. However, following adjustment for several covariates, the summary effect estimate attenuated to a difference of 3.16 points (95% CI 2.35–3.98) between breast-fed and non-breast-fed children, suggesting that other unmeasured confounders might explain the association. Although the authors of the meta-analysis attempted to minimize the effects of confounding by including only studies that adjusted for at least five covariates, many of the studies did not adjust for maternal intelligence and/or child stimulation.

However, given that most studies have been conducted in recent times and the known increased prevalence of breast-feeding in higher socioeconomic strata, mothers of breast-fed children in many studies may have tended to provide a more cognitively stimulating environment [28–30]. Additionally, mothers of breast-fed children may have been more likely to have higher IQs, which may also have been associated with their child's IQ [28–30]. Therefore, adequate adjustment for confounding needs to be made, but differences in SES and the home environment are difficult to control completely.

The association between duration of breast-feeding and child development scores, with simultaneous adjustment for positive parenting practices, maternal IQ, and other important covariates, has been examined in at least three prospective cohort studies [28–30]. In all three studies, an initial association vanished after adjusting for markers of maternal cognition and the home environment.

In summary, higher cognition scores in children who have been breast-fed may largely be attributable to confounding. In particular, important differences in SES, child stimulation, and maternal intelligence between mothers who do and do not breast-feed may account for the association [28–30]. Because it is inherently difficult to control for such differences, studies on the association between breast-feeding and child cognition must be interpreted with caution.

Asthma

Breast milk has been suggested to protect against childhood asthma by promoting gastrointestinal maturation and decreasing infant exposure to foreign dietary antigens, thereby decreasing the risk of sensitization [31]. Breast milk may also provide protection against lower respiratory tract infections, which may decrease inflammatory responses and prevent phenotypic changes within the lungs and hyperreactivity to airborne stimuli later in life. In a meta-analysis of 12 prospective studies, which included 8183 children aged 1.5 to 8.4 years, children who were breast-fed for 3 months or longer had a decreased risk of asthma compared with children breast-fed less than 3 months (OR = 0.70, 95% CI 0.60–0.81) [32]. The association was stronger in children with a history of atopy (OR = 0.52, 95% CI 0.35–0.79) than in children without family history of atopy (OR = 0.73, 95% CI 0.62–0.86). However, only about half of the studies controlled for confounding, and separate crude and adjusted estimates were not computed and compared to examine the role of confounding. More recently published studies in older children have been equivocal, with one suggesting no association between breast-feeding and asthma at age 14 [33], and another reporting an increased risk from ages 9 to 26 in children breast-fed for 4 weeks or longer versus 4 weeks or less [34].

Cardiovascular disease

Breast milk contains LCPUFAs [26], which form an important component of the vascular endothelium [35]. Breast-feeding, as opposed to formula-feeding, may also protect against insulin resistance [20, 21] and obesity later in life [23], although the magnitude of the association between infant feeding and obesity is likely small [24]. Blood pressure has been commonly investigated as a surrogate for CVD. The association between breast-feeding in infancy and blood pressure later in life (ranging from age 1 to 60 years) was examined in 17 503 participants in a meta-analysis of 14 studies [36]. Compared to non-breast-fed participants, breast-fed participants had a lower mean systolic blood pressure (mean difference = −1.4 mmHg, 95% CI −2.2 to −0.6). However, publication bias and confounding were suggested by subsequent analyses and are compelling explanations for any observed association between breast-feeding and blood pressure.

Breast cancer

Breast-feeding could hypothetically increase the risk of breast cancer by transmitting an oncogenic virus from mother to child [37]. In contrast, other hypothesized mechanisms suggest that breast-feeding might protect against the development of breast cancer. Compared with formula-fed infants, breast-fed infants have lower levels of circulating IGF-1 [19] and lower rates of weight and fat mass gain during the first year of life [17], both of which may decrease the risk of breast cancer [38]. Reports from the Boyd Orr Cohort, a prospective cohort of 4999 British participants born between 1918 and 1939, and the NHS I and II all suggested no associations of either having been breast-fed or the duration of having been breast-fed with risk of breast cancer later in life [38, 39]. In the NHS, no association was found when the analysis was restricted to women with a maternal history of breast cancer.

Type I diabetes

Breast-feeding may decrease the risk of Type I diabetes (TIDM) by delaying the introduction of cow's milk into the diet and preventing the development of β-cell autoantibodies [40]. Growth factors, cytokines, and other immunomodulatory factors present in breast milk may also prevent the development of TIDM by promoting the immunological maturity of the intestinal mucosal tissues of the infant [41]. In a meta-analysis of 14 studies, children who were breast-fed for less than 3 months had an increased risk of TIDM compared with children who were breast-fed for 3 months or longer (OR = 1.23, 95% CI 1.12–1.35) [42].

However, all of the studies had a case-control design and an overwhelming majority relied on maternal recall of infant diet. Prospective studies on the association of breast-feeding duration and islet autoantibodies in young, genetically predisposed children have been conflicting [43–45].

Type II diabetes

Breast-feeding may decrease the risk of TIIDM by protecting against insulin resistance [20, 21] and lowering the risk of obesity [23, 46], although the association between breast-feeding and obesity is likely small [24]. The association of having been breast-fed with risk of TIIDM was examined in a meta-analysis of 76 744 adolescents and adults from seven studies (including six cohort studies) [46]. Participants who were breast-fed in infancy had a lower risk of TIIDM later in life (OR = 0.61, 95% CI 0.44–0.85). No evidence for confounding existed in the three studies that measured and adjusted for birth weight, parental diabetes, SES, and individual or maternal body size. Further studies are needed to examine the role of duration and exclusivity of breast-feeding in the risk of TIIDM.

Benefits for mother

Breast cancer

Lactation may decrease the risk of maternal breast cancer by enhancing the differentiation of epithelial cells in the mammary duct [47]. Lactation for longer durations may also lower the number of lifetime ovulations, which has been hypothesized to decrease breast cancer risk [48], although the role of cumulative number of ovulatory cycles in the etiology of breast cancer has been questioned [49]. The excretion of carcinogens such as organochlorines through breast milk may decrease the risk of maternal breast cancer [50].

The association between lifetime duration of lactation and incidence of breast cancer was examined in a meta-analysis of 147 275 women from 47 studies [51]. Adjusting for study, age, parity, age at first birth, and menopausal status, the risk of breast cancer decreased by 4.3% for each 12-month increase in lifetime duration of lactation (95% CI 2.9–5.8). The magnitude did not differ by parity, age at birth of first child, age at diagnosis, family history of breast cancer, or menopausal status. The benefits of breast-feeding did not become substantial until women breast-fed for

19 to 30 months (relative risk [RR] = 0.89, floating standard error = 0.025). A significant limitation of this meta-analysis was that it excluded some of the largest studies for no apparent reason. Furthermore, the vast majority of studies had a case-control design, which is prone to bias.

At least three prospective studies (including two cohort studies and one nested case-control study) are available on the association between cumulative lactation duration and breast cancer. An association was found for extended durations only in a prospective cohort of 252 678 parous textile workers in Shanghai, China, who were aged 39 to 72 at the end of follow-up [52]. After adjusting for parity and age, having lactated for more than 3 years (but not shorter durations) was associated with reduced risk of breast cancer (RR for 37–48 months = 0.67, 95% CI 0.47–0.94; RR for ≥ 49 months = 0.61, 95% CI 0.43–0.87).

In contrast, no association was found for any duration of lactation and breast cancer in an NHS analysis of 89 887 U.S. parous nurses born from 1921 to 1945 and followed from 1986 to 1992 [53]. After adjusting for age, parity, age at first birth, age at menarche, and other confounders, no association was found between categories of lactation duration and breast cancer for either premenopausal (RR ≥ 24 months = 0.90, 95% CI 0.53–1.54) or postmenopausal women (RR for ≥ 24 months = 1.21, 95% CI 0.96–1.54). However, only 6% of the study population lactated for extended durations (i.e. ≥ 24 months).

In an Icelandic case-control study nested within a cohort of 80 219 women aged 20 to 90 years, participants who had no history of breast-feeding were excluded from a postpublication analysis because of concerns that an underlying medical condition may have increased their breast cancer risk [54]. In that analysis, in which lactation for 1 to 4 weeks was designated as the reference group, only women who lactated for more than 105 weeks had a decreased risk of breast cancer (OR for ≥ 105 weeks = 0.56, 95% CI 0.35–0.89). The association was stronger in women diagnosed before age 40 (OR for 53–104 weeks = 0.17, 95% CI 0.04–0.66; OR for ≥ 105 weeks = 0.23, 95% CI 0.02–2.17) than in women diagnosed after age 39 (OR for 53–104 weeks = 0.94, 95% CI 0.64–1.37; OR for ≥ 105 weeks = 0.62, 95% CI 0.38–0.99).

The epidemiological literature thus suggests that if lactation affects maternal breast cancer risk, prolonged lifetime durations would be required [52, 54]. This association was found in combined analyses of both premenopausal and postmenopausal women, although the association appeared to be stronger in younger women [54]. Even so, the results must be interpreted with caution because the association may be due to an underlying morphological breast structure that simultaneously increases risk of breast cancer and leads to inadequate milk supply [53]. Future studies should address the risk of breast cancer among women who cannot lactate versus women who choose not to breast-feed. Involution after lactation is a highly coordinated apoptotic process that may lead to malignant transformation if not regulated properly [55]. How this may affect women who cannot lactate, women who choose not to breast-feed, and women who use medication to suppress lactation needs to be established. More research is also warranted in populations for whom extended durations of lactation are common to clarify the role of age at diagnosis (i.e. premenopausal vs. postmenopausal) and exclusivity of breast-feeding.

Postpartum weight loss

A commonly held belief is that lactation helps mothers to lose weight more quickly postpartum. According to a La Leche League publication, breast-feeding may help some women to lose weight by mobilizing fat stores [56]. Lactation comes at a substantial metabolic cost that translates into an increased energy expenditure ranging from 595 to 670 k/cal day during the first 6 months postpartum [57]. However, in developed countries, where unlimited access to food is common, nursing mothers may be less likely to restrict their energy intake due to fears of impairing the ability to produce milk [58]. Additionally, an increase in prolactin during lactation may lead to increased appetite and increased energy intake in lactating mothers [59].

In a randomized trial of Honduran women, 141 primiparous mothers of term normal-weight infants who exclusively breast-fed for the first 4 months were randomized to exclusive breast-feeding or supplementing with solid foods [60]. Women randomized to exclusive breast-feeding lost significantly more weight between 4 and 6 months postpartum compared with women randomized to supplementation (−0.5 ± 1.6 vs. −0.1 ± 0.8 kg). However, these results may not be generalizable to industrialized nations because of unlimited access to food in developed countries.

The association between duration of exclusive breast-feeding and weight change from pre-pregnancy to postpartum was examined in a prospective cohort of 1538 primiparous and 2810 biparous participants in the NHS II who gave birth to a child between 1990 and 1991 [61]. After adjustment for age, physical activity in 1989, and physical activity change from 1989 to 1991, mothers who exclusively breast-fed for 1 or more months gained approximately 1 kg more compared with mothers who never breast-fed. Despite the relatively large sample size, there were several limitations to the NHS II analysis. First, the authors had to rely on the difference in weight following delivery relative to pre-pregnancy weight, making it difficult to differentiate between weight gain during pregnancy and weight change postpartum. Because women who gain more weight during pregnancy also lose more weight postpartum, weight gain during pregnancy would have to be adjusted for to assess the association between lactation and postpartum weight loss [58, 62]. Additionally, energy intake was not adjusted for, so that this particular analysis addressed the joint effects of lactation and differences in maternal caloric intake between breast-feeding and non-breast-feeding mothers.

Conversely, an association between lactation duration and postpartum weight loss was found in at least two small prospective cohort studies in which the authors measured actual postpartum weight change and accounted for dietary habits. In a prospective cohort of 46 California women, mothers who lactated for at least 12 months lost 2.0 kg more between 1 and 12 months postpartum compared with mothers who lactated for less than 3 months, independent of SES, age, ethnicity, maternal anthropometry, and infant sex and birth weight (−4.4 ± 3.4 kg vs. −2.4 ± 3.0 kg) [62]. Notably, women who intentionally dieted were excluded from this study. In another prospective cohort study ($n = 56$), conducted in Louisiana, mothers who lactated consumed significantly more kilocalories than mothers who did not lactate (2055 ± 435 kcal vs. 2005 ± 515 kcal) [63]. Women who exclusively breast-fed for 6 months lost significantly more weight from 3 to 6 months postpartum (−1.29 ± 0.64 kg) compared with mothers who partially breast-fed (−0.82 ± 0.65 kg) or did not breast-feed (−0.16 ± 0.85 kg) after adjusting for maternal age, parity, pre-pregnancy weight, energy intake, and energy expenditure exclusive of lactation.

In conclusion, null or small effect estimates have been found in most studies in which the association between duration of lactation and postpartum weight change was examined [62, 63]. Despite the high metabolic burden of lactation, increased energy intake in breast-feeding mothers remains the principal explanation for these findings. In studies in which an association was found, the magnitude was small.

Diabetes

Lactation may affect the risk of maternal diabetes through improvements in insulin and glucose homeostasis. Compared with nonlactating mothers, lactating mothers have higher total energy expenditure, higher carbohydrate utilization, and lower fasting insulin levels [64, 65]. Lactation may lead to decreased insulin resistance through preferential mobilization of glucose to the mammary gland for milk production [66].

In the NHS II, the association between lifetime duration of exclusive breast-feeding and incidence of TIIDM was examined in more than 73 000 U.S. parous nurses who were born between 1946 and 1965 and followed for 12 years from 1980 [67]. After adjusting for parity, BMI at age 18, diet, physical activity, and other established confounders, each additional year of exclusive breast-feeding over the lifetime was associated with a 12% decrease in risk of developing TIIDM (95% CI 6%–18%).

Similarly in the NHS, the association between lifetime duration of breast-feeding (whether exclusive or not) and incidence of TIIDM was examined in more than 83 000 U.S. parous nurses born from 1921 to 1945 and followed for 14 years from 1986 [67]. In an analytic model similar to that used in the NHS II analysis, each 1-year increase in lifetime duration of lactation was associated with a 4% decrease in risk of TIIDM after adjustment for confounders (95% CI 1%–8%).

A robust association between lactation and TIIDM was found in two studies [68]. However, results must be interpreted with caution and confirmed in further follow-up studies. Although clinical studies have found evidence to support a protective effect of lactation on glucose homeostasis [62, 65], failure to produce adequate milk for breast-feeding may be a marker for impaired glucose or lipid homeostasis or other health-related behaviors that may affect glucose or lipid homeostasis.

Cardiovascular disease

Lactation may affect several risk factors for coronary heart disease. Extended duration of lactation has been independently associated with improved glucose metabolism [64, 65] and decreased incidence of TIIDM [67], which may lower the risk of CVD. Lactation may also decrease the risk of CVD through improved lipid metabolism. Higher levels of high-density lipoprotein (HDL) have been reported in lactating women when compared with nonlactating women [68]. It has been hypothesized that an increased demand of triglycerides in the lactating breast may be met by increased mobilization of very low-density lipoproteins toward the mammary gland and the transfer of surface remnants to HDL.

The association between lactation and CHD has been examined in only one study. In the NHS, the association between duration of lactation and incidence of myocardial infarction (MI) and cardiac sudden death was analyzed in a prospective cohort of 92 648 parous women followed for 16 years from 1986 [69]. After adjustment for age, parity, early adult adiposity, family history, smoking, diet, exercise, and other confounders, women who had lactated for 23 months or more had a lower risk of developing MI and sudden death compared with women who did not lactate (RR = 0.81, 95% CI 0.67–0.98). However, no decreased risk of MI and sudden death was seen for women who lactated for shorter durations (>11–23 months RR = 0.91, 95% CI 0.80–1.04).

The association between lactation and hypertension has also been examined in only a few studies. In a prospective cohort of 106 584 parous Korean women followed for 6 years, lifetime lactation duration of as little as 1 to 6 months decreased the risk of hypertension by 10% (95% CI 0.87–0.93) independent of age, parity, obesity, smoking, alcohol use, physical exercise, and age at first pregnancy (RR for 4–6 months = 0.90, 95% CI 0.85–0.96; RR for 7–12 months = 0.92, 95% CI 0.87–0.98; RR for 13–18 months = 0.93, 95% CI 0.86–0.99) [70]. In the Coronary Artery Risk and Development in Young Adults Study (CARDIA), 109 parous U.S. women aged 24 to 42 years were followed for 3 years during which an interim conception and birth occurred. In CARDIA, no significant differences in change in systolic blood pressure and change in diastolic blood pressure from preconception levels existed between mothers who breast-fed and weaned their child and mothers who did not breast-feed [71]. Notably both the Korean Women's Health (mean = 32.2 years) and the CARDIA cohorts both consisted of relatively young women and had relatively short follow-up periods so that any long-term impact on blood pressure could not be evaluated.

Lactation may improve maternal cardiovascular health, although few studies exist. It remains unclear whether the changes in blood pressure will ultimately lead to long-term cardiovascular effects because hypertension studies have had short follow-up [70, 71]. Evidence for an association between lactation and CVD comes from the NHS, in which an inverse association between extended duration of lactation and MI and sudden death was found in a large prospective cohort with a long follow-up [69]. Further follow-up studies should examine the association in large cohorts for sufficiently long durations to confirm these results.

Conclusions

On the basis of the epidemiological evidence, breast-feeding is a modifiable risk factor for several maternal and child health outcomes. Evidence suggests that breast-feeding may reduce the risk of lower respiratory and gastrointestinal infections in infants and TIIDM later in life. Other data imply that breast-feeding may reduce the risk of maternal breast cancer, although only for extended durations of breast-feeding. Reports from a limited number of studies also suggest an important reduction in risk of maternal CVD and TIIDM with longer lifetime durations of lactation.

However, commonly held misconceptions about the benefits of breast-feeding persist. For example, any benefit for maternal breast cancer may be limited to the extended durations of breast-feeding more common in the developing world. Second, the difference in postpartum weight loss commonly reported in the literature with lactation may be clinically insignificant. Finally, the associations of breast-feeding with child cognition and obesity also commonly cited in the literature may be largely confounded by factors related to socioeconomic gradients, and it is unclear whether these relations can be attributed to residual or unmeasured confounding.

Although there is an extensive body of literature on the potential benefits of breast-feeding, several areas of research warrant further attention. First, the benefits of partial versus exclusive breast-feeding remain unknown for many health outcomes. Second, combining both women who choose not to breast-feed and women who cannot lactate in a reference group of women who do not breast-feed may obscure important differences. The inability to lactate may be associated with metabolic and structural characteristics linked to disease processes; conversely, the use of medication to suppress lactation may interfere with a coordinated apoptotic process. Finally, further research is warranted to identify ways to promote breast-feeding as a public health intervention. Large-scale trials of breast-feeding promotion such as PROBIT may help to establish the feasibility of such interventions, while evaluating their impact on maternal and child health outcomes.

References

1. Lawrence RA, and Lawrence RM, Breast-Feeding: A Guide for the Medical Profession, 5th edn (St. Louis, MO: Mosby, 1999).

2. Centers for Disease Control and Prevention, Breast-feeding Practices – Results from the National Immunization Survey (2007). Available at: http://www.cdc.gov/breast-feeding/data/NIS_data/data_2004.htm (accessed October 1, 2007).

3. Ross Laboratories Mothers' Survey,1965–2006, Columbus, OH. Wenjun Zhou, personal communication.

4. Jensen RG, and Lammi-Keefe CJ, Current status of research on the composition of bovine and human milk lipids. In: ed. Huang YS and Sinclair AJ, Lipids in Infant Nutrition (Champaign, IL: AOCS Press, 1998), pp. 168–91.

5. Foster LH and Sumar S, Infant formulas – a brief insight. Nutr Food Sci (1997), 97(3):112–116.

6. U.S. Department of Health and Human Services, Healthy People 2010: Objectives for Improving Health Volume 2, 2nd edn (Washington, DC: U.S. Government Printing Office, 2000). Available at: http://www.healthypeople.gov/document/tableofcontents.htm#Volume2 (accessed October 30, 2007).

7. Rothman KJ, and Greenland S, Modern Epidemiology, 2nd edn (Philadelphia: Lippincott-Raven, 1998).

8. World Health Organization, Indicators for Assessing Breast-Feeding Practices (1991). Available at: http://www.who.int/child-adolescent health/New_Publications/ NUTRITION/WHO_CDD_SER_91.14.pdf (accessed August 6, 2007).

9. Hanson LA, Session 1: Feeding and infant development breast-feeding and immune function. Proc Nutr Soc (2007), 66:384–96.

10. Kramer MS, Chalmers B, Hodnett ED, Sevkovskaya Z, Dzikovich I, and Shapiro S, et al., Promotion of Breast-feeding Intervention Trial (PROBIT): a randomized trial in the Republic of Belarus. JAMA (2001), 285:413–20.

11. Duncan B, Ey J, Holberg CJ, Wright AL, Martinez FD, and Taussig LM, Exclusive breast-feeding for at least 4 months protects against otitis media. Pediatrics (1993), 91:867–72.

12. Quigley MA, Kelly YJ, and Sacker A, Breast-feeding and hospitalization for diarrheal and respiratory infection in the United Kingdom Millennium Cohort Study. Pediatrics (2007), 119:e837–42.

13. WHO Collaborative Study Team on the Role of Breast-feeding on the Prevention of Infant Mortality, Effect of breast-feeding on infant and child mortality due to infectious diseases in less developed countries: a pooled analysis. Lancet (2000), 355:451–5.

14. Bhandari N, Bahl R, Mazumdar S, Martines J, Black RE, Bhan MK, et al., Effect of community-based promotion of exclusive breast-feeding on diarrhoeal illness and growth: a cluster randomised controlled trial. Lancet (2003), 361:1418–23.

15. Centers for Disease Control and Prevention, Does breast-feeding reduce the risk of pediatric overweight? (2007). Available at: http://www.cdc.gov/nccdphp/dnpa/nutrition/pdf/breast-feeding_r2p.pdf (accessed August 31, 2007).

16. Torgus J and Gotsch G, for La Leche League International, The Womanly Art of Breast-Feeding, 7th rev. edn (Schaumburg, IL: La Leche League International, 2004).

17. Heinig MJ, Nommsen LA, Peerson JM, Lonnerdal B, and Dewey KG, Energy and protein intakes of breast-fed and formula-fed infants during the first year of life and their association with growth velocity: the DARLING Study. Am J Clin Nutr (1993), 58:152–61.

18. Eriksson J, Forsen T, Tuomilehto J, Osmond C, and Barker D, Size at birth, childhood growth and obesity in adult life. Int J Obes Relat Metab Disord (2001), 25:735–40.

19. Chellakooty M, Juul A, Boisen KA, Damgaard IN, Kai CM, Schmidt IM, et al., A prospective study of serum insulin-like growth factor I (IGF-I) and IGF-binding protein-3 in 942 healthy infants: associations with birth weight, gender, growth velocity, and breast-feeding. J Clin Endocrinol Metab (2006), 91:820–6.

20. Lucas A, Sarson DL, Blackburn AM, Adrian TE, Aynsley-Green A, and Bloom SR, Breast vs bottle: endocrine responses are different with formula feeding. Lancet (1980), 1:1267–9.

21. Savino F, Costamagna M, Prino A, Oggero R, and Silvestro L, Leptin levels in breast-fed and formula-fed infants. Acta Paediatr (2002), 91:897–902.

22. Taveras EM, Rifas-Shiman SL, Scanlon KS, Grummer-Strawn LM, Sherry B, and Gillman MW, To what extent is the protective effect of breast-feeding on future overweight explained by decreased maternal feeding restriction? Pediatrics (2006), 118:2341–8.

23. Owen CG, Martin RM, Whincup PH, Smith GD, and Cook DG, Effect of infant feeding on the risk of obesity across the life course: a quantitative review of published evidence. Pediatrics (2005), 115:1367–77.

24. Michels KB, Willett WC, Graubard BI, Vaidya RL, Cantwell MM, Sansbury LB, et al., A longitudinal study of infant feeding and obesity throughout life course. *Int J Obes* (2007), **31**:1078–85.

25. Farquharson J, Jamieson EC, Abbasi KA, Patrick WJ, Logan RW, and Cockburn F, Effect of diet on the fatty acid composition of the major phospholipids of infant cerebral cortex. *Arch Dis Child* (1995), **72**:198–203.

26. Crawford, MA, The role of essential fatty acids in neural development: implications for perinatal nutrition. *Am J Clin Nutr* (1993), **57**(Suppl):703S–10S.

27. Anderson JW, Johnstone BM, and Remley DT, Breast-feeding and cognitive development: a meta-analysis. *Am J Clin Nutr* (1999), **70**:525–35.

28. Der G, Batty GD, and Deary IJ, Effect of breast feeding on intelligence in children: prospective study, sibling pairs analysis, and meta-analysis. *BMJ* (2006), **333**:945.

29. Jacobson SW, Chiodo LM, and Jacobson JL, Breast-feeding effects on intelligence quotient in 4- and 11-year-old children. *Pediatrics* (1999), **103**:e71.

30. Zhou SJ, Baghurst P, Gibson RA, and Makrides M, Home environment, not duration of breast-feeding, predicts intelligence quotient of children at four years. *Nutrition* (2007), **23**:236–41.

31. Oddy WH, A review of the effects of breast-feeding on respiratory infections, atopy, and childhood asthma. *J Asthma* (2004), **41**:605–21.

32. Gdalevich M, Mimouni D, and Mimouni M, Breast-feeding and the risk of bronchial asthma in childhood: a systematic review with meta-analysis of prospective studies. *J Pediatr* (2001), **139**:261–6.

33. Burgess SW, Dakin CJ, and O'Callaghan MJ, Breast-feeding does not increase the risk of asthma at 14 years. *Pediatrics* (2006), **117**:e787–92.

34. Sears MR, Greene JM, Willan AR, Taylor DR, Flannery EM, Cowan JO, et al., Long-term relation between breast-feeding and development of atopy and asthma in children and young adults: a longitudinal study. *Lancet* (2002), **360**:901–7.

35. Engler MM, Engler MB, Kroetz DL, Boswell KD, Neeley E, and Krassner SM, The effects of a diet rich in docosahexaenoic acid on organ and vascular fatty acid composition in spontaneously hypertensive rats. *Prostaglandins Leukot Essent Fatty Acids* (1999), **61**:289–95.

36. Martin RM, Gunnell D, and Smith GD, Breast-feeding in infancy and blood pressure in later life: systematic review and meta-analysis. *Am J Epidemiol* (2005), **161**:15–26.

37. Sarkar NH and Moore DH, On the possibility of a human breast cancer virus. *Nature* (1972), **236**:103–6.

38. Martin RM, Middleton N, Gunnell D, Owen CG, and Smith GD, Breast-feeding and cancer: the Boyd Orr cohort and a systematic review with meta-analysis. *J Natl Cancer Inst* (2005), **97**:1446–57.

39. Michels KB, Trichopoulos D, Rosner BA, Hunter DJ, Colditz GA, Hankinson SE, et al., Being breast-fed in infancy and breast cancer incidence in adult life: results from the two nurses' health studies. *Am J Epidemiol* (2001), **153**:275–83.

40. Vaarala O, Is type 1 diabetes a disease of the gut immune system triggered by cow's milk insulin? *Adv Exp Med Biol* (2005), **569**:151–6.

41. Harrison LC and Honeyman MC, Cow's milk and type 1 diabetes: the real debate is about mucosal immune function. *Diabetes* (1999), **48**:1501–7.

42. Norris JM and Scott FW, A meta-analysis of infant diet and insulin-dependent diabetes mellitus: do biases play a role? *Epidemiology* (1996), **7**:87–92.

43. Couper JJ, Steele C, Beresford S, Powell T, McCaul K, Pollard A, et al., Lack of association between duration of breast-feeding or introduction of cow's milk and development of islet autoimmunity. *Diabetes* (1999), **48**:2145–9.

44. Holmberg H, Wahlberg J, Vaarala O, Ludvigsson J, and the ABIS Study Group, Short duration of breast-feeding as a risk-factor for beta-cell autoantibodies in 5-year-old children from the general population. *Br J Nutr* (2007), **97**:111–16.

45. Ziegler AG, Schmid S, Huber D, Hummel M, and Bonifacio E, Early infant feeding and risk of developing type 1 diabetes-associated autoantibodies. *JAMA* (2003), **290**:1721–8.

46. Owen CG, Martin RM, Whincup PH, Smith GD, and Cook DG, Does breast-feeding influence risk of type 2 diabetes in later life? A quantitative analysis of published evidence. *Am J Clin Nutr* (2006), **84**:1043–54.

47. Russo J and Russo IH, Toward a physiological approach to breast cancer prevention. *Cancer Epidemiol Biomarkers Prev* (1994), **3**:353–64.

48. Henderson BE, Ross RK, Judd HL, Krailo MD, and Pike MC, Do regular ovulatory cycles increase breast cancer risk? *Cancer* (1985), **56**:1206–8.

49. Lipworth L, Bailey LR, and Trichopoulos D, History of breast-feeding in relation to breast cancer risk: a review of the epidemiologic literature. *J Natl Cancer Inst* (2000), **92**:302–12.

50. Dewailly E, Ayotte P, and Brisson J, Protective effect of breast feeding on breast cancer and body burden of carcinogenic organochlorines. *J Natl Cancer Inst* (1994), **86**:803.

51. Collaborative Group on Hormonal Factors in Breast Cancer, Breast cancer and breast-feeding: collaborative reanalysis of individual data from 47 epidemiological studies in 30 countries, including 50302 women with breast cancer and 96973 women without the disease. *Lancet* (2002), **360**:187–95.

52. Rosenblatt KA, Li Gao D, Ray RM, and Thomas DB, Re: History of breast-feeding in relation to breast cancer risk: a review of the epidemiologic literature. *J Natl Cancer Inst* (2000), **92**:942; author reply 943.

53. Michels KB, Willett WC, Rosner BA, Manson JE, Hunter DJ, Colditz GA, et al., Prospective assessment of breast-feeding and breast cancer incidence among 89,887 women. *Lancet* (1996), **347**:431–6.

54. Tryggvadottir L, Tulinius H, Eyfjord JE, and Sigurvinsson T, Breast-feeding and reduced risk of breast cancer in an Icelandic cohort study. *Am J Epidemiol* (2001), **154**:37–42.

55. Watson CJ, Post-lactational mammary gland regression: molecular basis and implications for breast cancer. *Expert Rev Mol Med* (2006), **8**:1–15.

56. Zahorick M and Webber V, Postpartum body image and weight loss. *New Beginnings* (2000), **17**:156–9. Available at:

http://www.llli.org/NB/NBSepOct00p156.html (accessed June 30, 2007).

57. Dewey KG, Energy and protein requirements during lactation. *Annu Rev Nutr* (1997), **17**:19–36.

58. Dewey KG, Impact of breast-feeding on maternal nutritional status. *Adv Exp Med Biol* (2004), **554**:91–100.

59. Janney CA, Zhang D, and Sowers M, Lactation and weight retention. *Am J Clin Nutr* (1997), **66**:1116–24.

60. Dewey KG, Cohen RJ, Brown KH, and Rivera LL, Effects of exclusive breast-feeding for four versus six months on maternal nutritional status and infant motor development: results of two randomized trials in Honduras. *J Nutr* (2001), **131**:262–7.

61. Sichieri R, Field AE, Rich-Edwards J, and Willett WC, Prospective assessment of exclusive breast-feeding in relation to weight change in women. *Int J Obes Relat Metab Disord* (2003), **27**:815–20.

62. Dewey KG, Heinig MJ, and Nommsen LA, Maternal weight-loss patterns during prolonged lactation. *Am J Clin Nutr* (1993), **58**:162–6.

63. Brewer MM, Bates MR, and Vannoy LP, Postpartum changes in maternal weight and body fat depots in lactating vs nonlactating women. *Am J Clin Nutr* (1989), **49**:259–65.

64. Butte NF, Hopkinson JM, Mehta N, Moon JK, and Smith EO, Adjustments in energy

expenditure and substrate utilization during late pregnancy and lactation. *Am J Clin Nutr* (1999), **69**:299–307.

65. Diniz JM and Da Costa TH, Independent of body adiposity, breast-feeding has a protective effect on glucose metabolism in young adult women. *Br J Nutr* (2004), **92**:905–12.

66. Jones RG, Ilic V, and Williamson DH, Physiological significance of altered insulin metabolism in the conscious rat during lactation. *Biochem J* (1984), **220**:455–60.

67. Stuebe AM, Rich-Edwards JW, Willett WC, Manson JE, and Michels KB, Duration of lactation and incidence of type 2 diabetes. *JAMA* (2005), **294**:2601–10.

68. Knopp RH, Walden CE, Wahl PW, Bergelin R, Chapman M, Irvine S, et al., Effect of postpartum lactation on lipoprotein lipids and apoproteins. *J Clin Endocrinol Metab* (1985), **60**:542–7.

69. Stuebe AM, Michels KB, Willett WC, Manson JE, and Rich-Edwards JW, Duration of lactation and incidence of myocardial infarction. *Am J Obstet Gynecol* (2006), **195**:S34.

70. Lee SY, Kim MT, Jee SH, and Yang HP, Does long-term lactation protect premenopausal women against hypertension risk? A Korean women's cohort study. *Prev Med* (2005), **41**:433–8.

71. Gunderson EP, Lewis CE, Wei GS, Whitmer RA, Quesenberry CP, and Sidney S, Lactation and changes in maternal metabolic risk factors. *Obstet Gynecol* (2007), **109**:729–38.

Specialized requirements

Teenage pregnancies

Annie S. Anderson and Wendy L. Wrieden

Key clinical messages

Teenage pregnancy is associated with poorer fetal and maternal outcomes including higher rates of low birth weight infants (< 2500 g) and neonatal deaths.

Nutritional requirements for pregnancy must meet the maternal and fetal needs of pregnancy plus the requirements for personal growth in the young mother.

Adolescent pregnancy growth is associated with greater weight gain, fat storage, and postpartum weight retention compared with older women but also a greater incidence of low birth weight babies.

In adolescence, high pre-pregnancy body mass index (BMI) and high weight gain during pregnancy independently confer dose-dependent increases in risk for macrosomia, primary cesarean delivery, labor induction, pregnancy-induced hypertension, preeclampsia, and gestational diabetes mellitus.

For younger adolescents, higher gestational weight gains are recommended, but this should be assessed on an individual basis according to pre-pregnancy weight.

Where possible, pregnant teenage women should be given individual counseling that focuses on motivation and skills for changing eating habits to help achieve appropriate dietary intake. Such counseling must take account of individual social and economic circumstances.

Access to financial support with food aid and practical advice appears to be a rational approach to help achieve dietary change, but the impact of such approaches on uptake and outcomes remains to be tested.

Introduction

Teenage pregnancy presents biological, social, and cultural challenges to young women as they strive to cope with the physiological and emotional demands of adolescent issues, fetal growth, and impending motherhood. At a global level, the nutritional issues of teenage

pregnancy vary enormously between the developed and developing world and are influenced by cultural norms, kinship, and social support.

Within Europe, the United Kingdom is often cited as having the highest teenage conception rate. In 2003, the rate was 42.3 per 1000 in England and Wales [1], but this is substantially lower than New Zealand or the United States [2], and in fact overall international comparisons suggest that the rate is moderate and has declined over the past 60 years. Lawlor and Shaw [2] noted that "over the same three to six decades the number of adolescents having sex has increased greatly (Wellings & Kane, 1999)[3] and the age at menarche has decreased (Whincup et al., 2001)" [4]. Thus, although the at-risk population has increased overall, declining conception rates indicate that teenagers must in fact be fairly competent at preventing unwanted pregnancies.

In the United States, approximately 900,000 teenagers become pregnant each year, and even with declining rates, it is estimated that more than 4 in 10 adolescent girls have been pregnant at least once before age 20 years. It should also be noted that approximately 25% of adolescent births are not first births [5]. Preliminary data for 2005 [6] show that the birth rate for teenagers declined by 2% in 2005, falling to 40.4 births per 1000 for those aged 15 to 19 years (the lowest ever recorded in the 65 years). The rate declined for teenagers 15 to 17 years to 21.4 births per 1000, but was essentially stable for older teenagers 18 to 19 years, at 69.9 per 1000 [6]. By contrast, in Brazil, the birth rate for adolescent mothers has increased from 8.0 per 1000 in 1980 to 9.1 per 1000 in 2000, now representing 19.4% of all births (cited by Gigante et al. [7]).

Teenage mothers are less likely to attain high levels of education, work experience, and financial stability. U.S. data suggest that as many as 83% of adolescents who give birth and 61% of those who have had abortions are from poor or low-income families and that

Table 12.1 Live births, stillbirths, and infant deaths by mother's age 2006

England and Wales			Number and rates				
	Number of births			Rates[a]			
Mother's age	Live births	Stillbirths	Stillbirth	Perinatal	Neonatal	Postnatal	Infant
All	669,514	3,603	5.4	7.9	3.4	1.4	4.8
Under 20	45,500	268	5.9	8.8	4.1	2.3	6.4
20–24	127,814	682	5.3	8.0	3.6	1.9	5.6
25–29	172,642	887	5.1	7.8	3.6	1.2	4.8
30–34	189,369	920	4.8	7.2	3.0	1.1	4.1
35–39	110,473	640	5.8	8.0	3.1	1.3	4.3
40 and over	23,716	206	8.6	12.0	4.4	1.4	5.9

Source: Office for National Statistics, Infant and perinatal mortality by biological and social factors 2006. *Health Stat Q* (2007), 36:84–91.
[a] Stillbirths and perinatal deaths per 1000 live births and stillbirths. Neonatal, postnatal, and infant deaths per 1000 live births.

at least one third of parenting adolescents are the children of adolescent parents.

Medical risks of teenage pregnancy

There is considerable evidence worldwide that teenage pregnancy is associated with increased maternal and fetal risk. For example, in the United States, the incidence of having a low birth weight (LBW) infant (< 2500 g) among adolescents is more than double the rate for adults, and the neonatal death rate (within 28 days of birth) is estimated to be almost 3 times higher. The mortality rate for the mother, although low, is twice that for the adult pregnant woman [8]. In England and Wales, women under 20 years have a greater risk of stillbirth, perinatal, neonatal, postnatal, and infant death compared with mothers aged 21 to 40 years (Table 12.1).

However, the incidence of teenage pregnancy and the impact on health may be most visible in the developing world. In a community-based, multicenter study of 93 356 married women, aged 15 to 45 years, from 23 districts in India, Oumachigui [9] reported that 40% to 80% of women married before age 18 years, and the incidence of teenage pregnancy was 66%. More recent research from a tertiary care teaching hospital in Varasi, India [10], reported that compared with adult controls, there were increased complications of teenage pregnancy including pregnancy-induced hypertension, preeclamptic toxemia, eclampsia, and premature onset of labor. Teenage mothers also had increased incidence of LBW, premature delivery, and neonatal morbidities (includ-

ing perinatal asphyxia, jaundice, and respiratory distress syndrome). Teenage pregnancy was also associated with higher fetal and neonatal mortality.

A range of biological factors has been associated with these unfortunate pregnancy outcomes, including poor nutritional status, low pre-pregnancy weight, maternal height, parity, and poor weight gain during pregnancy. These factors in turn are highly likely to have been influenced by social circumstances including poverty, poor social support, low educational levels, substance abuse (smoking and drugs), and poor uptake of antenatal services.

Nutritional requirements of adolescent pregnancy

Key characteristics of dietary habits in adolescence in developed countries have been described as unconventional meal patterns (particularly snacking), changing food consumption and choices (including a dominance of savory snacks, confectionery, and sweetened beverages), and concerns with body weight. It is recognized that many of these features reflect the need to express freedom from parental control and from adult tastes and lifestyles [11]. Adolescence is also a time where many experiment with tobacco, alcohol (often to excess), and other substances. It is also recognized that levels of psychological distress have increased among female adolescents in recent years because of increasing educational expectations and issues over personal identity [12], which may result in suboptimal health behavior choices. Additionally, peer influence

Table 12.2 Nutrient intakes recommended for teenage and nonteenage women

	Australian and New Zealand			United States		
	Recommended Dietary Intakes[a]			Recommended Dietary Allowances[b,c]		
	14–18 yr	19–30 yr	31–50 yr	≤18 yr	19–30 yr	31–50 yr
Energy (kcal)	Guidance given according to PAL and weight	Guidance given according to PAL and weight	Guidance given according to PAL and weight	2368, 2708, 2820[d]	2403, 2743, 2855[d]	2403, 2743, 2855[d]
Protein (g/day)	58	60	60	71	71	71
Vitamin A (μg/day)	700	800	800	750	770	770
Vitamin C (mg/day)	55	60	60	80	85	85
Folate (μg/day)	600	600	600	600	600	600
Iron (mg/day)	27	27	27	220	220	220
Calcium (mg/day)	1300	1000	1000	AI 1300	AI 1000	AI 1000
Zinc (mg/day)	10	11	11	12	11	11
Chromium (mg/day)	AI 30	AI 30	AI 30	AI 29	AI 30	AI 30

[a] Source: *Nutrient Reference Values for Australia and New Zealand: Including Recommended Dietary Intakes* (Department of Health and Ageing, National Health and Medical Research Council, 2006).
[b] Source: *Dietary Reference Intakes for Energy, Carbohydrate, Fiber, Fat, Fatty Acids, Cholesterol, Protein, and Amino Acids (Macronutrients)*, Food and Nutrition Board and Institute of Medicine (Washington, DC: National Academy Press, 2005).
[c] Source: *Dietary Reference Intakes for Vitamin A, Vitamin K, Arsenic, Boron, Chromium, Copper, Iodine, Iron, Manganese, Molybdenum, Nickel, Silicon, Vanadium, and Zinc*, Food and Nutrition Board and Institute of Medicine (Washington, DC: National Academy Press, 2000).
[d] PAL = physical activity levels. First, second, and third trimesters, respectively.

and peer group expectations contribute to a range of food and drink choices.

In the United Kingdom, the most recent large scale survey of young women, the National Diet and Nutrition Survey (NDNS) of Young People aged 4 to 18 years [13], reports that the dietary intake of teenage girls is far from desirable. As an indication of fruit and vegetable intake, during the 7-day recording period over which dietary intake was measured, 80% of 15- to 18-year-old girls had not eaten any citrus fruits, and 60% had not eaten any leafy green vegetables. Nonmilk extrinsic sugar intakes were also high, with as many as 83% of 11- to 14-year-old and 78% of 15- to 18-year-old girls above the maximum recommended intake, the main source being carbonated soft drinks. In addition, intakes of iron, calcium, and magnesium were particularly low in teenage girls with, for example, 51% of 11- to 14-year-olds and 50% of 15- to 18-year-olds consume less than the lower reference nutrient intake [14] for iron.

Pregnancy is a period of rapid growth and development of the fetus, with high physiological, metabolic, and emotional demands on the mother. Nutrient requirements for pregnancy (to meet the needs of increasing maternal tissue, fetal growth and development, and additional energy costs associated with increasing metabolism) have been identified by a number of scientific bodies (e.g. the 1991 Department of Health report [14]), but these do not always include allowances for the teenage mother, who may still have greater nutrient requirements for her own growth. For example, nutrient recommendations issued for the United States [15] and Australia [16] provide figures for pregnant women under 18, but these are in the main similar or lower than those given for older women except for calcium and phosphorus (see Table 12.2). However, this simply reflects the increased requirement for these nutrients by this age group and/or body size rather than any special need identified due to pregnancy per se. Special requirements may also be needed for women who are under- or overweight. Thus, an exact, personalized energy regimen may be difficult to estimate in clinical practice, and the reassurance provided by measurements of fetal growth are thus important.

Adequate nutrient intake during pregnancy is important to enable the fetus to grow and develop physically and mentally to full potential and will also affect adult nutritional status of the mother. There is evidence to show that growth in stature (as assessed by knee height measures) continues after menarche and during teenage pregnancy. This growth is associated with increased weight gain, fat storage, and greater postpartum weight retention [17]. Howie et al. [18] reported that 27% of adolescent mothers gained excessive weight (more than 40 pounds [18.4 kg]) during pregnancy compared with 18% of older women. A recent article from Brazil [7] has also reported that BMI of teenage mothers was 0.81 kg/m^2 higher than teenagers who had not become pregnant and was 1.58 kg/m^2 higher in those who had two teenage pregnancies. Despite this weight gain, adolescent mothers tend to give birth to infants with lower birth weights (by 150–200 g) than those of infants born to older women [19–21]. It has also been shown that growing adolescents have a surge in maternal leptin concentrations during the last trimester, which may reduce the rate of maternal fat breakdown during late pregnancy and thereby increase the mother's use of glucose for energy. This diminishes energy supply for fetal growth, accounting for higher maternal fat gains and lower birth weights among growing teenage pregnant women [22]. In recognition of the energy needs of the growing mother and growing baby, a higher gestational weight gain is recommended for young girls (especially if they are less than 2 years postmenarche) in the United States [23, 24] in an attempt to facilitate energy requirements.

An increasingly recognized concern for pregnant adolescence is high BMI. Groth [25] discussed categorization of BMI by Institute of Medicine (IOM) cutoffs used in recommendations for weight gain during pregnancy and the Centers for Disease Control and Prevention (CDC) BMI percentiles for classifying adolescent body size in 347 primiparous black adolescents. Using CDC centiles for adolescents, 24% of the sample were classified as at risk for overweight ($\geq$ 85th percentile and < 95th) or overweight ($\geq$ 95th percentile) compared with 19% using IOM cutoff points. These observations are a sharp reminder of the incidence of excess body weight in vulnerable adolescents but also a reminder that the IOM categories tend to classify more of this group as underweight (28%) compared with CDC categories (2%) and therefore they may be receiving inappropriate guidance for gestational weight gain, contributing to excess final weight and increased risk for overweight in the postpartum period.

Sukalich et al. [26] reported findings from a retrospective case-control study of 1498 overweight subjects (> 25 kg/m^2) who were aged younger than 19 years. This population-based study demonstrated that overweight adolescent women are at increased risk for a number of adverse perinatal and neonatal outcomes (which were independent of the presence of gestational diabetes mellitus or gestational weight gain). These outcomes included primary cesarean delivery, labor induction, pregnancy-induced hypertension, preeclampsia, and gestational diabetes mellitus. It is notable that an increased incidence of macrosomia and a decreased incidence of LBW infants and small-for-gestational-age infants were reported. Increasingly, pre-pregnancy BMI and weight gain during pregnancy independently confer dose-dependent increases for these risks.

The authors concluded that "obese women are at increased risk for adverse perinatal and neonatal outcomes and that youth does not ameliorate this effect." With rates of overweight increasing at all ages and adolescent pregnancy a continuing problem, overweight in the gravid adolescent is a pressing perinatal public health concern.

For the overweight or obese adolescent mother, appropriate weight gain recommendations are an important part of relevant counseling during pregnancy. Postpartum weight loss also becomes extremely desirable in relation to her own well-being, to meet the physical demands of parenting, to reduce the risk of obesity-related complications (hypertension, glucose intolerance, and congenital malformations) in further pregnancies [27], and to promote future family health.

It is, however, recognized that not all pregnant adolescent women gain high amounts of weight during pregnancy. Scholl et al. [28] demonstrated that adolescents with inadequate weight gain produced babies with a lower birth weight (180 g) and an increased prevalence of LBW overall. After adjusting for potential confounding variables, teenagers who went on to develop inadequate total weight gain for gestation had consumed 1878 kcal daily, versus 2232 kcal for teenagers with adequate total gain (p < 0.05). They also had significantly lower protein and carbohydrate intake. However, there was no direct effect of nutrient intake on birth weight, LBW, or preterm delivery. These findings suggest that the relationship between nutrient intake during pregnancy and birth weight may be indirect and moderated by weight gain during pregnancy.

Micronutrient depletion and pregnancy outcome

Poor maternal micronutrient status also is likely to influence pregnancy outcome. Poor maternal iron, zinc, and folate status has been associated with preterm births and intrauterine growth retardation, two outcomes for which teenage women are likely to be at high risk. A poor maternal folic acid status at conception may contribute to the poor reproductive outcomes in women. In young mothers, it is likely that other health behaviors (e.g. smoking and alcohol) will also affect folate status, and use of folic acid supplements is also likely to be less common. Data from the United States (http://www.cdc.gov/mmwr/preview/mmwrhtml/mm5701a3.htm) indicate that among all women of childbearing age, those aged 18 to 24 years had the least awareness regarding folic acid consumption (61%), the least knowledge regarding when folic acid should be taken (6%), and the lowest reported daily use of supplements containing folic acid (30%).

Iron-deficiency anemia is a prevalent problem among pregnant adolescents and is associated with preterm delivery and associated LBW. It is hypothesized that the excess preterm birth rate among teenage women may be related to poor maternal iron stores resulting from recent growth demands [29].

The circulating concentrations of other nutrients, such as zinc, vitamin A, vitamin B_6, and vitamin B_{12}, also decline during pregnancy, but the concentrations of those nutrients return to normal shortly after delivery, suggesting that they are less likely to be low in pregnant adolescents [22], although this is a topic of current investigation. For example, Maia et al. [30] reported that zinc and copper biochemical responses to pregnancy in adolescent women appeared qualitatively similar to those described in adult women, although they suggest that a poor maternal zinc status may limit the metabolic adaptation capacity of adolescent women during pregnancy.

Adolescent pregnancy is associated with increased risk for preterm birth and growth-restricted infants. Maternal nutrient depletion has been proposed as a possible cause of these poor pregnancy outcomes [22]. Low intake of food (total energy) is likely to affect the intake of all nutrients and have a significant impact on maternal nutritional status at conception, which in turn has the potential to influence pregnancy outcomes. Thus, it seems reasonable to surmise that individuals who are demonstrated to be at risk of poor nutritional status at conception because of recent maternal growth and/or inadequate food supply may benefit from receiving food and micronutrient supplements during pregnancy and in the postpartum period to improve overall nutritional status for adult health and future pregnancies.

Interventions to improve nutritional intake of teenage pregnant women

The nutritional needs of pregnant adolescents are the greatest at a time when it is often socially and culturally most difficult to achieve them. Dieting, skipping meals, snacking, eating away from home, consuming fast foods, and trying unconventional diets are challenges to achieving the nutrient dense diet required to optimize growth and development in the mother and child. Because of poor dietary habits in the preconception period, many young women start pregnancy with reduced nutrient stores and increased risk of nutritional deficiencies. It is recognized that up to 50% of all pregnancies are likely to be unplanned [31], and this is likely to be higher among adolescent women. Thus, although nutritional interventions for women are likely to have the greatest effect if delivered before conception and during the first 12 weeks, the practicalities of achieving this goal are substantially reduced in younger women.

Attempts to change dietary habits must move well beyond the provision of standard nutrition education and use culturally sensitive counseling strategies that take account of increased independence, busy schedules, search for self-identity, peer influence, group conformity, and body image dissatisfaction. Pregnancy has often been viewed as a time to promote dietary change [32]; however, Callins [33] wisely remarks that "although behaviour change in any age group presents a formidable challenge, it has the greatest potential for improving obstetric and neonatal outcomes in pregnant adolescents." She goes on to call for counseling support for overweight and obese adolescents before, during, and after pregnancy, making the important recommendation that psychological, environmental, socioeconomic, and educational factors should be incorporated into behavior change strategies. It is clear that there are unique opportunities for obstetricians to work in a "team organized, patient focused approach to decrease the adverse outcomes in subsequent pregnancies and decrease long term risk of chronic diseases." Hunt et al. [34] have commented that the nutritional component of standard prenatal care will not be sufficient to support positive dietary changes among pregnant adolescents and that it is likely that this population subgroup will require repeated exposure to both information and strategies that build motivation as well as skills for changing eating habits [35].

Ideally, all pregnant teenagers should have their dietary habits assessed and should be offered personal dietary counseling, which may include vitamin and mineral supplements if nutritional intake is below standard (or if appropriate nutritional status markers for pregnancy indicate primary deficiency). In addition, the weight-gain pattern should be monitored to ensure that energy intakes are sufficient to support a gain of about 0.4 kg (1 lb) per week in the second and third trimesters.

Interventions to improve dietary changes can act by affecting modifiable factors at an individual level, such as dietary knowledge, beliefs, and attitudes, and improving psychosocial components, such as self-efficacy. However, the long-term effect of these will ultimately be enhanced and facilitated by societal interventions that tackle the context and situation of the living environment and the balance between health promotion and food industry marketing. Successful health promotion campaigns such as those designed to improve folic acid uptake in the preconception period are known to be less effective in younger women [31]. Dietary interventions cannot tackle unmodifiable demographic characteristics such as socioeconomic status of women, but available income will both influence and be influenced by dietary interventions [36].

The improvement of nutrition and health is a major aim of the U.S. Special Supplemental Food Program for Women, Infants and Children (WIC), which provides federal grants to states for supplemental foods, health care referrals, and nutrition education for low-income pregnant, breast-feeding, and non-breast-feeding postpartum women and to infants and children up to age 5 who are found to be at nutritional risk (http://www.fns.usda.gov/wic). Although not specific to teenage women, the program is likely to have benefits for this group if they participate. The program has traditionally centered around five nutrients (protein, calcium, vitamin A, vitamin C, and iron). WIC funds are divided between supplemental foods (75% of funds) and nutrition education (one sixth of the administration funds) with food vouchers provided during pregnancy for cereal, juice, legumes, carrots, milk, cheese, eggs, and tuna. Participants receive food prescription vouchers, which can be exchanged at authorized WIC retailers in exchange for the foods specified on the voucher.

The choice of foods that vouchers can be used for reflects nutrient needs, although it should be noted that there may be increasing interest in promoting milk given recent findings that high milk consumption is associated with lower incidence of LBW babies across the general maternal population [37]. It is speculated that this may relate to water-soluble substances in milk that increase fetal growth (e.g. through increasing blood concentrations of insulin-like growth factor 1).

Nutrition education regulations define two main objectives – namely, to stress the relationship between proper nutrition and good health and to assist individuals at nutritional risk in achieving a positive change in food habits resulting in improved nutritional status.

In 2002, 11% of participants of WIC were pregnant women. Although there are few data available on the impact of WIC participation on adolescent pregnancy outcomes, participation in the program provides strong suggestive evidence that WIC has a positive impact on mean birth weight, the incidence of LBW, and several other birth outcomes. Although the inherent research errors of self-selection make it difficult to translate fully the available data, analysis has shown that the positive effects of the program can lead to savings in Medicaid [38], although the magnitude of effect has been questioned [39].

Another U.S. program that has demonstrated the achievement of changes in dietary awareness and empowering participants to change dietary practices is the Expanded Food and Nutrition Education Program (EFNEP; http://www.csrees.usda.gov/nea/food/efnep/about. html) [40]. This program, which has been running for many years, is a federally funded nutrition program aimed at assisting low-income youth and families (with young children) and ethnic minorities to acquire practical food knowledge, skills, attitudes, and behavior change (including money management and getting the most from health assistance programs) to help achieve nutritionally sound diets. As with WIC, it is not specific to teenage women (although some programs have been designed specifically for this target group) but is again likely to be useful for this vulnerable group overall. The program focuses on an experiential learning process; adult program participants learn how to make food choices to improve the nutritional quality of the meals they serve their families, and the youth program may also tackle wider health behaviors. Participants gain or enhance new skills in food production, preparation, storage, safety, and budgeting. EFNEP is delivered as a series of 10 to 12 or more lessons, often over several months, by paraprofessionals and volunteers and may include individually tailored home-education sessions [41]. The program has been shown to influence a range of food practices (including food budgeting, food safety, and food preparation) [42]. A number of EFNEP interventions have targeted pregnant adolescents with encouraging results on nutritional status, including weight gain during pregnancy [34].

In a review of interventions to improve diet and weight gain among pregnant adolescents undertaken to identify promising strategies for effective interventions, Nielson et al. [43] critically reviewed 27 articles including 13 controlled trials that specifically targeted pregnant adolescents and six that included this subgroup within the study population. Most examined birth weight and gestational weight gain, but none were concerned with risks of excessive weight gain. Positive outcomes were thought to be due to multidisciplinary team approaches supporting psychosocial needs, individualized counseling, home visits (and outreach to highest-risk teens), visual presentations and tracking of gestational weight gain, and support group work. In addition, the authors noted that only one study examined employed a theoretical framework, and they hypothesize that greater effects could be achieved by the application of behavior-change strategies that have been successfully utilized in wider population-based dietary intervention studies.

In the United Kingdom, there has been a long history of providing dietary advice during pregnancy, but the impact of this has rarely been rigorously assessed. Anderson et al. [44] undertook a minimal contact nutrition education intervention program and demonstrated that nutrition knowledge can be increased through education programs, but this has little impact on dietary behaviors. More intensive dietary counseling for pregnant women indicates that nutrient intake can be improved during pregnancy, but there is no consistent evidence that nutrition counseling has an impact on rates of LBW, gestational age, or length of birth. However, Doyle et al. [45], in a nonrandomized trial in London, demonstrated that intervention women who received multiple episodes of nutrition counseling alone or with two types of food supplement given during second and third trimesters had significantly greater mean birth weight compared with women in the control population

Little work has been undertaken on interventions aimed at improving access to healthy diets, food affordability and availability, and practical issues such as food skills in adolescent women. One published study from University of Dundee evaluated the feasibility of a cooking skills program led by midwives in a community setting for teenage pregnant women. The program [46] incorporated seven informal food-preparation sessions and opportunities for discussion of food and health matters (including food safety and well-being in pregnancy). Although the midwives found the package easy to follow and use, only 16 (of the 120 invited) women attended the course, and the authors concluded that alternative methods of delivering and evaluating such a package should be investigated.

Following a revision of the Welfare Foods scheme in the United Kingdom, a new food-based nutrition intervention scheme ("Starting Well") is currently rolling out from the Department of Health across the United Kingdom for teenage pregnant women (< 18 years), low-income pregnant women, and young families [47]. During pregnancy, eligible women will receive vouchers for £2.80 per week, which can be used for milk, fresh fruits, and vegetables, and free supplements containing vitamin C, vitamin D, and folic acid; advice will be available in relation to practical aspects of healthy eating. Although the scheme has some similarities to the U.S. programs described earlier, the total monetary value of vouchers is considerably less, and the advice program has yet to be described in systematic detail. It is also important to note that current policy work lacks robust evidence that such initiatives are likely to have a significant effect on dietary intakes during pregnancy and subsequent maternal and fetal health outcomes. The scheme should now be evaluated for such outcomes. There is considerable skepticism about the small monetary value of the food vouchers [31]. In addition, an analysis of how successful such initiatives might be in an environment that promotes excess consumption has not been undertaken, and this might be particularly relevant with respect to weight gain in overweight pregnant teenage women. Clearly, this scheme needs careful evaluation and monitoring of process, impact, and outcomes.

A window on the realities of dietary intake, food choices, poverty, and life for the pregnant teenager is provided in a recent report by the Maternity Alliance [48], highlighting the day-to-day problems of trying to attain a modest but adequate diet on a limited budget. Clearly much work is being undertaken to pro-mote healthy food choices during pregnancy, but further research is necessary to produce an evidence base to inform program development and to ensure that the most vulnerable infants and women in society are given the best possible nutritional reserves for future health [49].

References

1. Office for National Statistics, Conceptions in England and Wales 2003. *Health Stat Q* (2005), **26**:58–61

2. Lawlor DA and Shaw M, Teenage pregnancy rates: high compared with where and when. *R Soc Med* (2004), **97**:121–3.

3. Wellings K and Kane R, Trends in teenage pregnancy in England and Wales: how can we explain them? *J R Soc Med* (1999), **92**:277–82.

4. Whincup PH, Gilg JA, Odoki K, Taylor SJC, and Cook DC, Age of menarche in contemporary Britain teenagers: survey of girls born between 1982–1986. *BMJ* (2001), **322**:1095–6.

5. Kirby D, Emerging Answers; Research Findings on Programs to Reduce Teen Pregnancy (Washington, DC: National Campaign to Prevent Teen Pregnancy, 2001).

6. Hamilton BE, Martin JA, and Ventura SJ, Births preliminary data for 2005. *Natl Vit Stat Rep* (2006), **55**:11.

7. Gigante DP, Rasmussen KM, and Cesar GV, Pregnancy increases BMI in adolescents of a population based birth cohort. *J Nutr* (2005), **135**:74–80.

8. Klein JD and the Committee on Adolescence, Adolescent pregnancy: current trends and issues. *Paediatrics* (2005), **116**:281–6.

9. Oumachigui A, Pre-pregnancy and pregnancy nutrition and its impact on women's health. *Nutr Rev* (2002), **60**:S64–7.

10. Kumar A, Singh T, Basu S, Pandey S, and Bhargava V, Outcome of teenage pregnancy. *Ind J Paed* (2007), **74**:927–31.

11. Anderson AS, Macintyre S, and West P, Dietary patterns among adolescents in the West of Scotland. *Br J Nutr* (1994), **71**:111–22.

12. Sweeting H & West P, Female and stressed: changing patterns of psychological distress over time. *J Child Psychol Psychiatry* (2003), **44**:399–411.

13. Gregory J, Lowe S, Bates CJ, Prentic A, and Jackson LV, National diet and nutrition Survey: young people aged 4 to 18 years (London: The Stationery Office, 2000).

14. Department of Health (U.K.), Report on Health and Social Subjects 41. Dietary Reference Values for food energy and nutrients for the United Kingdom (Lodnon: HMSO, 1991).

15. Insel P, Turner RE, and Ross D, *Nutrition*, 2nd edn (Subury, MA: Jones and Bartlett, 2004).

16. Australian Government Ministry, of Health, *Nutrient Reference Values for Australia and New Zealand Including Recommended Dietary Intakes* (2006).

17. Scholl TO, Hediger ML, Schall JI, Mead JP, and Fischer RL, Maternal growth during adolescent pregnancy. *JAMA* (1995), **274**:26–7.

18. Howie LD, Parker JD, and Schoendorf KC, Excessive weight gain patterns in adolescents. *J Am Diet Assoc* (2003), **103**:1653–7.

19. Scholl TO, Hediger ML, and Ances IG, Maternal growth during pregnancy and decreased infant birth weight. *Am J Clin Nutr* (1990), **51**:790–3.

20. Scholl TO, Hediger ML, Ances IG, Belsky DH, and Salmon RW, Weight gain during pregnancy in adolescence: predictive ability of early weight gain. *Obstet Gynecol* (1990), **75**:948–53.

21. Nielsen JN, Gittelsohn J Anliker J, and O'Brien K, Interventions to improve diet and weight gain among pregnant adolescents and recommendations for future research. *J Am Diet Assoc* (2006), **106**:1825–40.

22. King JC, The risk of maternal nutritional depletion and poor outcomes increases in early or closely spaced pregnancies. *J Nutr* (2003), **133**:1732S–6.

23. Institute of Medicine, Nutrition during Pregnancy Part 1: Weight Gain (Washington, DC: National Academies Press, 1990).

24. Gutierrez Y and King JC, Nutrition during teenage pregnancy. *Pediatr Ann* (1993), **22**:99–108.

25. Groth SG, Are the Institute of Medicine recommendations for gestational weight gain appropriate for adolescents? *J Obstet Gynecol Neonatal Nurs* (2007), **36**:21–7.

26. Sukalich S, Mingione MJ, and Glantz JC, Obstetric outcomes in overweight and obese adolescents. *Am J Ob Gyn* (2006), **195**:851–5.

27. Galtier-Dereure F, Boegner C, and Bringer J, Obesity and pregnancy: complications and cost. *Am J Clin Nutr* (2000), **71**:1242S–8S.

28. Scholl TO, Hediger ML, Khoo CS, Healey MF, and Rawson NL, Maternal weight gain, diet and infant birth weight: correlations during adolescent pregnancy. *J Clin Epidemiol* (1991), **44**: 423–8.

29. Scholl TO and Reilly T, Anemia, iron and pregnancy outcome. *J Nutr* (2000), **130**:443S–7S.

30. Maia PA, Figueiredo RCB, Anastacio AS, Da Silviera CLP, and Donagelo CM, et al. Zinc and copper metabolism in pregnancy and lactation of adolescent women. *Nutrition* 2007, **23**:248–53.

31. National Institute for Health and Clinical Excellence, (2007) Guidance for midwives, health visitors, pharmacists and other primary care services to improve the nutrition of pregnant and breastfeeding mothers and children in low income households Programme Guidance

Development. Available at: http://www.nice.org.uk/ guidance/index.jsp?action= byID&o=11677#keydocs

32. Anderson AS, Pregnancy as a time for dietary change. *Proc Nutr Soc* (2001), **60**:497–504.

33. Callins KR, Sizing up our teens. *Am J Obstetr Gynecol* (2007), **196**:6e7.

34. Hunt DJ, Stoecker BJ, Hermann JR, Kopel BL, Williams GS, and Claypool PL, Effects of nutrition education programs on anthropometric measurements and pregnancy outcomes of adolescents. *J Am Diet Assoc* (2002), **102**:S100–2.

35. Hoelscher A, Evans A, Parcel GS, and Kelder SH, Designing effective nutrition interventions for adolescents. *J Am Diet Assoc* (2002), **102**(Suppl 3):S52–S63.

36. Anderson AS, Nutrition interventions in low income women. *Proc Nutr Soc* (2007), **66**:25–32

37. Olsen SF, Halldorsson T, Walter WC, and NUTRIX Consortium, Milk consumption during pregnancy is associated with increased infant size at birth: prospective cohort study. *Am J Clin Nutr* (2007), **86**:1104–10.

38. Fox MK, Hamiliton W, and Lin BH, Effects of Food Assistance and Nutrition Programs on Nutrition and Health: Volume 3, Literature Review. Food and Rural Economic Development, Economic Research Service, U.S. Department of Agriculture (2004). Available at: http://www.ers.usda.gov/ publications/fanrr19–3.

39. U.S. Department of Agriculture, Economic Research Service, Informing Food and Nutrition Assistance Policy, 10 Years of Research at ERS MP-1598 (2007). Available at: http://www.ers.usda. gov/Publications/MP1598.

40. Expanded Food and Nutrition Education Program, FY 2001, Program Impacts (2001). Available at: http://www.reeusda. gov/f4hn/efnep,htm.

41. Bowering J, Morrison MA, Lowenburg RL, and Tirado N, Role of EFNEP (Expanded Food and Nutrition Education Program) aides in improving diets of pregnant women. *J Nutr Educ* (1976), **8**:111–17.

42. Arnold CG and Sobal J, Food practices and nutrition knowledge after graduation from the Expanded Food and Nutrition Education Program (EFNEP). *J Nutr Educ* (2000), **32**:130–8.

43. Nielson J, O'Brien K, Witter FR, Chang SC, Mancini J, Nathanson MS, et al., (2006) High gestational weight gain does not improve birth weight in a cohort of African American adolescents. *Am J Clin Nutr* **84**:183–9.

44. Anderson AS, Campbell D, and Shepherd R, Influence of dietary advice on nutrient intake during pregnancy. *Br J Nutr* (1995), **73**:163–77.

45. Doyle W, Wynn AHA, Crawford MA, and Wyn SW, Nutritional counselling and supplementation in the second and third trimester of pregnancy, a study in a London population. *J Nutr Med* (1992), **3**:249–256.

46. Wrieden WL and Symon A, The development and pilot evaluation of a nutrition education intervention program for pregnant teenage women (food for life). *J Hum Nutr Diet* (2003), **16**:67–71.

47. Department of Health, Healthy Start (2008). Available at: http://www.dh.gov.uk/en/ Healthcare/Maternity/ Maternalandinfantnutrition/ DH_4112476.

48. Burchett H and Seeley A, Good Enough to Eat? The Diets of Pregnant Teenagers (London: The Maternity Alliance and the Food Commission, 2003). Available at: http://www.foodcomm.org.uk/ Too_good_to_eat.PDF.

49. Anderson AS, Nutrition and pregnancy – motivations and interests. *J Hum Nutr Diet* (2003), **16**:65–6.

13 Vegetarians and vegans during pregnancy and lactation

Rana Conway and Adrienne Cullum

Introduction

A number of studies have been used to assess the adequacy of consuming a vegetarian diet during pregnancy. A small number of studies have compared pregnancy outcomes for different types of vegetarians with those of nonvegetarians. A limited amount of data have also been gathered on the nutrient intakes of vegetarians during pregnancy. However, there is little good evidence regarding nutrient status (e.g. hemoglobin or serum vitamin B_{12} levels) during pregnancy or lactation, therefore studies of nonpregnant vegetarians are useful.

Figure 13.1 summarizes the main categories of vegetarian diets. Being vegetarian while pregnant or lactating cannot be assumed to be risky. For example, women may benefit from higher intakes of fruit and vegetables and whole grain, and lifestyles associated with a vegetarian diet: they may be more active, less likely to smoke or binge drink, and less likely to be obese or have diabetes [1]. The balance of benefits and risks of a vegetarian pregnancy is likely to depend on how restrictive the diet is. The reasons for following a vegetarian diet may also play a part; in developed countries people choose to be vegetarian or vegan for a variety of reasons including health, ethical concerns, and religious beliefs. Risks associated with vegetarian diets are more likely for those on more restrictive regimes – both those following a more extreme vegan diet and those following a lacto-ovo (LOV) vegetarian diet, but on a restrictive choice of foods. In addition, the diets of affluent vegetarians in Europe or the United States are likely to be very different in quality from those of deprived vegetarians in South Asia.

The prevalence of women of childbearing age following a vegetarian diet is likely to vary substantially between developed and developing countries. Although in some countries, such as Brazil and China, the total numbers of vegetarians are thought to be negligible, the worldwide population of individuals surviving on a largely (if not exclusively) vegetarian diet may be high due to poverty and economic reasons. In India, 20% to 30% of the total population are thought to be vegetarian for religious reasons, but substantial additional numbers may seldom eat meat because of economic reasons. In developed countries, such as the United States and United Kingdom, between 2% and 7% of the population are vegetarian, the figures varying depending on who sponsors and collects the data and how dietary intakes are assessed. A significant amount of the population may not classify themselves as vegetarian but eat fish but not meat, eat meat rarely, or avoid red meat but not other types of meat [2]. For example, the U.K. Food Standards Agency Consumer Attitudes Survey 2007 [3] found that 7% of all respondents (i.e. all age groups and both sexes combined) claimed to follow a vegetarian diet, and a further 5% claimed to be "partly vegetarian."

In developed countries, more women than men tend to be vegetarian, and vegetarians tend to be of higher educational or socioeconomic status, less likely to have children, and more likely to be under 40 years of age [2]. There are also likely to be differences between ethnic groups. In the United Kingdom, people of nonwhite ethnic origin are more likely to describe themselves as vegetarian than white respondents (15% vs. 6% of white respondents) [3].

Because of the substantial differences in prevalence between countries, the available evidence, and the differences in specific dietary recommendations between countries, this chapter focuses primarily on evidence, guidance, and recommendations from developed countries, particularly the United Kingdom.

Clinical approach

There is no national, evidence-based, clinical guidance on vegetarian pregnancy or lactation. In England, the National Institute for Health and Clinical Excellence

- Lacto-ovo vegetarians (LOVs) avoid meat, poultry and fish but consume milk, dairy and eggs.
- Vegans consume no food of animal origin.
- Macrobiotics consume whole-grain cereals, especially brown rice, plus vegetables, beans, sea vegetables, and miso soup. Other foods including fruit and fish are eaten occasionally, and dairy and eggs are avoided.
- Individuals describing themselves as semivegetarian may restrict their intake of red meat, poultry and/or fish.

Figure 13.1 Categories of vegetarian diets.

(NICE) has issued guidance on maternal and child nutrition [4], postnatal care [5], and antenatal care [6]; although these do not specifically address vegetarian pregnancy, the recommendations apply in general. The Dietary Guidelines for Americans 2005 briefly mention how the population guidelines can be adapted to a vegetarian diet [7].

Because there is no specific dietary guidance for vegetarian women during pregnancy and lactation, standard dietary advice – such as guidance on preconceptual intake of folic acid, avoidance of alcohol, avoidance of certain foods to prevent risk of food poisoning (such as soft cheese), and intake of sufficient fiber and water to prevent constipation (as that issued by, for example, the Department of Health, Food Standards Agency, and National Institute for Health and Clinical Excellence in England and the Centers for Disease Control and Prevention in the United States) – will need to be adapted.

Both health professionals and women themselves are likely to have concerns about following a vegetarian diet during pregnancy or lactation. However, the issues they rate as important may differ substantially. Although a vegetarian diet is often associated with a healthier lifestyle, health professionals should not assume that vegetarian pregnant women have better (or worse) diets than average or are necessarily following standard dietary (and other) advice for pregnancy and lactation.

Health professional concerns

Pregnancy outcome

In the United Kingdom, lower birth weights have been reported among Hindu vegetarians than either Muslim nonvegetarians or European nonvegetarians [8, 9]. However, although differences between Hindus and Europeans remain significant after adjustment for length of gestation, sex of infant, maternal height and weight, and parity, those between Hindus and Muslims do not. The effect of vegetarianism alone cannot be concluded from these studies because pregnancy outcome may have been affected by genetic differences between the ethnic groups. A more recent study comparing Caucasian LOV, fish eaters, and nonvegetarians found no significant differences in birth weight, length of gestation, birth length, or head circumference [10]. Smaller studies in the United States similarly found no differences between the birth weights of LOVs and nonvegetarians.

A tendency toward lower birth weights has been reported among vegans in the United Kingdom [11]. However, this was not found to be the case among members of a vegan commune in Tennessee, where pregnant women routinely received multivitamin and mineral supplements and advice about increasing protein intake [12]. Studies of women following a macrobiotic diet in the United States and the Netherlands have reported lower birth weights [13, 14]. In both countries it was found that women following the most restrictive macrobiotic diets, for example, those eating dairy foods and fish less than once per week, were more likely to have smaller babies. These studies highlight that although women following very restrictive vegetarian diets are nutritionally vulnerable, even those on vegan or macrobiotic diets can be reassured that it is possible to have a good nutrient intake while still adhering to their dietary principles.

Those studying pregnant vegetarians have speculated that lower birth weights (where observed) may be related to lower energy or protein intake or inadequate iron, zinc, vitamin B_{12}, or essential fatty acid status.

Energy and macronutrients

Vegetarians, on average, have a lower body mass index (BMI, kg/m^2) than nonvegetarians [15]. This is probably because of the higher fiber content and lower energy density of vegetarian diets. Indeed, it has also been speculated that some young women may adopt a vegetarian diet as a means of weight reduction or control. Although this is not an issue for the average vegetarian, it should be considered for some severely underweight vegetarians or vegetarian women who are gaining little weight during pregnancy, and handled appropriately. Because vegetarian diets, and vegan diets in particular, can be bulky it may be appropriate to encourage more energy-dense, but also nutrient-rich foods such as avocados, nuts and seeds, dried fruit, and fortified breakfast cereals.

The protein intake of vegetarians is usually lower than that of nonvegetarians [15] but adequate for pregnancy [10, 16]. LOVs can meet many of their protein requirements through dairy produce. However, by eating a more varied diet with foods such as beans and lentils as well, their intake of iron, fiber, and B vitamins will also be increased. Vegans tend to have lower protein intakes than LOVs and need to consume a variety of protein sources to meet their essential amino acid requirements. Eating cereal foods (such as bread, rice, and pasta) as well as peas, beans, and lentils should be encouraged.

Vegetarians usually have a higher carbohydrate intake than nonvegetarians, and they tend to consume more unrefined carbohydrates and have a higher fiber intake as well [10, 15, 17]. Although high fiber intakes are an advantage as far as pregnancy-associated constipation is concerned, very high intakes can reduce absorption of essential minerals such as iron and zinc. The addition of bran to meals is not recommended, and consumption of unrefined cereal products occasionally may be advantageous.

Iron

An increased risk of iron-deficiency anemia is a common concern in relation to pregnant vegetarians. Studies of nonpregnant women have generally found similar iron intakes among LOVs as nonvegetarians [15], and this is also true in pregnancy [10]. Studies of vegans have found they usually have higher intakes of iron than nonvegetarians. However, this iron is non-hem iron, which is less easily absorbed than hem iron derived from meat. Studies of iron status have consistently shown LOVs to have lower serum ferritin levels than nonvegetarians [15, 17, 18], and they appear to be more likely to be diagnosed with anemia during pregnancy [10].

Despite these findings and anecdotal evidence of anemia among vegetarians, routine iron supplementation is not advisable, because there is some evidence that in nonanemic women it may be detrimental [19]. Instead, vegetarians, like other pregnant women, should be prescribed iron supplements only if blood tests demonstrate a need for them. However, it is worth

Table 13.1 Nutrients that may be of concern in vegetarian diets and good food sources for different types of vegetarians

Nutrient	LOVs	All vegetarians
Protein	Milk, cheese, yogurt, eggs	Beans, peas, lentils, soy milk, tofu, nuts, and nut butters
Iron	Eggs	Fortified breakfast cereals, dried fruit such as apricots and raisins, whole-grain cereals including bread, brazil nuts, almonds, broccoli and peas, beans, and lentils
Calcium	Milk, yogurt, cheese	Green vegetables including cabbage and broccoli, and fortified soy products
Zinc	Hard cheeses	Whole grains, nuts, seeds, legumes, and soy products
Vitamin B_{12}	Milk, yogurt, cheese, eggs	Fortified soy products and yeast extract (e.g. Marmite).
Vitamin D	Egg yolk	Fortified margarines, soy milks, and breakfast cereals
Iodine	Dairy products	Seaweed (small amounts), iodized salt, and fortified soy milk

LOV = lacto-ovo vegetarians.

noting that some multivitamin and mineral supplements for pregnancy contain low doses of iron that will help women meet their daily requirements. If supplemental iron is required, some women may prefer to take a natural iron supplement, such as Spatone (http://www.spatone.com), which appears to be better absorbed than ferrous sulphate and causes fewer gastrointestinal symptoms [20]. Advice regarding intake of dietary iron may benefit all vegetarians. There are many good vegetarian sources of iron (Table 13.1), and iron absorption can be increased considerably by consuming these with a good source of vitamin C, which can be found in many fruits, fruit juices, and vegetables. In addition, tea should not be taken an hour before or after a meal because it contains iron-binding polyphenols, which inhibit absorption.

Folate

LOVs generally have higher folate intakes than nonvegetarians. Pregnant LOVs in Germany have been found to have higher serum and red cell folate concentrations than women following an average Western diet [21]. Although vegetarian women of childbearing age are at lower risk of folate deficiency, they should still be strongly encouraged to follow standard advice to take a daily supplement of folic acid from preconception until the 12th week of pregnancy to reduce the risk of neural tube defects [4].

Vitamin D

The dietary sources of vitamin D are limited (they are predominantly of animal origin and include oily fish, fortified margarines, and some fortified breakfast cereals, smaller amounts are found in red meat and egg yolk), and the main source is the synthesis following exposure of the skin to sunlight [22]. There is long-standing advice in the United Kingdom (recently reiterated by Scientific Advisory Committee on Nutrition [22] and NICE [4]) that all pregnant and breast-feeding women should consider taking a daily supplement of vitamin D (10 μg) to ensure their own requirement is met and to build adequate fetal stores. However, uptake of vitamin D supplementation in the United Kingdom is low, and vitamin D deficiency has reemerged as a public health concern, particularly for women and children from South Asian and Afro-Caribbean groups [4]. Concern about maternal and infant vitamin D deficiency has also been raised in other countries in recent years, including Australia [23] and the United States [24].

It has been suggested that low meat intake or a vegetarian diet may increase risk of rickets or osteomalacia. However, it remains unclear whether observed associations are due to dietary, religious, or cultural practices because studies have focused on particular groups of Asian vegetarians [25]. All vegetarian and vegan women, particularly those with a restrictive diet and who are at greatest risk of deficiency (are obese, have limited skin exposure to sunlight, or are of South Asian, African, Caribbean, or Middle Eastern descent [4]), should be encouraged to follow advice to take a vitamin D supplement during pregnancy and while breast-feeding.

Vitamin B_{12}

Vitamin B_{12} is found naturally only in foods of animal origin, and consequently lower intakes are found among vegetarians, both nonpregnant and pregnant [10, 15, 26]. A study of pregnant women in the Netherlands found that LOVs were at increased risk of vitamin B_{12} deficiency. On the basis of serum vitamin B_{12} levels and plasma total homocysteine levels, it was found that 22% of LOVs were vitamin B_{12} deficient compared with 3% of nonvegetarians [26]. Elevated methylmalonic aciduria (an indicator of vitamin B_{12} deficiency) has also been found among breast-feeding vegetarian women and their infants [27].

Vitamin B_{12} is required for the uptake of folate by cells, and vitamin B_{12} deficiency is considered an independent risk factor for neural tube defects [28]. In pregnant LOVs, red blood cell folate levels have been shown to be positively correlated with serum B_{12} concentrations, suggesting that inadequate vitamin B_{12} is limiting the efficiency of folate utilization for some [21]. If vegetarians have a good intake of dairy products and eggs, they should get enough vitamin B_{12}. However, vegans need to consume fortified foods daily or take a supplement. Certain fermented soy products (e.g. tempeh and miso) and marine vegetables are considered by some to be good sources of vitamin B_{12}. However, up to 90% of the levels measured in these foods may be inactive analogues [29].

Calcium

The calcium intake of vegetarians depends largely on their intake of dairy products. LOVs tend to have similar calcium intakes to nonvegetarians, but vegans usually have substantially lower intakes [15, 17, 18]. A German study of vegan women recently found calcium intakes to be 81% of recommended levels [30]. A study of women following a macrobiotic diet in the United States found calcium intakes were approximately half those of nonvegetarians during pregnancy [27]. Breast milk calcium levels were not reduced [27] but the implications for the mother's bone health are unclear.

Zinc

LOVs have been found to have lower zinc intakes than nonvegetarians during pregnancy in some [10], but not all [16, 31], studies. There is concern that a vegetarian's higher intake of fiber and phytate may reduce bioavailability, but LOVs have not been found to have lower serum zinc levels [16, 21, 31].

Iodine

Low iodine intakes and status have been reported among vegans, because the main dietary sources of iodine are meat, fish, and dairy products [32, 33]. There is limited evidence regarding iodine status during pregnancy and lactation, but to ensure an adequate intake, vegans need to regularly include foods fortified with iodine or take a supplement.

Women's concerns

On top of the usual concerns that many women have during pregnancy and lactation, vegetarian women may be concerned about the impact of standard advice – such as the advice on food safety and nut consumption – on their dietary choices. Some women may feel guilty about avoiding animal products during pregnancy, may be concerned whether their body can "cope," and may have experienced pressure from their family, friends, or health professionals to change their dietary habits. As for many women, pregnancy and lactation may also raise long-standing issues about, for example, their weight and body image. Although there is no evidence-based guidance addressing these concerns, there is no shortage of advice for women online – entering "vegetarian pregnancy" into the Google Internet search engine resulted in 18 700 hits (as of May 2008). However, the quality and consistency of advice are highly variable. Providing women with information about trusted, reliable sources of information on diet and nutrition – such as the U.S. Department of Agriculture and the Food Standards Agencies in the United Kingdom and Australia – may be a useful first step. If women are looking for additional information specific to vegetarians, they could be directed to the Vegetarian or Vegan Societies in the United Kingdom.

Cravings and aversions

Although it is reported that meat is one of the foods that many women report developing an aversion to during pregnancy [34, 35], vegetarian women have also reported craving meat [10]. Women may be concerned that craving meat means their body is not able to "cope" without meat or that it signifies that they are deficient in nutrients contained in meat such as iron, vitamin B_{12}, or protein. Other common cravings or aversions may include foods that make a significant contribution to the diets of vegetarian women including eggs (aversion [36]) and dairy products (craving [36] or aversion [34]).

Women can be assured that there is little evidence of a direct relationship between a food craving and nutrient deficiency [37]; other factors – such as changes in hormone levels affecting taste and smell, mood and emotional responses to foods, and inadvertent control of pregnancy symptoms and concerns for the growing fetus – are more likely to be the cause. Specific food-based advice may best be focused on ensuring that women continue to eat a wide variety of foods, that any aversions or cravings do not result in their diet becoming yet more restricted, and that alternative foods are suggested as necessary.

Some vegetarian or vegan women may decide to introduce meat or other animal products to their diet for one reason or another during pregnancy or lactation. Again, advice should ensure that women continue to eat a wide variety of foods.

Peanuts and other nuts

The frequency and quantity of nut consumption are higher in vegetarian (particularly vegan) populations than nonvegetarian populations [38]. Vegetarian pregnant and lactating women may be concerned about how the impact of standard advice on peanut consumption may affect the quality of their diets. In the United Kingdom, the Food Standards Agency recommends that women who have a family history of allergic diseases (asthma, eczema, food allergies, etc.) avoid eating peanuts during pregnancy and breast-feeding and avoid introducing peanuts into the child's diet before 3 years of age. Committee on toxicity of chemicals in food, consumer products and the environment (2008). Statement on the review of the 1998 COT recommendations on peanut avoidance. http://cot.food.gov.uk/pdfs/cotstatement200807peanut.pdf. Unlike the U.K. advice, the American Academy of Pediatrics (AAP)[39] extends its advice to tree nuts (such as almonds and cashews) for women who are breast-feeding. This would seem prudent, given that between 30% and 50% of children with peanut allergy (around 1.5% of children,) will have a sensitization or allergy to tree nuts [40]. There is currently some scientific uncertainty about whether young children should avoid peanuts to escape sensitization or instead should eat peanuts to induce early oral tolerance and thus prevent peanut allergy. However, although there are major studies under way to resolve this issue [41], it is prudent for women to adhere to the existing advice.

The AAP [39] makes clear that its advice is based on the fact that nuts are not an essential food and their avoidance will not lead to nutritional problems. However, this assertion is based on a standard, Western diet; for some vegan women, nuts may make a significant contribution to their energy and protein intake and a useful contribution to their iron intake. Women with a family history of allergies can be advised that alternative sources of protein include soy products, tempeh, seeds, beans, and pulses. The U.K. Committee on Toxicity has highlighted that although peanut allergic individuals may also clinically react to tree nut allergens, they generally do not react to other legumes, such as green peas, soy beans, kidney beans, and lentils [42].

Although nut avoidance may be prudent for some women, those without a family history of allergies should be reassured that avoidance is not necessary for them.

Impact of food safety advice

Given that cheese and eggs may be important "staples" in their everyday diet, LOVs may be concerned about how standard food safety advice on the consumption of these foods during pregnancy might affect their dietary choices. Most developed countries recommend that to avoid the risk of listeria (which is more common in pregnancy and can lead to premature delivery, miscarriage, stillbirth, or serious health problems for the newborn), pregnant women should avoid soft mold-ripened cheeses, such as camembert and brie, blue-veined cheeses (whether pasteurized or unpasteurized), and any unpasteurized dairy products. Because cooking kills listeria, cooked dishes (served piping hot) that contain these cheeses do not need to be avoided. Vegetable paté should also be avoided. Women can be assured that hard cheeses (such as cheddar), feta, ricotta, mascarpone, cream cheese, cottage cheese, processed cheese, and cheese spread can be eaten safely during pregnancy, as can live or bio yogurt, probiotic drinks, fromage frais, crème fraiche, and sour cream.

Other pertinent advice for vegetarian women is the importance of thoroughly washing any fruits, vegetables, and pre-prepared salad leaves to reduce the risk of toxoplasmosis. Owing to the risk of salmonella, women are advised to avoid raw and partially cooked eggs and products that may contain them. In practice, this is likely to mean being cautious about home- or restaurant-cooked foods such as homemade mayonnaise, salad dressing, or some desserts; products purchased from grocers will generally have been made with pasteurized egg. Although there is advice not to give children aged under 1 year honey, there is no need for pregnant or lactating women to avoid it.

Soy

Many meat and dairy substitutes (such as tofu, textured vegetable protein, soy milk, and tempeh) are made from (or contain) soy beans. Soy naturally contains phytoestrogens, which can (weakly) mimic or block the action of the human hormone, estrogen. It has been hypothesized that pregnant women who eat soy might affect the future fertility of their babies. However, the U.K. Food Standards Agency highlights that this theory is based on animal studies, and there have not been any reports of problems in countries such as Japan where the traditional diet includes soy [43] and average consumption is around 65 g per person per day (mainly from tofu and miso) [44]. There has also been a single study that found an association between maternal vegetarian diet and hypospadias [45]. The Food Standards Agency states that there is no need for pregnant women to avoid soy products if they are eaten as part of a healthy balanced diet.

Women hoping to obtain omega-3 from soy products are likely to be disappointed. Although 7% to 8% of the fat contained in soy beans is α-linolenic acid (ALA; omega-3), soya products, which mostly contain the isolated protein or protein concentrates and are nearly fat free (such as defatted soya milks, flours, and textured vegetable protein (TVP), are not good sources of these fatty acids. Furthermore partial hydrogenation of soya oils reduces α-linolenic acid by 50% to 80% [44].

Supplements

Vegetarian and vegan women may be more likely than their peers to take dietary supplements [46]. In this light, key advice should ensure that any supplements they are taking contain folic acid and vitamin D and do not contain vitamin A – in line with standard dietary advice for pregnant women. As discussed earlier, a supplemental vitamin B_{12} may be advisable for vegan women, especially if they do not consume fortified products.

Some vegetarian and vegan women may seek advice on the importance of consuming fish or taking fish oil supplements during pregnancy because of the proposed association between maternal omega-3 fatty acid consumption and cognitive function in childhood [47]. Long-chain omega-3 fatty acids found in fish oils, particularly docosahexaenoic acid (DHA), are required for the normal development of the retina and central nervous system [48], and it has been suggested that pregnant and lactating women should aim to achieve a daily intake of 200 mg of DHA [47]. However, the evidence for such an association is limited. In addition, many fish oil supplements contain high amounts of vitamin A (although this is not necessarily stated on the label), which can cause birth defects.

Plant foods generally contain no naturally occurring long-chain polyunsaturated fatty acids. Long-chain omega-3s can be synthesized from the shorter-chain omega-3 α-linolenic acid found in certain seeds, including flaxseed (linseed), walnut, rapeseed (canola), and soy-bean oils, but only to a limited extent. Levels of cord plasma and cord artery phospholipid DHA, and also breast milk DHA, have been found to be lower among Hindu vegetarians than nonvegetarians [11]. The long-term health implications for the infant of these differences in fatty acid intake and status are unclear. Several brands of omega-3 and -6 supplements, suitable for vegetarians, are available. These generally contain a combination of plant oils including flaxseed oil and oil of evening primrose and advertise benefits to brain and general fetal and infant development. However, there is a lack of evidence to support such claims. A study in the Netherlands found that supplementation with ALA during pregnancy failed to improve neonatal DHA status [49]. Another study, in the United States, found that 20 g supplements of flax seeds during pregnancy did not increase the DHA content of breast milk [50].

Part of the problem is that vegetarians tend to have higher intakes of omega-6 fatty acids, including arachidonic acid, which reduces the synthesis of DHA from ALA by competing for the desaturase enzymes. Reducing the ratio of LA to ALA is therefore advisable [48] and can be achieved by consuming less corn and sunflower oils. High intakes of trans fats also appear to interfere with the conversion of AA to DHA [48] and should be avoided. Supplements containing preformed DHA, derived from algal oils and suitable for vegetarians, are also now available. Initial trials show dose-dependent increases in plasma phospholipid and erythrocyte DHA levels [51], suggesting that they may be a better option for vegetarians wishing to supplement their diets with omega-3 fatty acids. Although fish is obviously not a normal part of vegetarian diets some women describing themselves as vegetarians may include it in their diets either occasionally or regularly. Women who have no objection to fish should be given the general advice to consume oily fish (e.g. salmon, sardine, mackerel) once or twice a week.

Conclusions

Vegetarian diets can vary enormously in quality, and it cannot be assumed that a woman describing herself as vegetarian has a diet that is any better or worse than average. The degree of risk largely depends on how restrictive an individual's diet is. Although the evidence base is limited, there are specific issues health professionals should consider when advising vegetarian women during pregnancy or lactation. Because there are no specific evidence-based or clinical guidelines for vegetarian and vegan women, the best starting point is to adapt existing guidance for all women.

Because health professionals' and women's key concerns may not tally, it is important to discuss with a woman her individual concerns. Most LOV women can be reassured that, with some careful planning, their diets should be adequate. For those who are following more restrictive diets (such as those who do not consume dairy products daily or eggs on a regular basis), more effort will be required to ensure their nutrient requirements are met. For such women, consumption of fortified foods and/or supplements is recommended to ensure adequate intakes of iron, calcium, iodine, and vitamins B_{12} and D.

This work represents the views of the authors only and may not reflect the views of the National Institute for Health and Clinical Excellence.

References

1. Sabate J, The public health risk to benefit ratio of vegetarian diets: changing paradigms. In: ed. Sabate J, Vegetarian Nutrition, CRC Series in Modern Nutrition (Boca Raton, FL: CRC, 2001), pp. 19–30.

2. Sabate J, Ratzin-Turner RA, and Brown JE, Vegetarian Diets: Descriptions and Trends. In: ed. Sabate J, Vegetarian Nutrition, CRC Series in Modern Nutrition (Boca Raton, FL: CRC, 2001), pp. 3–18.

3. Food Standards Agency, *Consumer Attitudes to Food Standards: Wave 8.* UK final Report. (London: Food Standards Agency, 2008).

4. *Improving the Nutrition of Pregnant and Breastfeeding Mothers and Children in Low Income Households.* NICE Public Health Guidance 11 (2008). Available at: http://www.nice.org.uk/PH011.

5. *Routine Postnatal Care of Women and Their Babies.* NICE Clinical Guidance 37 (2006). Available at: http://www.nice.org.uk/CG037

6. *Antenatal Care: Routine Care for Healthy Pregnant Women.* NICE Clinical Guideline 62 (2008). Available at: www.nice.org.uk/CG062.

7. U.S. Department of Health and Human Services and US Department of Agriculture, *Dietary Guidelines for Americans* (2005). Available at: http://www.health.gov/DietaryGuidelines.

8. McFadyen IR, Campbell-Brown M, Abrhan R, North WRS, and Haines AP, Factors affecting birth weight in Hindus, Moslems and Europeans. *Br J Obstet Gyn* (1984), **91**:968–72.

9. Reddy S, Sanders TAB, and Obeid O, The influence of maternal vegetarian diet on essential fatty acid status of the newborn. *Eur J Clin Nutr* (1994), **48**:358–68.

10. Drake R, Reddy S, and Davies J, Nutrient intake during pregnancy and pregnancy outcome of lacto-ovo-vegetarians, fish-eaters and non-vegetarians. *Vegetarian Nutr Int J* (1998), **2**:45–52.

11. Sanders TAB and Reedy S, The influence of a vegetarian diet on the fatty acid composition of human milk and the essential fatty acid stats of the newborn. *J Pediatr* (1992), **120**:S71–7.

12. Furman T and Morgan B. The effect s of a vegan diet on pregnancy outcome. In: ed. Horwitz C, *Advances in Diet and Nutrition* (London: Libby, 1985), pp. 320–3.

13. Dwyer JT, Palombo T, Thorne H, Valadian I, and Reed RB, Preschoolers on alternate life-style diets. Associations between size and dietary indexes with diets limited in types of animal foods. *J Am Diet Assoc* (1978), **72**:264–70.

14. Dagnelie PC, van Staveren WA, van Klaveren JD, and Burema J, Do children on macrobiotic diets show catch-up growth? *Eur J Clin Nutr* (1988), **42**:1007–16.

15. Key TJ, Appleby PN, and Rosell MS, Health effects of vegetarian and vegan diets. *Proc Nutr Soc* (2006), **65**:35–41.

16. King JCC, Stein T, and Doyle M, Effect of vegetarianism on zinc status of pregnant women. *Eur J Clin Nutr* (1981), **34**:1049–55.

17. Ball M and Bartlett MA, Dietary intake and iron status of Australian vegetarian women. *Am J Clin Nutr* (1999), **70**:353–8.

18. Alexander D, Ball MJ, and Mann J, Nutrient intakes and haematological status of vegetarians and age-sex matched omnivores. *Eur J Clin Nutr* (1994), **48**:538–46.

19. Ziaei S, Norrozi M, Fag hihsadeh S, and Jafarbegloo E, A randomized placebo-controlled trial to determine the effect of iron supplementation on pregnancy outcome in pregnant women with haemoglobin > or = 13.2g/dl. *Br J Obstet Gynecol* (2007), **114**:684–8.

20. Halksworth G, Moseley L, Carter K, and Worwood M, Iron absorption from Spartone (a natural mineral water) for prevention of iron deficiency in pregnancy. *Clin Lab Haematol* (2003), **25**:227–311.

21. Koebnick C, Heins UA, Hoffmann I, Dagneli PC, and Leitzmann C, Folate status during pregnancy in women is improved by long-term high vegetable intake compared with the average western diet. *J Nutr* (2001), **131**:733–9.

22. Scientific Advisory Committee on Nutrition, Update on vitamin D (London: TSO, 2007).

23. Nowson CA, Diamond TH, Pasco JA, Mason RS, Sambrook PN, and Eisman JA, Vitamin D in Australia. Issues and recommendations. *Aust Fam Physician* (2004), **33**:133–8.

24. Hollis BW and Wagner CL, Nutritional vitamin D status during pregnancy: reasons for concern. *CMAJ* (2006), **174**:1287–90.

25. National Institute for Health and Clinical Excellence Maternal and Child Nutrition Programme, *Review 7: The Effectiveness and Cost-Effectiveness of Interventions to Promote an Optimal Intake of Vitamin D to Improve the Nutrition of Pre-conceptual, Pregnant and Post-partum Women and Children, in Low Income Households* (2008). Available at: http://www.nice.org.uk/nicemedia/pdf/MCNReview7VitaminD.pdf.

26. Koebnick C, Hoffmann I, Dagnelie PC, Heins UA, Wickramasinghe SN, Ratnayaka ID, et al., Long-term ovo-lacto vegetarian diet impairs vitamin B12 status in pregnant women. *J Nutr* (2004), **134**:3317–26.

27. Specker BL, Nutritional concerns of lactating women consuming

vegetarian diets. *Am J Clin Nutr* (1994), **59**(Suppl):1182S–6S.

28. Kirke PN, Molloy AM, Daly LE, Burke H, Weir DG, and Scott JM, Maternal plasma folate and vitamin B-12 are independent risk factors for neural tube defects. *Q J Med* (1993), **86**:703–8.

29. Herbert V, Vitamin B12: plant sources, requirements, and assay. *Am J Clin Nutr* (1988), **28**:852–8.

30. Waldmann A, Koschizke JW, Leitzmann C, and Hahn A, Dietary intakes and lifestyle factors of a vegan population in Germany: results from the German vegan study. *Eur J Clin Nutr* (2003), **58**:947–55.

31. Abu-Assal MJ and Craig WJ, The zinc status of pregnant vegetarian women. *Nutr Rep Int* (1984), **29**:485–94.

32. Lightowler HJ, Davies GJ, and Trevan MD, Iodine intake and iodine deficiency in vegans as assessed by the duplicate-portion technique and urinary iodine excretion. *Br J Nutr* (1998), **80**:529–35.

33. Krajcovicová-Kudláčková M, Bucko K, Klimes I, and Seboko E, Iodine deficiency in vegetarians and vegans. *Ann Nutr Metab* (2003), **47**:183–5.

34. Lawson CC, LeMasters GK, and Wilson KA, Changes in caffeine consumption as a signal of pregnancy. *Reprod Toxicol* (2004), **18**:625–33.

35. Hook EB, Dietary cravings and aversions during pregnancy. *Am J Clin Nutr* (1978), **31**:1355–62.

36. Williamson CS, Nutrition in pregnancy. *Br Nutr Foundation*

Nutr Bull (2006), **31**:28–59.

37. Pressman P and Clemens R, Are food cravings the body's way of telling us that we are lacking certain nutrients? *Sci Am* (May 23, 2005). Available at: http://www.sciam.com/article.cfm?id=are-food-cravings-the-bod&topicID=3&catID=3.

38. Sabate J, Nut consumption, vegetarian diets, ischemic heart disease risk, and all-cause mortality: evidence from epidemiologic studies. *Am J Clin Nutr* (1999), **70**:500S–3S.

39. American Academy of Pediatrics, Committee on Nutrition, Hypoallergenic infant formulas. *Pediatrics* (2000), **106**: 346–9.

40. Clark AT and Ewan PW, The development and progression of allergy to multiple nuts at different ages. *Pediatr Allergy Immunol* (2005), **16**:507–11.

41. Food Standards Agency, *Peanut Allergy* (2008). Available at: http://www.fsascience.net/2008/01/23/giving_advice_when_the_science_is_uncertain.

42. Committee on Toxicity of Chemicals in Food, Consumer Products and the Environment, Peanut Allergy (London: Department of Health, 1998).

43. Food Standards Agency, *Eat Well, Be Well: Pregnancy* (2008). Available at: http://www.eatwell.gov.uk/asksam/agesandstages/pregnancy/?lang=en#A219879

44. Messina V, Mangels R, and Messina M, Dietician's Guide to Vegetarian Diets: Issues and

Applications, 2nd edn (Sudbury, MA: Jones & Bartlett, 2004).

45. North K, Golding J, and the ALSPAC Study Team, A maternal vegetarian diet in pregnancy is associated with hypospadius. *BJU Int* (2000), **85**:107–13.

46. Ball MJ and Bartlett MA, Dietary intake and iron status of Australian vegetarian women. *Am J Clin Nutr* (1999),**70**:353–8.

47. Koletzko B, Cetin I, and Brenna JT for the Perinatal Lipid Intake Working Group, Dietary fat intakes for pregnant and lactating women. *Br J Nutr* (2007), **98**:873–7.

48. Sanders TAB, Essential fatty acid requirements of vegetarians in pregnancy, lactation, and infancy. *Am J Clin Nutr* (1999), **70**:555S–9S.

49. de Groot RHM, Hornstra G, van Houwelingen AC, and Roumen F, Effect of α-linolenic acid supplementation during pregnancy on maternal and neonatal polyunsaturated fatty acid status and pregnancy outcome. *Am J Clin Nutr* (2004), **79**:251–60.

50. Francois CA, Connor SL, Bolewicz LA, and Connor WA, Supplementing lactating women with flaxseed oil does not increase docosahexaenoic acid in their milk. *Am J Clin Nutr* (2003), **77**:226–33.

51. Arterburn LM, Oken HA, Hoffman JP, Baily-Hall E, Chung G, Rom D, et al., Bioequivalence of docosahexaenoic acid from different algal oils in capsules and in a DHA-fortified food. *Lipids* (2007), **42**:1011–24.

Hyperemesis in pregnancy

James D. Paauw and Alan T. Davis

Introduction

Nausea and vomiting during pregnancy are extremely common, presenting in 50% to 90% of all gravidas [1]. The most common presentation of this complex is between the fourth and seventh weeks of pregnancy, when 70% of those affected develop symptoms [2]. Vomiting abates in 90% of cases by the 16th week of pregnancy [2]. A more severe variant associated with greater morbidity, hyperemesis gravidarum (pernicious vomiting of pregnancy), affects between 0.3% and 2% of pregnancies [3–5]. Definitions of hyperemesis gravidarum (HG) vary considerably, but HG is best described as vomiting in pregnancy that is sufficiently severe to produce weight loss, dehydration, starvation ketoacidosis, alkalosis from loss of hydrochloric acid in vomitus, and hypokalemia [6]. A transient rise in liver enzymes is seen in 15% to 25% of women who are hospitalized with HG [7]. Although the etiology of HG has not been identified, a number of factors have been suggested as contributory, including high or rapidly rising serum concentrations of serum chorionic gonadotropin or estrogens [8], seropositivity to *Helicobacter pylori* [9, 10], thyrotoxicosis [11, 12], upper gastrointestinal dysmotility [13], and psychological factors [14, 15]. Eating disorders have also been associated with HG [16, 17]. Goodwin has postulated that nausea and vomiting during pregnancy is not a single condition but a syndrome with multiple potential etiologies, such as vestibular mechanism, "background" gastrointestinal motility dysfunction, or hormonal sensitivity, among others, each of which may respond to a different targeted therapy [18].

The diagnosis of HG is made clinically after exclusion of other causes. Onset of HG usually occurs between the 4th and 10th weeks of gestation, with associated progressive weight loss ($\geq$ 5% of pre-pregnant body weight), ketosis, and dehydration in association with abnormal serum electrolytes, including hyponatremia, hypochloremia, and hypokalemia.

Hypersalivation, or ptyalism, is typical [19]. Elevated serum concentrations of hepatic enzymes and salivary amylase are not uncommon findings in HG, and abnormalities in thyroid function are seen in approximately 60% of patients [20–23].

A number of maternal complications have been associated with HG, including those related to the physiology of vomiting, such as Mallory-Weiss syndrome, esophageal rupture, retinal hemorrhage, pneumothorax, aspiration pneumonia, and splenic avulsion [24–26]. Possibly the most dangerous nutritional consequence related to HG is Wernicke's encephalopathy, which is a rare but potentially devastating complication caused by a deficiency of thiamine, an essential cofactor in carbohydrate metabolism. In the presence of HG, thiamine deficiency is typically precipitated by provision of glucose without concurrent thiamine supplementation. In a recent review of the 49 reported cases of HG-related Wernicke's encephalopathy, 46.9% manifested all three of the classic triad of confusion (63.3%), ocular signs (95.9%) and symptoms (57.1%), and ataxia (81.6%) [27]. The mean gestational age at the presentation of these signs and symptoms was 14.3 weeks, after a mean duration of 7.7 weeks of nausea and vomiting. Diagnosis is made clinically but can be rapidly confirmed by magnetic resonance imaging. Complete remission occurred in only 28.6% of patients, with symptom resolution requiring months. Permanent impairments were common. The overall pregnancy loss rate (spontaneous and planned abortions) in HG patients with Wernicke's encephalopathy was 47.9%. The authors recommended provision of supplemental thiamine in prolonged vomiting of pregnancy, especially before initiation of intravenous hydration or parenteral nutrition, and prompt thiamine replacement if neurologic symptoms develop in patients with HG. Other nutrition-related complications associated with HG, although uncommon, include coagulopathy as a result of vitamin K deficiency and peripheral neuropathy caused by deficiency of either vitamin B_6 or B_{12} [28, 29].

The existence of economic consequences to HG has also been established, with some authors attempting to quantify these effects. In patients with HG, 12% discontinued employment altogether in one Swedish study, and one third (of 363 subjects) lost an average of 62 hours of work between gestational Days 39 through 84 in a prospective investigation [30, 31].

Treatment of hyperemesis gravidarum

Appropriate fluid, electrolyte, and vitamin resuscitation is the initial treatment for HG. This regimen includes generous supplementation of thiamine, as well as vitamin B_6 (pyridoxine), which, although usually given in conjunction with antihistamines, has been found to ameliorate nausea and vomiting of pregnancy by itself [32]. Adjunct pharmaceutical therapy to relieve nausea and vomiting commonly includes promethazine, prochlorperazine, chlorpromazine, meclizine, droperidol-diphenhydramine, and metoclopramide. Extensive data show lack of teratogenic effects with histamine H_1 receptor blockers (promethazine and cyclizine), phenothiazines (chlorpromazine and prochlorperazine), and dopamine antagonists (metoclopramide and domperidone) [33, 34]. Although evidence exists for a better pregnancy outcome from the use of antihistamines in HG, there is a consensus that withholding the use of these agents until after the first 10 weeks of pregnancy is best. The literature contains a number of stepwise drug regimens for the treatment of HG, all with some variation. A reasonable approach for the first line of therapy for HG consists of rehydration and maintenance of fluid status, as necessary, with intravenous fluids, thiamine supplementation, and choice of pyridoxine or promethazine as the antiemetic agent, with prochlorperazine serving as a second-line antiemetic therapy [35]. Patients with HG who fail these therapies are determined to have resistant HG, and a number of pharmaceuticals and modalities are being studied in the further treatment of this group. Metoclopramide has become a common alternative to conventional antiemetics, either alone or in combination with other agents, with promising enough results to consider it as a second-line antiemetic. In one prospective trial, 174 women with first trimester singleton pregnancies associated with severe nausea and vomiting were assessed for subjective response and number of emesis episodes after being randomized to a 3-day trial with one of three treatments: pyridoxine-metoclopramide, promethazine, or prochlorperazine. Despite an initial lack of difference in pretreatment symptoms, the women taking pyridoxine-metoclopramide reported improved subjective response and fewer emesis episodes than those subjects receiving either of the two monotherapy treatments [36]. Continuous subcutaneous metoclopramide resulted in complete symptom resolution in 64% of subjects in a large retrospective study of HG patients from a national database. Most of the side effects that were reported by approximately 30% of the subjects were considered to be mild, and the therapy had the added benefit of allowing for outpatient treatment in most cases [37]. Odansetron is also frequently used in refractory HG, although it is not thought to be more effective than promethazine [38].

Several newer antiemetics have been tried in the treatment of resistant HG with some success, although so far only in a few small studies. In a case series of six women treated for resistant HG with levomepromazine, good symptomatic control was achieved in each case [35]. Five of the pregnancies progressed to the birth of live-born infants with no evidence of congenital anomaly, and the sixth pregnancy culminated in an intrauterine death with no external or ultrasound evidence of congenital anomaly. Another case series reported the use of mirtazapine within the intravenous fluid support for approximately 1 week in three patients with severe HG who had previously failed conventional treatment, including promethazine and metoclopramide [39]. All responded to mirtazapine within 24 hours, with resumption of diet within a few days of initiation of this treatment. Each was reported to have no relapse of symptoms throughout the pregnancy and delivered healthy newborns. Such early results are promising in the development of these newer antiemetic agents as second-line drugs for the treatment of resistant HG. Large-scale prospective randomized trials need to be undertaken to validate the efficacy of these therapies.

Considerable discussion has centered on the use of corticosteroids for the treatment of the symptoms of HG. The genesis of this approach lies in the successful use of this modality for the treatment of nausea and vomiting due to cancer chemotherapy-induced emesis. Although some success has been reported, the literature is variable with regard to the type, dose, schedule, and route of corticosteroids to be employed in the treatment of HG, as well as outcome measures. Most studies to date seem to validate some usefulness of corticosteroids in symptomatic relief of nausea and vomiting in HG. One week of daily 40 mg oral prednisolone, or its intravenous equivalent as hydrocortisone for those intolerant of the oral medication, led to an improved sense of well-being, appetite, and weight gain compared with placebo controls and a trend toward improved nausea and vomiting [40]. A short course of oral methylprednisolone with a 2-week taper has been found to be more effective than promethazine in effecting resolution of symptoms and resumption of eating, with the advantage of completing treatment in an outpatient setting [41]. Pulsed high-dose intravenous hydrocortisone was found to be significantly more effective than regularly scheduled intravenous metoclopramide in reducing vomiting episodes and in preventing readmission in women with intractable hyperemesis [42]. Conversely, intravenous methylprednisolone followed by a prednisone taper did not reduce the need for later rehospitalization compared with placebo controls in women with HG who had failed outpatient therapy when both groups were also receiving promethazine and metoclopramide [43]. When promethazine was compared with low-dose prednisolone over 10 days, despite an early (48-hour) advantage with promethazine, after completion of treatment, the group receiving prednisolone experienced less nausea and fewer episodes of vomiting than the promethazine group [44]. Both low-dose and high-dose corticosteroids appear to bestow some treatment advantage over other single entities in reducing symptoms, as well as possibly limiting rehospitalization. However, the differences seem to dissipate when corticosteroids are used concurrently with other agents. One caveat is that the presence of weight loss may be a determining factor in predicting success of corticosteroids in prompting resolution of symptoms in severe HG. Women who have lost more than 5% of pre-pregnant weight uniformly manifest a successful response to corticosteroids [45].

Because there is a high recurrence in subsequent pregnancies in women who have previously experienced HG, some clinicians advocate the use of preemptive treatment in pregnant women with a past history of HG. Women with previous HG who were identified before a subsequent planned pregnancy were prospectively assigned to preemptive therapy beginning anywhere from before conception to up to 7 weeks gestation and were found to be significantly less symptomatic than a control group [46]. The authors concluded that preemptive therapy appears to be effective in preventing HG in subsequent pregnancies.

Several alternative therapies have been promoted for use in patients with HG. There have been a number of preliminary studies looking at the efficacy of ginger in reducing the nausea and vomiting of pregnancy. Although data are insufficient to recommend ginger universally and there are concerns about product quality due to the limited regulation of dietary supplements, several literature reviews have suggested that ginger appears to be a fairly low-risk and effective treatment for nausea and vomiting associated with pregnancy in patients not responding to traditional first-line therapies [47, 48]. Although these authors recommend further study of ginger, there has been vigorous dissent for this suggestion on the grounds that dietary supplements cannot be assumed to be safe for the embryo or fetus and that ginger, although possibly effective, offers no advantage compared with medications for which safety for the fetus has received more extensive evaluation [49]. Despite this objection, the American College of Obstetrics and Gynecology guidelines currently recommend ginger as worth trying for nausea and vomiting of pregnancy. In a study of the related issue of Internet advice offered by "medical herbalists" on the use of ginger, raspberry, and juniper in the nausea and vomiting of pregnancy, the authors concluded that "the advice offered is misleading at best and dangerous at worst," with frequent omission of any mention of potential side effects [50]. Two studies have found that multivitamins given at conception help reduce the severity of nausea and vomiting of pregnancy [51, 52]. These data offer a potential treatment option for planned pregnancies in women with a past history of HG. Finally, in an intriguing study of acupuncture plus acupressure in women with HG, twice weekly sessions for 2 weeks was equally as effective as metoclopramide with vitamin B_{12} in reducing nausea intensity and vomiting, as well as improving the rate of food intake [53]. Although it bears noting that metoclopramide also was given only twice weekly for 2 weeks, acupuncture was found to be significantly more effective than drugs in improving ability to function in routine daily activities.

A representative summary of current treatment options is shown in Table 14.1, with the general order of choice of treatment listed from top to bottom and

Table 14.1 Current treatment options for hyperemesis gravidarum

First-line therapy

Intravenous fluids, electrolytes, thiamine

Pyridoxine

Promethazine

Second-line therapy

Prochlorperazine

Metoclopramide, intravenous or subcutaneous

With or without pyridoxine

Pharmacotherapy in refractory hyperemesis gravidarum

Odansetron

Corticosteroids

2-week oral prednisolone/methylprednisolone (if initially tolerant)

Intravenous hydrocortisone with oral taper (if initially intolerant)

Levomepromazine

Mirtazapine

Alternative therapy in refractory hyperemesis gravidarum

Ginger

Acupuncture/acupressure

the most commonly accepted therapies listed higher in each category.

Hyperemesis gravidarum and nutrition

It has been understood for some time that women suffering from HG are at high risk for malnutrition, whether monitored by percentage of body loss or by serum markers of nutriture [54, 55]. The risks of maternal malnutrition in pregnancy and associated complications, both maternal and fetal, are well known, and the literature is replete with these. The controversy regarding malnutrition in HG relates not to its existence but to its effect on the outcome of pregnancy. There has been an ongoing debate over whether HG has any effect on pregnancy outcome and, if so, the magnitude of that effect. Inherent in this debate is whether the nature and extent of therapy and, in particular, nutrition intervention, ameliorates an effect of HG on pregnancy outcome. It is clear that maternal weight loss should be minimized in HG, because it is an independent predictor of poor fetal outcome [55]. Conflicting data exist in the literature with regard to an association between HG and birth weight. A num-

ber of authors have found no relationship [3, 56–58], whereas other researchers describe evidence of a negative effect of HG on infant birth weight [4, 59, 60]. Several studies have shown that when confounding variables can be included in a multivariate analysis of the data, an initial apparent relationship of HG to reduced birth weight can be excluded [61, 62]. However, infants born to hyperemetic mothers have a significantly lower gestational age as well as a significantly longer length of hospital stay than infants born to control mothers [61]. These outcomes support the need for aggressive treatment of HG during pregnancy, including nutrition support, where indicated.

In situations in which the symptomatology and associated malnutrition of HG become severe, nutrition intervention beyond manipulation of oral intake is necessitated. The American Society of Parenteral and Enteral Nutrition (ASPEN) clinical guidelines strongly encourage the use of nutrition support in pregnant women who are at increased risk of the complications of malnutrition and to improve outcome for both mother and infant [63]. Reports of enteral nutrition as a therapeutic modality for HG appeared contemporary to the first reports, in the early 1980s, of the use of parenteral nutrition in the treatment of HG, but it appears to have fallen out of comparative favor, mainly because of concerns of poor tolerance and promotion of recurrent symptoms [64, 65]. The use of enteral nutrition in the treatment of HG underwent a resurgence in the 1990s, not only as a source of nutrition but as a modality to alleviate the nausea and vomiting of HG [66–68]. The nasogastric route seems to be the most effective route of enteral nutrition in reducing the nausea and vomiting of HG in patients in whom these symptoms are associated with the consumption of food [66]. It is thought that smell and tactile sensations promote the symptoms of nausea and vomiting in these patients, such that bypassing the oral cavity with a nasogastric tube minimizes these gustatory and olfactory cues. In a detailed report of seven women with meal-related nausea and vomiting of HG, nasogastric feeds successfully alleviated these symptoms within 24 hours in each subject [68]. Oral liquids were tolerated within 2 to 5 days of feeding tube placement, and all patients were discharged within 8 days of initiation of enteral nutrition (mean = 4.6 days), six on outpatient enteral nutrition. All patients were eventually able to discontinue enteral nutrition prior to delivery (mean = 43 days). The authors stress that the key to successful enteral nutrition in HG is patient stabilization with appropriate hydration and electrolyte balance first. In follow-up to this report, van de Ven noted that an iso-osmotic solution is recommended in this situation, with periodic aspiration of the stomach to prevent gastric retention and pulmonary aspiration [69].

Because the presence of a long-term nasogastric tube may be somewhat onerous to a patient, a gastrostomy tube can be placed instead. The first two reported cases of percutaneous endoscopic gastrostomy (PEG) in conscious pregnant women supported the safety of this modality as well as favorable maternal and fetal outcomes [70].

Jejunal feeding may be necessary in HG patients who are intolerant of gastric feeding. Nasojejunal tubes can be placed either endoscopically or fluoroscopically with appropriate shielding [71, 72]. Patients with HG refractory to standard treatment with intravenous fluids and antiemetics undergoing nasojejunal feeding had relatively rapid improvement in nausea and vomiting and were able to have their feeding tubes removed when they were well enough to take more than 1000 calories orally (4–21 days) [71]. Several case reports of the use of PEG with a jejunal port (PEGJ) have demonstrated that this technique is a safe, effective, and relatively cost-effective intervention for severe refractory HG [73, 74].

There has been some debate over which technique (nasogastric tube, PEG, or PEGJ) is the preferred route of enteral nutrition in patients with severe refractory nausea and vomiting of HG [75, 76]. Inherent with enteral nutrition by PEGJ is the necessity of giving feedings in a continuous or cyclic fashion to avoid the usual jejunal intolerance of bolus feeding. In the current absence of prospective, randomized controlled trials, it makes empiric sense to first give a trial of nasogastric enteral nutrition in patients with refractory HG. If symptoms improve but prolonged enteral nutrition becomes necessary, a PEG should be considered for longer-term support. However, if there is intolerance for nasogastric feedings, a trial of nasojejunal feedings would be prudent before placing a PEGJ. In the face of the complete failure of enteral nutrition, initiation of parenteral nutrition would become necessary.

The use of parenteral nutrition in pregnancy, in general, and in HG, specifically, has been reported for more than 25 years, with successful outcomes [77–80]. However, it is clear that the use of parenteral nutrition in pregnancy is associated with a variety of maternal complications, including infection, venous thrombo-

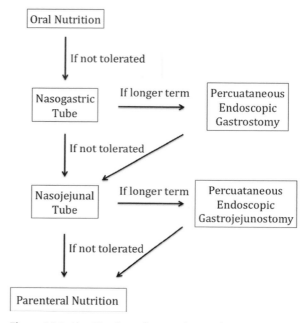

Figure 14.1 Algorithm for preference of route of nutrition support in hyperemesis gravidarum.

sis, pneumothorax, intrahepatic cholestasis, placental fatty infiltration, and catheter dislodgement [80, 81]. At least one maternal-fetal death has been reported as a complication of parenteral nutrition in pregnancy [82]. The complication rate of parenteral nutrition in pregnancy can be reduced by the use of peripherally inserted central catheters (PICC), but the incidence of line-related sepsis alone, which is generally independent of type of venous catheter used, is approximately 25% [80, 83]. In addition, the HG patient is at high risk for central catheter-related thromboembolism through a combination of the elevated coagulopathy factors associated with pregnancy and dehydration contributing to venous stasis. In nonpregnant adult patients, the incidence of Doppler ultrasound–detected PICC-related upper extremity venous thrombosis was found to be 62% in patients not prophylaxed with anticoagulants and remained 23% in those who were prophylaxed with some type of anticoagulation [84]. These are not insignificant values given that pregnant patients are almost certainly at a higher risk of venous thromboembolic disease than the general population. Given the risk of complications related to use of parenteral nutrition in pregnancy, as well as the previously noted significant cost differential relative to enteral nutrition, parenteral nutrition should be used only under established, documented criteria in patients with HG. These criteria include weight loss over a time period of at least 4 weeks, failed conservative therapy (including intravenous hydration and a variety of antiemetic medications), and persistent laboratory findings, such as serum electrolyte abnormalities and hypoalbuminemia [83]. In addition, patients should have failed all earlier steps in the decision-making tree shown earlier. Parenteral nutrition in HG should be considered a "therapy of exclusion," that is, resorted to only after all other options have been exhausted. Figure 14.1 summarizes the preferences for the route of nutrition support in a treatment algorithm.

References

1. Broussard CN and Richter JE, Nausea and vomiting of pregnancy. *Gastroenterol Clin North Am* (1998), **27**:123–51.

2. Gadsby R, Barnie-Adshead AM, and Jager C, A prospective study of nausea and vomiting during pregnancy. *Br J Gen Pract* (1993), **43**:245–8.

3. Fairweather DV, Nausea and vomiting in pregnancy. *Am J Obstet Gynecol* (1968), **102**:135–7.

4. Kallen B, Hyperemesis during pregnancy and delivery outcome: a registry study. *Eur J Obstet Gynecol Reprod Biol* (1987), **26**:291–302.

5. Bashiri A, Newmann L, Maymon E, and Katz M, Hyperemesis gravidarum: epidemiologic features, complications and outcome. *Eur J Obstet Gynecol Reprod Biol* (1995), **63**:135–8.

6. Cunningham FG, Gant NF, Leveno KJ, Gilstrap LC III, Hauth JC, and Wenstrom KD, et al., *Williams Obstetrics* (New York: McGraw-Hill, 2001), p. 1275.

7. Morali GA and Braverman DZ, Abnormal liver enzymes and ketonuria in hyperemesis gravidarum. A retrospective view of 80 patients. *J Clin Gastroenterol* (1990), **12**:303–5.

8. Goodwin TM, Hershman JM, and Cole L, Increased concentration of the free beta-subunit of human chorionic gonadotropin in hyperemesis gravidarum. *Acta Obstet Gynecol Scand* (1994), **73**:770–2.

9. Frigo P, Lang C, Reisenberger K, Heinz K, and Hirschl AM, Hyperemesis gravidarum associated with *Helicobacter pylori* seropositivity. *Obstet Gynecol* (1998), **91**:615–17.

10. Jacoby EB and Porter KB, *Helicobacter pylori* infection and persistent hyperemesis gravidarum. *Am J Perinatol* (1999), **16**:85–8.

11. Boullion R, Naesens M, van Assche FA, De Keyser L, De Moor P, Renaer M, et al., Thyroid function in patients with hyperemesis gravidarum. *Am J Obstet Gynecol* (1982), **143**:922–6.

12. Valbo A and Jerve F, A study of thyroid hormones in women suffering from vomiting in pregnancy. *Acta Eur Fertil* (1987), **18**:381–3.

13. Riezzo G, Pezzolla F, Darconza G, and Giorgio I, Gastric myoelectric activity in the first trimester of pregnancy: a cutaneous electrogastrographic study. *Am J Gastroenterol* (1992), **87**:702–7.

14. Katon WJ, Ries RK, Bokan LA, and Kleinman A, Hyperemesis gravidarum: a biopsychological perspective. *Int J Psychiatry Med* (1980), **10**:151–62.

15. Iancu I, Kotler M, Spivak B, Radvak M, Weizman A, Psychiatric aspects of hyperemesis gravidarum. *Psychother Psychosom* (1994), **64**:143–9.

16. Lingham R and McCluskey S, Eating disorders associated with hyperemesis gravidarum. *J Psychosom Res* (1996), **40**:231–4.

17. Hiroi H, Kugu K, Hoshino H, Kozuma S, and Takesani Y, Hyperemesis gravidarum associated with thyrotoxicosis and a past history of an eating disorder. *Arch Gynecol Obstet* (2001), **265**:228–330.

18. Goodwin TM, Nausea and vomiting of pregnancy: an obstetric syndrome. *Am J Obstet Gynecol* (2002), **186**:S184–9.

19. Eliakim R, Abulafia O, and Sherer DM, Hyperemesis gravidarum: a current review. *Am J Perinatol* (2000), **17**:207–18.

20. Wallstedt A, Riley CA, Shaver D, et al., Prevalence and characteristics of liver dysfunction in hyperemesis gravidarum. *Clin Res* (1990), **38**:970–2.

21. Robertson C, and Millar H, Hyperamylasemia in bulimia nervosa and hyperemesis gravidarum. *Int J Eat Disorder* (1999), **26**:223–7.

22. Goodwin TM, Hyperemesis gravidarum. *Clin Obstet Gynecol* (1998), **41**:597–605.

23. Weng MT, Wei SC, Wong JM, and Chang TC, Hyperemesis gravidarum presenting as jaundice and transient hypothyroidism complicated with acute pancreatitis. *J Formosan Med Assoc* (2005), **104**:194–7.

24. Woolford TJ, Birzgalos AR, Lundell C, and Farrington WT, Vomiting in pregnancy resulting in oesophageal perforation in a 15 year old girl. *J Laryngol Otol* (1993), **107**:1059–60.

25. Schwartz M and Rossoff L, Pneumomediastinum and bilateral pneumothoraces in a patient with hyperemesis gravidarum. *Chest* (1994), **106**:1904–6.

26. Nyugen M, Deitel M, and Lacy E, Splenic avulsion in a pregnant patient with vomiting. *Can J Surg* (1995), **38**:464–5.

27. Chiossi G, Neri I, Cavazutti M, Basso G, and Facchinetti F, Hyperemesis gravidarum complicated by Wernicke encephalopathy: background, case report, and review of the literature. *Obstetr Gynecol Surv* (2006), **61**:255–68.

28. Robinson JN, Banerjee R, and Thiet MP, Coagulopathy secondary to vitamin K deficiency in hyperemesis gravidarum. *Obstet Gynecol* (1998), **92**:673–5.

29. Welsh A, Hyperemesis, gastrointestinal and liver disorders in pregnancy. *Curr Obstet Gynecol* (2005), **15**:123–31.

30. Jarnfelt-Samisoe A, Samisoe G, and Verlinder GM, Nausea and vomiting in pregnancy: a contribution to its epidemiology. *Gynecol Obstet Invest* (1983), **16**:221–9.

31. Gadsby R, Barnie-Adshead AM, and Jagger C, A prospective study of nausea and vomiting during pregnancy. *Br J Gen Pract* (1993), **43**:245–8.

32. Sahakian V, Rouse D, Sipes S, Rose N, and Niebyl J, Vitamin B6 is effective therapy for nausea and vomiting of pregnancy: a randomized double blind placebo controlled study. *Obstet Gynecol* (1991), **78**:33–6.

33. Broussard CN and Richter JE, Nausea and vomiting of pregnancy. *Gastrenterol Clin North Am* (1998), **27**:23–151.

34. Nelson-Piercy C, Treatment of nausea and vomiting of pregnancy. *Drug Safety* (1998), **19**:155–64.

35. Heazell AEP, Langford N, Judge JK, Heazell MA, and Downey GP, The use of levomepromazine in hyperemesis gravidarum resistant to drug therapy – a case series. *Reprod Toxicol* (2005), **20**:569–72.

36. Bsat FA, Hoffman DE, and Seubert DE, Comparison of three outpatient regimens in the management of nausea and vomiting in pregnancy. *J Perinatol* (2003), **23**:531–5.

37. Buttino L Jr, Coleman SK, Bergauer NK, Gambon C, and Stanziano GJ, Home subcutaneous metoclopramide therapy for hyperemesis gravidarum. *J Perinatol* (2000), **20**:359–62.

38. Sullivan CA, Johnson CA, Roach H, Martin RW, Stewart DK, and Morrison JC, A pilot study of intravenous ondansetron for hyperemesis gravidarum. *Am J Obstet Gynecol* (1996), **174**:1565–8.

39. Guclu S, Gol M, Dogan E, and Saygili U, Mirtazapine use in resistant hyperemesis gravidarum: report of three cases and review of the literature. *Arch Gynecol Obstet* (2005), **272**:298–300.

40. Nelson-Piercy C, Fayers P, and de Swiet M, Randomised, double-blind, placebo-controlled trial of corticosteroids for the treatment of hyperemesis gravidarum. *Br J Obstet Gynaecol* (2001), **108**:9–15.

41. Safari HR, Alsulyman OM, Gherman RB, and Goodwin TM, Experience with oral methylprednisolone in the treatment of refractory hyperemesis gravidarum. *Am J Obstet Gynecol* (1998), **178**:1054–8.

42. Bondok RS, El Sharnouby NM, Eid HE, and Abd Elmaksoud AM, Pulsed steroid therapy is an effective treatment for intractable hyperemesis gravidarum. *Crit Care Med* (2006), **34**:2781–3.

43. Yost NP, McIntire DD, Wians FH, Ramin SM, Balko JA, and Leveno KJ, A randomized, placebo-controlled trial of corticosteroids for hyperemesis due to pregnancy. *Obstet Gynecol* (2003), **102**:1250–4.

44. Ziaei S, Hosseiney FS, and Faghihzadeh S, The efficacy of low dose prednisolone in the treatment of hyperemesis gravidarum. *Acta Obstet Gynecol Scand* (2004), **83**:272–5.

45. Moran P and Taylor R, Management of hyperemesis gravidarum: the importance of weight loss as a criterion for steroid therapy. *Q J Med* (2002), **95**:153–8.

46. Koren G and Maltepe C, Pre-emptive therapy for severe nausea and vomiting of pregnancy and hyperemesis gravidarum. *J Obstet Gynecol* (2004), **24**:530–3.

47. Boone SA and Shields KM, Treating pregnancy-related nausea and vomiting with ginger. *Ann Pharmacother* (2005), **39**:1710–13.

48. Borrelli F, Capasso R, Aviello G, Pittler MH, and Izzo AA, Effectiveness and safety of ginger in the treatment of pregnancy-induced nausea and vomiting.

Obstet Gynecol (2005), **105**:849–56.

49. Marcus DM and Snodgrass WR, Effectiveness and safety of ginger in the treatment of pregnancy-induced nausea and vomiting. *Obstet Gynecol* (2005), **106**:640.

50. Ernst E and Schmidt K, Health risks over the Internet: advice offered by "medical herbalists" to a pregnant woman. *Wien Med Wochen* (2002), **152**:190–2.

51. Czeizel AE, Dudas I, Fritz G, Técsöi A, Hanck A, and Kunovits G, The effect of periconceptual multivitamin-mineral supplementation on vertigo, nausea and vomiting in the first trimester of pregnancy. *Arch Gynecol Obstet* (1992), **251**:181–5.

52. Emelianova S, Mazzotta P, Einarson A, and Koren G, Prevalence and severity of nausea and vomiting of pregnancy and effect of vitamin supplementation. *Clin Invest Med* (1999), **22**:106–10.

53. Neri I, Schiapparelli P, Biasi I, Benedetto C, and Facchinetti F, Acupuncture versus pharmacological approach to reduce hyperemesis gravidarum discomfort. *Minerva Ginecol* (2005), **57**:471–5.

54. Schulman PK, Hyperemesis gravidarum: an approach to the nutritional aspects of care. *J Am Diet Assoc* (1982), **80**:577–8.

55. Jarnfelt-Samisoe A, Erikkson B, Waldenstrom J, and Samisoe G, Some new aspects on emesis gravidarum. Relations to clinical data, serum electrolytes, total protein and creatinine. *Gynecol Obstet Invest* (1985), **19**:174–86.

56. Brandes JM, First trimester nausea and vomiting as related to outcome of pregnancy. *Obstet Gynecol* (1967), **30**:427–31.

57. Tierson FD, Olsen FL, and Hook EB, Nausea and vomiting of pregnancy and association with pregnancy outcome. *Am J Obstet Gynecol* (1986), **155**:1017–22.

145

58. Hallak M, Tsalamandris K, Dombrowski MP, Isada NB, Pryde PG, and Evans MI, Hyperemesis gravidarum: effects on fetal outcome. *J Reprod Med* (1996), 41:871–4.

59. Gross S, Librach C, and Cecutti A, Maternal weight loss associated with hyperemesis gravidarum: a predictor of fetal outcome. *Am J Obstet Gynecol* (1989), **160**: 906–9.

60. Chin RKH and Lao TT, Low birth weight and hyperemesis gravidarum. *Eur J Obstet Gynecol Reprod Biol* (1988), 28:179–83.

61. Paauw JD, Bierling S, Cook CR, and Davis AT, Hyperemesis gravidarum and fetal outcome. *J Parenter Enter Nutr* (2005), **29**:93–6.

62. Vilming B and Nesheim BI, Hyperemesis gravidarum in a contemporary population in Oslo. *Acta Obstet Gynecol Scand* (2000), **79**:640–3.

63. ASPEN Board of Directors and the Clinical Guidelines Task Force, Guidelines for the use of parenteral and enteral nutrition in adult and pediatric patients. *J Parenter Enter Nutr* (2002), 26(Suppl):S1–139.

64. Smith CV, Rufleth P, Phelan JP, and Nelson KJ, Long-term enteral nutrition support in the pregnant woman with diabetes: a report of 2 cases. *Am J Obstet Gynecol* (1981), 141:180–3.

65. Levine MG and Esser D, Total parenteral nutrition and the treatment of severe hyperemesis gravidarum: maternal nutritional effect and fetal outcome. *Obstet Gynecol* (1988), 72:102–7.

66. Boyce RA, Enteral nutrition in hyperemesis gravidarum: a new development. *J Am Diet Assoc* (1992), **92**:733–6.

67. Gulley RM, Vander Ploeg N, and Gulley JM, Treatment of hyperemesis with nasogastric feeding. *Nutr Clin Pract* (1993), 8:33–35.

68. Hsu JJ, Clark-Glena R, Nelson DK, and Kim CH, Nasogastric enteral feeding in the management of hyperemesis gravidarum. *Obstet Gynecol* (1996), **88**:343–6.

69. van de Ven CJM, Nasogastric enteral feeding in hyperemesis gravidarum. *Lancet* (1997), 349:445–6.

70. Godil A and Chen YK, Percutaneous endoscopic gastrostomy for nutrition support in pregnancy associated with hyperemesis gravidarum and anorexia nervosa. *J Parenter Enter Nutr* (1998), **22**:238–41.

71. Vaisman N, Kaidar R, Levin I, and Lessing JB, Nasojejunal feeding in hyperemesis gravidarum – a preliminary study. *Clin Nutr* (2004), **23**:53–7.

72. Cimbalik C, Paauw JD, and Davis AT, Pregnancy and lactation. In: ed. Gottschlich MM, *Science & Practice of Nutrition Support: Case-Based Core Curriculum*, 2nd edn, (Silver Spring, MD: ASPEN, 2007).

73. Serrano P, Velloso A, Garcia-Luna PP, Pereira JL, Fernández Z, Ductor MJ, Castro D, et al., Enteral nutrition by percutaneous endoscopic gastrojejunostomy in severe hyperemesis gravidarum: a report of two cases. *Clin Nutr* (1998), **17**:135–9.

74. Irving PM, Howell RJS, and Shidrawi RG, Percutaneous endoscopic gastrostomy with a jejunal port for severe hyperemesis gravidarum. *Eur J Gastroenterol Hepatol* (2004), **16**:937–9.

75. Garcia-Luna PP, Serrano P, and Velloso A, PEG and PEG-J for nutrition support in pregnancy. *J Parenter Enter Nutr* (1999), 23:367–8.

76. Godil A and Chen YK, Response to Garci-Luna, et al. *J Parenter Enter Nutr* (1999), 23:368.

77. Hew LR and Deitel M, Total parenteral nutrition in gynecology and obstetrics. *Obstet Gynecol* (1980), **55**: 464–8.

78. Seifer DM, Silberman H, Cantanzarite V, et al. Total parenteral nutrition in obstetrics. *JAMA* (1985), **253**:2073–5.

79. Kirby DF, Fiorenza V, and Craig RM, Intravenous nutrition support during pregnancy. *J Parenter Enter Nutr* (1988), 12:72–80.

80. Russo-Stieglitz KE, Levine AB, Wagner BA, and Armenti VT, Pregnancy outcome in patients requiring parenteral nutrition. *J Maternal Fetal Med* (1999), 8:164–7.

81. Martin R and Blackburn GL, Principles of hyperalimentation during pregnancy. In: ed. RL Berkowitz, *Critical Care of the Obstetric Patient* (New York: Churchill Livingstone, 1983), pp. 149–63.

82. Greenspoon JS, Masaki DI, and Kurz CR, Cardiac tamponade in pregnancy during hyperalimentation. *Obstet Gynecol* (1989), **73**: 465–6.

83. Folk JJ, Leslie-Brown HFM, Nosovitch JT, Silverman RK, and Aubry RH, Hyperemesis gravidarum. Outcomes and complications with and without total parenteral nutrition. *J Reprod Med* (2004), **49**:497–502.

84. Paauw JD, Borders H, Ingalls N, Boomsta S, Lambke B, Goldsmith A, and Davis AT, The incidence of PICC line associated thrombosis with and without the use of prophylactic anti-coagulants. *J Parenteral Enteral Nutr* 2008 (in press).

Multiple pregnancy

Barbara Luke

In 2004, there were 139,494 infants born from multiple pregnancies in the United States, the highest number ever recorded [1]. Since 1980, there has been a 93% increase in the incidence of twins and a 544% increase in triplet and higher-order multiples (quadruplets and quintuplets). The primary factors contributing to this change have been the widespread use and availability of infertility treatments, in combination with the trend of childbearing at older ages. Although infants of multiple births account for only approximately 3% of all live births, they are disproportionately represented among the preterm (< 37 weeks, 16%), very preterm (< 32 weeks, 22%), low birth weight (< 2500 g, 32%), and very low birth weight (< 1500 g, 27%) infant populations. The average birth weight and gestational age is 3316 g at 38.7 weeks for singletons, compared with 2333 g at 35.2 weeks for twins, 1700 g at 32.1 weeks for triplets, 1276 g at 29.7 weeks for quadruplets, and 1103 g at 28.4 weeks for quintuplets [1]. An estimated 19% of all neonatal intensive care unit days are associated with multiple pregnancies [2].

The population of women pregnant with multiple gestations is distinctly different from the average pregnant woman in the United States (Table 15.1). Over the past 20 years, there has been a growing trend in delaying pregnancy; this pattern is magnified among women pregnant with multiples. Although the percent of women aged 35 and older having a singleton baby has increased threefold since 1980, the percent having twins has increased nearly fourfold, and those having triplets or higher-order births nearly sixfold [1]. Although older maternal age may be associated with better financial and social resources, from a physiological perspective, the special nutritional demands of a multiple pregnancy have important implications for the mother's future health. For example, when a woman has a multiple pregnancy in her 40s or 50s, she may be within only a few years of menopause, and the substantial calcium drain may increase her risk for osteoporosis [3].

Multiple pregnancy represents a state of magnified nutritional requirements, resulting in a greater nutrient drain on maternal resources and an accelerated depletion of nutritional reserves. The accelerated starvation that occurs in pregnancy is exaggerated with a multiple gestation, particularly during the second half of pregnancy, with more rapid depletion of glycogen stores and resultant metabolism of fat between meals and during an overnight fast. A reduced glucose stream from mother to fetus results in slower fetal growth and smaller birth size, as well as a higher risk of preterm labor and preterm birth. For this reason, diet therapy with a diabetic regimen of 20% of calories from protein, 40% of calories from carbohydrate, and 40% of calories from fat may be particularly useful. Iron-deficiency anemia has also been linked to preterm delivery and other adverse pregnancy outcomes. Maternal iron status, in addition to the amount and pattern of gestational weight gain, is an important factor associated with fetal growth and length of gestation in twin pregnancies. Supplementation with calcium, magnesium, and zinc, as well as multivitamins and essential fatty acids, may also reduce pregnancy complications and improve postnatal health for infants born from a multiple gestation. Diet therapy for women pregnant with multiples is an important component of effective prenatal care. The majority of studies to date have evaluated the effects of nutritional factors on the course and outcome of singleton pregnancies; the body of literature on multiple gestations is growing, but there are still many gaps in our knowledge of normal and abnormal physiological changes and effective interventions. The following chapter summarizes current research on maternal pregravid weight, gestational weight gain, carbohydrate metabolism, iron status, and vitamin and mineral intake on fetal growth and length of gestation in singletons and, when known, in twin and triplet gestations.

Table 15.1 Live births by maternal age, birth order, and plurality, United States, 1980, 1990, and 2004

Birth order and year	Number of births by maternal age (years)							Percent of births maternal age (year)		
	All Ages	<20	20–24	25–29	30–34	35–39	≥40	≥30	≥35	≥40
First births										
1980	1 545 604	435 333	605 183	371 859	112 964	18 241	2 024	8.6	1.3	0.1
1990	1 689 118	401 900	515 455	465 458	230 612	66 541	9152	18.1	4.5	0.5
2004	1 630 921	336 783	483 752	395 784	279 884	110 418	24 300	25.4	8.3	1.5
All births										
1980	3 612 258	562 330	1 226 200	1 108 291	550 354	140 793	24 290	19.8	4.6	0.7
1990	4 158 212	533 483	1 093 730	1 277 108	886 063	317 583	50 245	30.2	8.8	1.2
2004	4 112 052	422 043	1 034 454	1 104 485	965 663	475 606	109 801	37.8	14.2	2.6
Plurality and year singletons										
1980	3 478 715	545 958	1 184 408	1 064 764	526 049	134 294	23 242	19.7	4.5	0.7
1990	4 061 319	525 793	1 072 431	1 246 144	860 478	307 498	48 975	30.0	8.8	1.2
2004	3 972 558	415 327	1 010 421	1 069 417	924 160	450 733	102 500	37.2	13.9	2.6
Twins										
1980	68 339	7 212	21 374	22 712	12 944	3559	538	24.9	6.0	0.8
1990	93 865	7 605	20 945	30 020	24 466	9587	1242	37.6	11.5	1.3
2004	132 219	6 629	23 602	33 315	38 751	23 088	6834	51.9	22.6	5.2
Triplets and more										
1980	1337	83	385	474	321	67	7	29.5	5.5	0.5
1990	3028	85	354	944	1119	498	28	54.3	17.4	0.9
2004	7275	87	431	1753	2752	1785	467	68.8	31.0	6.4
All multiples										
1980	69 676	7295	21 759	23 186	13 265	3626	545	25.0	6.0	0.8
1990	96 893	7690	21 299	30 964	25 585	10 085	1270	38.1	11.7	1.3
2004	139 494	6716	24 033	35 068	41 503	24 873	7301	52.8	23.1	5.2

Carbohydrate metabolism

Pregnancy is a state of accelerated starvation, resulting in lower fasting glucose levels and an exaggeration of the insulin response to eating. In twin pregnancies, these changes are magnified, particularly during the second half of pregnancy, with significantly lower maternal serum glucose and insulin concentrations and higher plasma concentrations of β-hydroxybutyrate compared with maternal concentrations in singleton pregnancies, indicating more rapid depletion of glycogen stores and resultant metabolism of fat between meals and during an overnight fast [4]. Both fasting and ketonuria have been linked to an increase in preterm labor and preterm delivery, a phenomenon termed the "Yom Kippur effect" [5]. A reduced glucose stream from mother to fetus results in slower fetal growth, smaller birth size, and an increased risk of fetal growth restriction [6]. The diet therapy we have used successfully in both twin and triplet pregnancies is based on the diabetic regimen of three meals and three snacks per day (Table 15.2). We have found in studies with both twins and triplets [7, 8] that diet therapy with 20% of calories from protein, but a lower percentage of calories from carbohydrate (40%) for better glycemic control, and a higher percentage of calories from fat

Table 15.2 Body mass index (BMI)-specific dietary recommendations for twin gestations

BMI Group	Under weight	Normal weight	Over weight	Obese
BMI range	<19.8	19.8–26.0	26.1–29.0	>29.0
Calories	4000	3500	3250	3000
Protein (20% of calories)	200 g	175 g	163 g	150 g
Carbohydrate (40% of calories)	400 g	350 g	325 g	300 g
Fat (40% of calories)	178 g	156 g	144 g	133 g
Exchanges (servings) per day				
Dairy	10	8	8	8
Grains	12	10	8	8
Meat and meat equivalents	10	10	8	6
Eggs	2	2	2	2
Vegetables	5	4	4	4
Fruits	8	7	6	6
Fats and oils	7	6	5	5

Adapted from Luke B, Brown MB, Misiunas R, Anderson E, Nugent C, van de Ven C, Burpee B, Gogliotti S. Specialized prenatal care and maternal and infant outcomes in twin pregnancy. *Am J Obstet Gynecol* (2003), 189:934–8.

(40%), to provide additional calories with less bulk, are most effective. The emphasis is also on the use of low glycemic index carbohydrates to prevent wide fluctuations in blood glucose concentrations.

Iron status

Iron-deficiency anemia is also significantly associated with preterm delivery [9–11]. Serum ferritin levels, which are lowered with iron deficiency and elevated in the presence of infection, have also been linked to prematurity. Extremes of maternal serum ferritin levels measured early in the second trimester (15–17 weeks), as well as elevated levels at 24, 26, or 28 weeks, have been associated with preterm birth [12, 13]. Elevated third trimester serum ferritin levels are significantly associated with preterm and very preterm birth, with iron-deficiency anemia and poor maternal nutritional status underlying the relationship [13]. Dietary sources of iron are preferable, particularly hem-iron-rich sources such as red meat, pork, poultry, fish, and eggs, because of better absorption and utilization, their positive effect on non-hem-iron bioavailability, and their high quality and quantity of protein and other nutrients. The inclusion of non-hem-iron sources is

encouraged as well, such as iron-fortified breads and grains, vegetables, and nuts.

The few studies that have evaluated iron status in multiple pregnancies have reported lower hemoglobin levels in the first and second trimesters, higher rates of iron-deficiency anemia, and even residual iron-deficiency anemia in the infants, up to 6 months of age [14–16]. Hediger and Luke [17] reported that by the third trimester, lower levels of serum ferritin (indicating better volume expansion) were significantly associated with pregravid body mass index (BMI) and rate of weight gain to 20 weeks. Serial measures of iron status (hemoglobin [Hgb], hematocrit [Hct]) and measures of maternal nutritional status, including weight gain, were collected for 293 twin pregnancies. As in singleton pregnancies, levels of Hgb and Hct declined through the first trimester to a nadir at 20 to 24 weeks. Consistent with greater volume expansion in twin pregnancies, the levels were even lower in the second trimester than for singleton pregnancies. By the third trimester, lower levels of serum ferritin (indicating better volume expansion) were associated with pregravid BMI (-0.50 ± 0.21 µg/l per kg, $p = 0.02$) and rate of weight gain to 20 weeks (-11.6 ± 5.0 µg/l per kg weight gain, $p = 0.02$). As shown in prior studies, both maternal pregravid BMI and rate of weight gain before 20 weeks are consistently strong predictors of twin birth weight outcomes. Mean levels by trimester were as follows:

	First Trimester	Second Trimester	Third Trimester
Hemoglobin	12.8 g/dL	11.3 g/dL	11.0 g/dL
Hematocrit	37.3%	32.8%	32.0%
Ferritin	56.6 µg/L	34.3 µg/L	12.2 µg/L

Iron status during pregnancy has also been linked to fetal programming and the development of chronic disease. Low maternal hemoglobin is strongly related to the development of a large placenta and high placental:birth weight ratio, which is seen as predictive of long-term programming of hypertension and cardiovascular disease. Because the iron demands of pregnancy may exceed 1 g, with nearly half this amount in the red cell mass increase in blood volume, the maternal preconceptional and early pregnancy iron status are extremely important. Severe maternal iron-deficiency anemia leads to placental adaptive hypertrophy, a fall in the cortisol metabolizing system, and increased susceptibility to hypertension in later life.

Calcium, magnesium, and zinc supplementation

Calcium, magnesium, and zinc have been identified by the World Health Organization as having the most potential for reducing pregnancy complications and improving outcomes [18, 19]. Results of calcium supplementation trials among high-risk women have been promising, with significant reductions in preterm deliveries among teenagers and women with low-calcium diets [20, 21]. Magnesium may have a neuroprotective role, particularly for the premature infant. Although maternal zinc nutriture has been significantly related to length of gestation, infection, and risk of premature rupture of membranes [22, 23], clinical trials of zinc supplementation have yielded equivocal results [24]. A trial that randomly supplemented only women with plasma zinc levels below the median reported an increase in length of gestation of approximately 0.5 week and an increase in birth weight (approximately half of which was explained by the longer duration of gestation) [25]. Scholl et al. [26] reported that a low dietary zinc intake during singleton pregnancy ($\leq$ 6 mg/day or < 40% of the Recommended Dietary Allowance [RDA] for pregnancy) was associated with an increased incidence of iron-deficiency anemia at entry to care, a lower use of prenatal supplements during pregnancy, and a higher incidence of inadequate weight gain during pregnancy, as well as an increased risk of low birth weight, preterm delivery, and early preterm delivery. The joint effect of iron-deficiency anemia at entry to care and a low dietary zinc intake during pregnancy increased the risk of preterm delivery fivefold.

Multivitamin and multimineral supplementation

Ideally, pregnant women should get the level and range of required nutrients through a balanced diet. National dietary surveys indicate, however, that adult women fail to meet the RDAs for five nutrients: calcium, magnesium, zinc, and vitamins E and B_6 [27]. In addition, prenatal use of vitamin-mineral supplements among low-income women has been shown to reduce the risks of preterm delivery and low birth weight, particularly if initiated during the first trimester [28]. Supplementation in excess of twice the RDA should be avoided because of the potential for birth defects. The fat-soluble vitamins, particularly vitamins A and D, are the most potentially toxic during pregnancy. The pediatric and obstetric literature includes case reports of kidney malformations in children whose mothers took between 40 000 and 50 000 IU of vitamin A during pregnancy. Even at lower doses, excessive amounts of vitamin A may cause subtle damage to the developing nervous system, resulting in serious behavioral and learning disabilities in later life. The margin of safety for vitamin D is smaller for this vitamin than for any other. Birth defects of the heart, particularly aortic stenosis, have been reported in both humans and experimental animals with doses as low as 4000 IU, which is 10 times the RDA during pregnancy. These recommendations are for singleton pregnancies but are applicable to multiple pregnancies as well.

Essential fatty acid requirements

There is an established maternal drain of the essential fatty acids during pregnancy, particularly during multiple gestation [29, 30]. Additional supplementation with omega-3 fatty acids, which are vital for neurological and retinal development, may be particularly beneficial during pregnancy for both the mother and

Table 15.3 Optimal rates of maternal weight gain and cumulative gain by pregravid body mass index (BMI) status

Pregravid BMI	Rates of weight gain (kg/week)			Cumulative weight gain (kg)		
	0–20 weeks	20–28 weeks	29 weeks–delivery	To 20 weeks	To 28 weeks	To 36–38 weeks
Underweight (BMI < 19.8)	0.57–0.79	0.68–0.79	0.57	11.3–15.9	16.8–22.2	22.7–28.1
Normal weight (BMI 19.8–26.0)	0.45–0.68	0.57–0.79	0.45	9.1–13.6	13.6–20.0	18.1–24.5
Overweight (BMI 26.1–29.0)	0.45–0.57	0.45–0.68	0.45	9.1–11.3	12.7–16.8	17.2–21.3
Obese (BMI >29.0)	0.34–0.45	0.34–0.57	0.34	6.8–9.1	9.5–13.6	13.2–17.2

Results are from models controlling for diabetes and gestational diabetes, preeclampsia, smoking during pregnancy, parity, placental membranes, and fetal growth before 20 weeks.
Adapted from Luke B, Hediger ML, Nugent C, Newman RB, Mauldin JG, Witter FR, O'Sullivan MJ. Body mass index specific – weight gains associated with optimal birthweights in twin pregnancies. *J Reprod Med* (2003), 48:217–24.

her developing baby. Populations with a higher intake of omega-3 fatty acids have significantly lower rates of preterm delivery and low birth weight [31]. Infants whose mothers had higher omega-3 fatty acid levels at birth demonstrated better cognitive development [32]. One of the newest prenatal supplements incorporates omega-3 fatty acids in its formulation (Duet DHA by StuartNatal).

Maternal weight gain

The pattern of maternal weight gain has been shown to be as important as total weight gain in its effect on birth weight in both singleton and twin pregnancies. Although the increase in fetal weight is greatest during the third trimester (after 28 weeks), gains during mid-gestation (either second trimester or 20–28 weeks) have the strongest association with birth weight. In singletons, Abrams and Selvin [33] demonstrated that birth weight increased in each trimester by 18 g, 33 g, and 17 g, respectively, per kilogram per week of maternal weight gain. Scholl et al. [34] reported that weight gains to 20 weeks and to 28 weeks were most strongly related to birth weight, contributing 22 to 24 g to birth weight per kilogram per week of maternal weight gain. In addition, a low rate of weight gain or a poor pattern of weight gain is associated with an increased risk of preterm birth. Studies in twins by our research team have shown similar results, with low weight gains consistently associated with reduced birth weights. Early and mid-gestation weight gains exert an even greater effect on twin birth weight, with gains to 20 weeks, between 20 and 28 weeks, and from 28 weeks to birth increasing birth weights by 65 g, 37 g, and 16 g, respectively, per kilogram per week of maternal weight gain [35–37].

BMI-specific weight gain guidelines are associated with the best intrauterine growth and subsequent birth weights, and longer length of gestation [38, 39], but studies among women pregnant with singletons [40, 41] and twins [42] have reported that more than one fourth of women receive no advice regarding weight gain. Among women who do receive guidance, for more than one third of women, the advice they receive is inappropriate [40]. We have developed BMI-specific guidelines for twins based on optimal rates of fetal growth and birth weights between the singleton 50th percentile and twin 90th percentile at 36 to 38 weeks (2700–2800 g)[43] (Table 15.3).

The effect of higher weight gain before 20 or 24 weeks on twin and triplet birth weight is most pronounced among infants of underweight gravidas [35, 44]. This early weight gain may reflect the acquisition of maternal nutrient stores, particularly the deposition of body fat [45]. In addition, levels of fat-mobilizing hormones, such as follicle-stimulating hormone (FSH) and human placental lactogen (hPL), may be higher in normal-weight and overweight women, as well as in women with dizygotic twin pregnancies [46]. Therefore, underweight women with low early weight gain may be lacking appropriate nutrient reserves (including maternal stored fat) as well as adequate levels of hormones to mobilize those nutrient stores that are available, resulting in a high incidence of fetal growth restriction. Higher early gains may be particularly important in multiple pregnancies for two distinct reasons. First, pregnancy is usually much shorter for multiple gestations, by as much as 4 to 12 weeks, thereby shortening the period for intrauterine growth. As shown by Williams et al. [47], the peak rate of growth in weight for multiples occurs at about 31 weeks compared with 33 weeks for singletons. Second, higher gains during early gestation may influence the structural and functional development of the placenta [48]. In multiple pregnancies, the placenta ages more quickly, shortening the gestational period during which it can most effectively transfer nutrients to the developing fetuses. Higher gains during early gestation may therefore initially benefit placental structure and function, and subsequently augment fetal growth through more effective placental function as well as the transfer of a higher level of nutrients.

In their analysis of 1138 triplet pregnancies, Elster et al. [49] reported several factors to be predictive of higher average fetal weight for a given gestational age, including male sex, older maternal age, maternal height, pregravid weight and weight gain, and parity. These investigators also reported that length of gestation correlated with maternal age, parity, and weight gain. Maternal weight gain was even more strongly associated with outcomes in triplets than in twins, and gains in different periods of gestation affected birth weight, birth-weight-for-gestation (birth weight z score), and length of gestation as demonstrated in a study of 144 triplets by Luke et al. [7]. Regression analyses indicated that the most significant

periods of maternal weight gain for average triplet birth weight were from conception to 20 weeks and between 20 and 28 weeks (351 g/kg/week, $p = 0.001$, and 247 g/kg/week, $p = 0.001$, respectively); for average triplet birth weight, z scores were between 20 and 28 weeks (1.17 SD units/kg/week, $p < 0.0001$); and for length of gestation from 28 weeks to delivery (10.1 days/kg/week, $p < 0.0001$).

Key clinical points

- The primary factor contributing to the rise in multiple births has been the widespread use and availability of infertility treatments, in combination with the trend of childbearing at older ages.
- The average birth weight at gestational age is 3316 g at 38.7 weeks for singletons, compared with 2333 g at 35.2 weeks for twins, 1700 g at 32.1 weeks for triplets, 1276 g at 29.7 weeks for quadruplets, and 1103 g at 28.4 weeks for quintuplets.
- The accelerated starvation is exaggerated with a multiple gestation, and therefore diet therapy with a diabetic regimen of 20% of calories from protein, 40% of calories from carbohydrate, and 40% of calories from fat is particularly effective.
- The pattern of maternal weight gain has been shown to be as important as total weight gain in its effect on birth weight in both singleton and twin pregnancies. BMI-specific weight gain guidelines are associated with the best intrauterine growth and subsequent birth weights, as well as longer length of gestation.

References

1. Martin JA, Hamilton BE, Sutton PD, Ventura SJ, Menacker F, and Munson ML, *Births: Final Data for 2004. National Vital Statistics Reports*, vol. 55, no. 1 (Hyattsville, MD: National Center for Health Statistics, 2006).

2. Ross MG, Downey CA, Bemis-Heys R, Nguyen M, Jacques DL, and Stanziano G, Prediction by maternal risk factors of neonatal intensive care admissions: evaluation of >59,000 women in national managed care programs. *Am J Obstetr Gynecol* (1999), **181**:835–42.

3. Okah FA, Tsang RC, Sierra R, Brady KK, and Specker BL, Bone turnover and mineral metabolism in the last trimester of pregnancy: effect of multiple gestation. *Obstet Gynecol* (1996), **88**:168–73.

4. Casele HL, Dooley SL, and Metzger BE, Metabolic response to meal eating and extended overnight fast in twin gestation. *Am J Obstet Gynecol* (1996), **175**:917–21.

5. Kaplan M, Eidelman AI, and Aboulafia Y, Fasting and the precipitation of labor: the Yom Kippur effect. *JAMA* (1983), **250**:1317–18.

6. Caruso A, Paradisi G, Ferrazzani S, Lucchese A, Moretti S, and Fulghesu AM, Effect of maternal carbohydrate metabolism on fetal growth. *Obstet Gynecol* (1998), **92**:8–12.

7. Luke B, Nugent C, van de Ven C, Martin D, O'Sullivan MJ, Eardley S, et al., The association between maternal factors and perinatal outcomes in triplet pregnancies. *Am J Obstet Gynecol* (2002), **187**:752–7.

8. Luke B, Brown MB, Misiunas R, Anderson E, Nugent C, van de Ven C, et al., Specialized prenatal care and maternal and infant outcomes in twin pregnancy. *Am J Obstet Gynecol* (2003), **189**: 934–8.

9. Scholl TO, Hediger ML, Fischer RL, and Shearer JW, Anemia vs iron deficiency: increased risk of preterm delivery. *Am J Clin Nutr* (1992), **55**:985–8.

10. Klebanoff MA, Shiono PH, Selby JV, Trachtenberg AI, and Graubard BI, Anemia and spontaneous preterm birth. *Am J Obstet Gynecol* (1991), **164**:59–63.

11. Siega-Riz A, Adair LS, and Hobel CJ, Maternal hematologic changes during pregnancy and the effect of iron status on preterm delivery in a West Los Angeles population. *Am J Perinatol* (1998), **15**:515–22.

12. Tamura T, Goldenberg RL, Johnston KE, Cliver SP, and Hickey CA, Serum ferritin: A predictor of early spontaneous preterm delivery. *Obstet Gynecol* (1996), **87**:360–5.

13. Scholl TO, High third-trimester ferritin concentration: associations with very preterm delivery, infection, and maternal nutritional status. *Obstet Gynecol* (1998), **92**:161–6.

14. Spellacy WN, Handler A, and Ferre CD, A case-control study of 1,253 twin pregnancies from a 1982–1987 prenatal data base. *Obstet Gynecol* (1990), **75**:168–71.

15. Blickstein I, Goldchmit R, and Lurie S, Hemoglobin levels during twin vs singleton pregnancies. *J Reprod Med* (1995), **40**:47–50.

16. Ben Miled S, Bibi D, Khalfi N, Blibech R, Gharbi Y, Castalli R, Khrouf N, Iron stocks and risk of anemia in twins. *Arch Inst Pasteur Tunis* (1989), **66**:221–41.

17. Hediger ML and Luke B, Hemodynamics and maternal weight gain in twin pregnancies. Presented at the American Public Health Association meeting, Chicago, IL, November 9–11, 1999.

18. Gülmezoglu AM, de Onis M, and Villar J, Effectiveness of interventions to prevent or treat impaired fetal growth. *Obstet Gynecol Survey* (1997), **6**:139–49.

19. Kulier R, de Onis M, Gülmezoglu AM, and Villar J, Nutritional interventions for the prevention of maternal morbidity. *Int J Gynecol Obstet* (1998), **63**: 231–46.

20. Villar J, Gülmezoglu AM, and de Onis M, Nutritional and antimicrobial interventions to prevent preterm birth: a review of randomized controlled trials. *Obstet Gynecol Survey* (1998), **53**:575–85.

21. Belizán JM, Villar J, Gonzalez L, Campodonico L, and Bergel E, Calcium supplementation to prevent hypertensive disorders of pregnancy. *N Engl J Med* (1991), **325**:1399–405.

22. Neggers YH, Cutter GR, Acton RT, Alvarez JO, Bonner JL, Goldenberg RL, et al. A positive association between maternal serum zinc concentration and birth weight. *Am J Clin Nutr* (1990), **51**:678–84.

23. Sikorski R, Juszkiewicz T, and Paszkowski T, Zinc status in women with premature rupture of membranes at term. *Obstet Gynecol* (1990), **76**:675–7.

24. Cherry FF, Sandstead HH, Rojas P, Johnson LK, Baston HK, and Wang XB, Adolescent pregnancy: associations among body weight, zinc nutriture, and pregnancy outcome. *Am J Clin Nutr* (1989), **50**:945–54.

25. Goldenberg RL, Tamura T, Neggers Y, Copper RL, Johnston KE, DuBard MB, and Hauth JC, The effect of zinc supplementation on pregnancy outcome. *JAMA* (1995), **274**:463–8.

26. Scholl TO, Hediger ML, Schall JI, Fischer RL, and Khoo C-S, Low zinc intake during pregnancy: its association with preterm and very preterm delivery. *Am J Epidemiol* (1993), **137**:1115–24.

27. Enns CW, Goldman JD, and Cook A, Trends in food and nutrient intakes by adults: NFCS 1977–78, CSFII 1989–91, and

CSFII 1994–95. *Fam Econ Nutr Rev* (1997), **10**:2–15.

28. Scholl TO, Hediger ML, Bendich A, Schall JI, Smith WK, and Krueger PM, Use of multivitamin/mineral prenatal supplements: influence on the outcome of pregnancy. *Am J Epidemiol* (1997), **146**:134–41.

29. Foreman-van Drongelen MM, Zeijdner EE, van Houwelingen AC, Kester AD, Al MD, et al., Essential fatty acid status measured in umbilical vessel walls of infants born after a multiple pregnancy. *Early Hum Dev* (1996), **46**:205–15.

30. Zeijdner EE, van Houwelingen AC, Kester ADM, and Hornstra G, Essential fatty acid status in plasma phospholipids of mother and neonate after multiple pregnancy. *Prostaglandins Leukot Essent Fatty Acids* (1997), **56**:395–401.

31. Olsen SF and Secher NJ, Low consumption of seafood in early pregnancy as a risk factor for preterm delivery: prospective cohort study. *BMJ* (2002), **324**:447–50.

32. Colombo J, Kannass KN, Shaddy DJ, Kundurthi S, Maikranz JM, Anderson CJ, et al., Maternal DHA and the development of attention in infancy and toddlerhood. *Child Dev* (2004), **75**:1254–67.

33. Abrams B and Selvin S, Maternal weight gain pattern and birth weight. *Obstet Gynecol* (1995), **86**:163–9.

34. Scholl TO, Hediger ML, Ances IG, Belsky DH, and Salmon RW, Weight gain during pregnancy in adolescents: predictive ability of early weight gain. *Obstet Gynecol* (1990), **75**:948–53.

35. Luke B, Minogue J, Witter FR, Keith LG, and Johnson TRB, The ideal twin pregnancy: patterns of weight gain, discordancy, and length of gestation. *Am J Obstet Gynecol* (1993), **169**:588–97.

36. Luke B, Gillespie B, Min S-J, Avni M, Witter FR, and O'Sullivan MJ, Critical periods of maternal weight gain: effect on twin birthweight. *Am J Obstet Gynecol* (1997), **177**:1055–62.

37. Luke B, Min S-J, Gillespie B, Avni M, Witter FR, Newman RB, et al., The importance of early weight gain on the intrauterine growth and birthweight of twins. *Am J Obstet Gynecol* (1998), **179**:1155–61.

38. Schieve LA, Cogswell ME, and Scanlon KS, An empiric evaluation of the Institute of Medicine's pregnancy weight gain guidelines by race. *Obstet Gynecol* (1998), **91**:878–84.

39. Caulfield LE, Stoltzfus RJ, and Witter FR, Implications of the Institute of Medicine weight gain recommendations for preventing adverse pregnancy outcomes in black and white women. *Am J Public Health* (1998), **88**: 1168–74.

40. Cogswell ME, Scanlon KS, Fein SB, and Schieve LA, Medically advised, mother's personal target, and actual weight gain during pregnancy. *Obstet Gynecol* (1999), **94**:616–22.

41. Taffel SM and Keppel KG, Advice about weight gain during pregnancy and actual weight gain. *Am J Public Health* (1986), **76**:1396–9.

42. Luke B, Keith L, and Keith D, Maternal nutrition in twin gestations: weight gain, cravings and aversions, and sources of nutrition advice. *Acta Genet Med Gemellol* (1997), **46**:157–66.

43. Luke B, Hediger ML, Nugent C, Newman RB, Mauldin JG, Witter FR, and O'Sullivan MJ, Body mass index specific-weight gains associated with optimal birthweights in twin pregnancies. *J Reprod Med* (2003), **48**:217–24.

44. Lantz ME, Chez RA, Rodriguez A, and Porter KB, Maternal weight gain patterns and birth weight outcome in twin gestations. *Obstet Gynecol* (1996), **87**:551–6.

45. Taggart NR, Holiday RM, and Billewicz WZ, Changes in skinfolds during pregnancy. *Br J Nutr* (1967), **21**:439–51.

46. MacGillivray I and Campbell DM, The physical characteristics and adaptations of women with twin pregnancies. In: Twin Research: Clinical Studies (New York: Alan R. Liss, 1978), pp. 81–6.

47. Williams RL, Creasy RK, Cunningham GC, Hawes WE, Norris FD, Tashiro M, Fetal growth and perinatal viability in California. *Obstet Gynecol* (1982), **59**:624–32.

48. Young M, Placental factors and fetal nutrition. *Am J Clin Nutr* (1981), **34**:738–43.

49. Elster AD, Bleyl JL, and Craven TE, Birth weight standards for triplets under modern obstetric care in the United States, 1984–1989. *Obstet Gynecol* (1991), **77**:387–93.

Specialized requirements

Mineral and vitamin supplementation before, during, and after conception

Y. Ingrid Goh

Adequate quantities of vitamins and minerals are essential for the development of the embryo, fetus, and neonate. These substances are involved in cell growth and differentiation and are central components of cell structure, cell signaling, protein translation, enzymes, catalytic enzyme sites, and enzymatic reactions. Together, these processes are critical for organ development in the fetus. The critical period of organogenesis occurs at 20 to 60 days gestation [1, 2]. The brain, however, is especially vulnerable to nutritional insults because it develops through the entire course of pregnancy and after birth. Deficiencies in vitamins and minerals may result in a disruption of normal development, leading to undesirable outcomes such as increased rates of spontaneous abortion, congenital malformation, or fetal death. This chapter highlights the importance of vitamin and mineral supplementation before, during, and after conception. It is important to note that although the following studies discuss the use of multivitamins, multivitamins vary in composition from study to study, which may have an overall influence on the effects.

The importance of multivitamin supplementation during pregnancy dates back to the 1960s, when a case-control study by Smithells demonstrated that prenatal multivitamin supplementation was protective against neural tube defects (NTDs) [3]. A large cohort study by Milunsky et al. also observed a decreased incidence of NTDs (1.1/1 000 multivitamin supplemented vs. 3.5/1 000 unsupplemented) [4]. Several studies published by Czeizel et al. indicate that folic acid–containing multivitamins are associated with a decreased risk of NTDs [5, 6]. However, the most significant trial demonstrating this relationship was a multicenter randomized double-blinded trial headed by the United Kingdom Medical Research Council [7]. In this study 1817 women who had previously delivered a child with an NTD were randomized to one of four treatments: folic acid (4 mg), folic acid (4 mg) and a multivitamin, multivitamin without folic

acid, or no supplementation. Supplementation commenced 1 month before conception and continued through the first 12 weeks of pregnancy. Supplementation with multivitamin containing folic acid resulted in 3 of 256 (1.17%) children with NTD, whereas no supplementation resulted in 11 of 260 (4.23%) children born with NTD [7]. A 72% protective effect was associated with folic acid supplementation (relative risk [RR] = 0.28, 95% confidence interval [CI] 0.12–0.71) [7]. A meta-analysis of the available literature observed that folic acid–containing multivitamins resulted in an odds ratio (OR) = 0.67, 95% CI 0.58–0.77 in case-control studies and an OR = 0.52, 95% CI 0.39–0.69 in cohort and randomized controlled studies (Table 16.1) [8].

Multivitamin supplementation has also been associated with decreased risk for other congenital malformations including oral clefts and congenital heart defects (CHDs) [6, 9–11]. A retrospective study of women who delivered a child with oral cleft observed a 3.1% incidence in the multivitamin-supplemented mothers, whereas a 4.8% incidence was observed in unsupplemented mothers [9]. Another case-control study observed a 50% decrease in cleft palate with cleft lip (OR = 0.5, 95% CI 0.36–0.68) and a 27% decrease in cleft palate without cleft lip (OR = 0.73, 95% CI 0.46–1.2) with multivitamin supplementation [12]. A meta-analysis of the available literature observed that supplementation with prenatal multivitamins resulted in an OR = 0.76, 95% CI 0.62–0.93 of cleft palate in case-control studies and an OR = 0.42, 95% CI 0.06–2.84 in cohort and randomized controlled studies (Table 16.1) [8]. This was similar for oral cleft with or without cleft palate: OR = 0.63, 95% CI 0.54–0.73 in case-control studies and OR = 0.58, 95% CI 0.28–1.19 for cohort and randomized controlled studies (Table 16.1) [8]. These protective effects were confirmed by a meta-analysis in which vitamin supplementation was associated with reduction in the incidence of cleft lip and palate (RR = 0.51, 95%

Table 16.1 Dietary reference intakes recommended for pregnant individuals

	Case-control	Cohort and randomized control trial
Neural tube defect	OR = 0.67, 95% CI 0.58–0.77	OR = 0.52, 95% CI 0.39–0.69
Cleft palate	OR = 0.76, 95% CI 0.62–0.93	OR = 0.42, 95% CI 0.06–2.84
Cleft lip without palate	OR = 0.63, 95% CI 0.54–0.73	OR = 0.58, 95% CI 0.28–1.19
Urinary tract anomalies	OR = 0.48, 95% CI 0.30–0.76	OR = 0.68, 95% CI 0.35–1.31
Cardiovascular defects	OR = 0.78, 95% CI 0.67–0.92	OR = 0.61, 95% CI 0.40–0.92
Limb defects	OR = 0.57, 95% CI 0.38–0.85	OR = 0.25, 95% CI 0.05–1.15
Congenital hydrocephalus	OR = 0.37, 95% CI 0.24–0.56	OR = 1.54, 95% CI 0.53–4.50

From Goh YI, Bollano E, Einarson TR, Koren G, Prenatal multivitamin supplementation and rates of congenital anomalies: a meta-analysis. *J Obstet Gynaecol Can* (2006), 28:680–9.

CI 0.32–0.95), cleft palate (RR = 1.19, 95% CI 0.43–3.28), and all clefts (RR = 0.55, 95% CI 0.32–0.95) in prospective studies; cleft lip and palate (RR = 0.77, 95% CI 0.65–0.90), cleft palate (RR = 0.80, 95% CI 0.6–0.93), and all clefts (RR = 0.78, 95% CI 0.71–0.85) in case-control studies [13].

Several studies by Czeizel et al. observed that folic acid–containing multivitamins decreased the occurrence of CHDs (RR = 0.48, 95% CI 0.23–1.03) in one study and (OR = 0.60, 95% CI 0.38–0.96) in another [6, 14]. Botto et al. observed decreased rates as well (RR = 0.48, 95% CI 0.20–0.89) [15]. Prenatal multivitamin supplementation was specifically associated with a decreased occurrence of heart defect (OR = 1.8, 95% CI 1.4–2.4), tricuspid atresia (OR = 5.2), obstructive defects (OR = 2.7), transposition of great arteries (OR = 1.9), and ventral septal defect (OR = 1.8) compared with unsupplemented mothers [16]. A meta-analysis of the available literature observed that supplementation with prenatal multivitamins resulted in a decreased association of cardiovascular defects in both case-control studies (OR = 0.78, 95% CI 0.67–0.92) and cohort and randomized controlled studies (OR = 0.61, 95% CI 0.40–0.92) [8].

Studies investigating the effects of prenatal multivitamin supplementation on urinary tract development observed a 78% reduced risk for urinary tract anomalies compared with the unsupplemented group (RR = 0.22, 95% CI 0.05–0.99) [17]. A retrospective case-control study observed that supplementation in the first trimester was associated with an 85% reduction in risk of having a child with urinary tract anomalies (OR = 0.15, 95% CI 0.05–0.43); the most noticeable decrease was that of hydronephrosis (OR = 0.12, 95% CI 0.04–0.38) [18]. A reduction in stenosis/atresia

of the pelvic-ureteric junction was observed in children born to women who took prenatal multivitamins (OR = 0.19, 95% CI 0.04–0.86) [6]. A meta-analysis of the available literature observed that supplementation with prenatal multivitamins resulted in an OR = 0.48, 95% CI 0.30–0.76 in case-control studies, and OR = 0.68, 95% CI 0.35–1.31 in cohort and randomized controlled studies [8].

Czeizel et al. observed that the incidence of limbs defects was lower in women who supplemented with multivitamins compared with unsupplemented women [5]. Shaw et al. also observed that supplementation with multivitamins was associated with a 35% decrease in limb defects (OR = 0.65, 95% CI 0.43–0.99) [11]. A meta-analysis of the available literature observed that supplementation with prenatal multivitamins resulted in an OR = 0.48, 95% CI 0.30–0.76 in case control studies, and OR = 0.57, 95% CI 0.38–0.85 in cohort and randomized controlled studies [8].

The literature regarding the relationship of prenatal multivitamin supplementation and omphalocele, pyloric stenosis, and imperforate anus is limited. One case-control study observed that multivitamin supplementation was associated with a 60% reduction in nonsyndromic omphalocele (OR = 0.4, 95% CI 0.2–1.0) [19]. A study by Czeizel et al. observed a lower incidence of hyperpyloric stenosis in women with prenatal multivitamin supplementation compared with women without supplementation [5]. This protective effect, however, was not observed by Correa-Villaseñor et al. [20]. One study observed that prenatal multivitamin supplementation was associated with a 50% decrease in imperforate anus [21].

Prenatal multivitamin supplementation has also been associated with decreasing the risk for pediatric cancers [22–24]. Several studies have been published associating prenatal multivitamin supplementation with the decrease of pediatric brain tumors. Preston-Martin et al. were the first to observe this relationship (OR = 0.6, p = 0.12) [22]. These results were supported by findings by Bunin et al. (OR = 0.56, p = 0.02) [25]. Primitive neuroectodermal tumors (PNET), specifically, were noted to decrease with prenatal multivitamin supplementation (OR = 0.38, p = 0.005) [25]. An additional study by this group further noted that supplementation was associated with a decreased risk of astrocytoma [26]. Further confirmation of these findings of decreased PNET and astrocytoma was observed in the studies by Preston-Martin et al. [23] An international study of more than 1 000 women observed that prenatal multivitamin supplementation in the first two trimesters of pregnancy was associated with a decreased risk for brain tumors in children aged under 5 years (OR = 0.7, 95% CI 0.5–0.9) [24]. Moreover, a greater reduction was observed when supplementation occurred over all three trimesters of pregnancy (OR = 0.5, 95% CI 0.3–0.8) [24]. A retrospective population-based study observed that prenatal multivitamin supplementation was associated with a decreased risk of medulloblastomas [27]. A meta-analysis of the available literature observed that folic acid containing multivitamins resulted in an OR = 0.73, 95% CI 0.60–0.88 for pediatric brain tumors [28].

Some studies have also suggested that prenatal multivitamins decrease the risk for acute lymphoblastic leukemia (ALL) [29, 30]. A case-control study by Sarasua and Savitz observed that prenatal multivitamin supplementation was associated with a decreased risk for ALL [29]. A decrease in ALL was also observed in a case-control study by Wen et al. (OR = 0.7, 99% CI 0.5–1.0) [30]. Ross et al. also noted that multivitamin supplementation was associated with a decreased risk for ALL (OR = 0.51, 95% CI 0.30–0.89). A meta-analysis of the available literature observed that folic acid–containing multivitamins resulted in an OR = 0.61, 95% CI 0.50–0.74 for ALL [28].

Prenatal multivitamin supplementation has also been associated with a decreased risk for neuroblastoma [31, 32]. A case-control study by Michalek et al. reported a decreased risk for neuroblastoma (OR = 0.28, 95% CI 0.03–0.69) [31], as did a case-control study by Olshan et al. (OR = 0.6, 95% CI 0.4–0.9) [32]. A meta-analysis of the available literature observed that folic acid–containing multivitamins

resulted in an OR = 0.53, 95% CI 0.42–0.68 for neuroblastoma [28].

Prenatal multivitamin has been shown to have benefits for both human immunodeficiency virus (HIV)-infected women and their babies. A double-blinded trial demonstrated that HIV-1-infected women receiving multivitamins had a higher hemoglobin concentration than women who did not receive multivitamins (p = 0.07) [33]. In addition, they had a 63% lower risk of macrocytic anemia (RR = 0.37, 95% CI 0.18–0.79, p = 0.01), and children also had reduced risk of anemia [33]. Supplementation was also associated with a decreased incidence of low birth weight (RR = 0.82; 95% CI 0.70–0.95; p = 0.01), lower rates of fetal death (RR = 0.87; 95% CI 0.72–1.05; p = 0.15), reduction in the risk of a birth size that was small for gestational age (RR = 0.77; 95% CI 0.68–0.87; p < 0.001), increase in Psychomotor Development Index score of 2.6 in children aged 6 to 18 months (95% confidence interval 0.1–5.1), reduction in the development of hypertension during pregnancy (RR = 0.62, 95% CI 0.40–0.94, p = 0.03), reduction in maternal mortality, reduction in risk of progression of HIV to Stage IV disease, and reduction in early-child mortality among immunologically and nutritionally comprised women [34–37].

There are different risk groups for vitamin deficiency in pregnancy, including genetic factors and concomitant medications. Genetic factors that may result in malabsorption of vitamins and minerals include genetic mutations; maternal disease including liver, renal, cancer, gastrointestinal, diabetes, and cancer; concomitant medications; and interactions with other vitamins and minerals. Drugs that may alter maternal levels of multivitamins include methotrexate and valproic acid.

Women actively planning pregnancy should supplement with a prenatal multivitamin. Supplementation to prevent birth defects has been shown to be cost-effective [38–41]. Supplementation should commence approximately 3 to 4 months before the planned pregnancy to permit the body to achieve protective levels of vitamins and minerals such as folate. This, however, may be difficult because 50% of pregnancies are unplanned [42]. A possible solution to this dilemma is to encourage women of childbearing potential to incorporate multivitamin supplementation into their daily routine.

Some women believe that multivitamin supplementation is required only in the first trimester of

Table 16.2 Dietary reference intakes recommended for pregnant individuals

Micronutrient	Dietary reference intakes
Vitamin A (retinol)	770 µg/day
Vitamin B$_1$ (thiamine)	1.4 mg/day
Vitamin B$_2$ (riboflavin)	1.4 mg/day
Vitamin B$_3$ (niacin)	18 mg/day
Vitamin B$_5$ (pantothenic acid)	6 mg/day
Vitamin B$_6$ (pyridoxine)	1.9 mg/day
Vitamin B$_9$ (folate)	600 µg/day
Vitamin B$_{12}$ (cobalamin)	2.6 mg/day
Vitamin C (ascorbic acid)	85 mg/day
Vitamin D	5 µg/day
Vitamin E (tocopherol)	15 mg/day

Source: Dietary Reference Intakes: Recommended Intakes for Individuals (PDF 87 KB) (Washington, DC: Food and Nutrition Board, Institute of Medicine, National Academy of Sciences, 2004). Available at: http://www.iom.edu/Object.File/Master/21/372/0.pdf.

pregnancy. This is untrue. Supplementation should, as previously mentioned, commence before pregnancy and continue through the entire pregnancy and during lactation. It is true that the first trimester is a critical time for structural formation of the fetus. However, during the second and third trimesters, the brain of the fetus is continually forming, and the fetus itself is growing at a rapid pace. As such, adequate macronutrient supply during the entire pregnancy is necessary. Moreover, supplementation should continue after pregnancy into the period of lactation. In cases in which the mother is unable to attain a well-balanced diet (e.g. for medical, socioeconomic, physical, or emotional reasons), multivitamin supplementation will assist her in achieving a balance of vitamins and minerals regardless of her dietary habits. For instance, calcium and vitamin D will assist in the maintenance of bone mineral density. Supplementing with multivitamins will also help replenish nutrients necessary for the production of blood to replenish blood that is lost during delivery. Moreover, multivitamin supplementation during lactation will ensure that the baby is being breast-fed milk containing sufficient nutrients (Table 16.2).

The formulations of prenatal multivitamins usually vary between manufacturers; however, they generally comprise a combination including vitamin A (beta-carotene and/or acetate), vitamin B$_1$ (thiamine),

vitamin B$_2$ (riboflavin), vitamin B$_3$ (niacin), vitamin B$_5$ (pantothenic acid), vitamin B$_6$ (pyridoxine), vitamin B$_9$ (folic acid), vitamin B$_{12}$ (cyanocobalamin), vitamin C (ascorbic acid), vitamin D, vitamin E, calcium, chromium, copper, iodine, iron, magnesium, manganese, molybdenum, selenium, and zinc (Table 16.2). The following sections review their importance during pregnancy.

Vitamin A

Vitamin A is a fat-soluble, antioxidant vitamin that is important in growth, epithelial tissue proliferation, and vision. Vitamin A is an important component of photoreceptor cells, and as such it is important for the development of the eyes. Vitamin A deficiency results in irreversible impairment or loss of vision in 250 000 to 500 000 preschool-aged children in the Third World annually [43, 44]. Vitamin A and its synthetic congeners, the retinoids, have been proven to be active human teratogens. The minimum teratogenic dose during pregnancy has not been established, and thus doses exceeding the recommended daily amount (RDA) should be avoided. Vitamin A is transported and stored in a nontoxic protein-bound form. Congenital malformations are seen only when the storage capacity of 25 000 to 50 000 IU is exceeded. High exposure of vitamin A in utero can result in retinoid syndrome. This is characterized by central nervous system malformation, cardiovascular malformations, and musculoskeletal abnormalities [45]. A study comparing women consuming 8 000 to 25 000 IU with those who had less than 5 000 IU vitamin A daily observed no increased risk for malformations (OR = 0.73, 95% CI 0.27–1.96) or cranial neural crest defects (OR = 1.09, 95% CI 0.24–4.98) compared with the control group [46]. Conversely, a study by Rothman et al. reported that women who ingested more than 10 000 IU per day of vitamin A supplements had an increased risk for delivering a child with a congenital malformation [47]. Dietary sources of vitamin A include animal-derived products such as eggs, liver, meat, and fruits and vegetables containing beta-carotene.

Vitamin B$_1$ (thiamine)

Vitamin B$_1$ is a water-soluble vitamin essential for metabolism of carbohydrates as well as for nerve and heart function. Pregnant women have substantially greater than normal need for vitamin B$_1$ [48]. Deficiency in this vitamin may arise from inadequate dietary intake, increased dietary requirements, hyperemesis gravidarum, and malabsorption due to gastrointestinal disorders, alcohol abuse, HIV, genetic factors, or drugs [49]. Lower vitamin B_1 content in blood cells has been observed in fetuses with severe intrauterine growth retardation versus controls [50, 51]. Dietary sources of vitamin B_1 include cereal products, brewer's yeast, meat, poultry, and legumes.

Vitamin B_2 (riboflavin)

Vitamin B_2 is a water-soluble vitamin that is essential for the metabolism of carbohydrates and amino acids. It also integral for tissue respiration and indirectly maintains erythrocyte integrity. Riboflavin has been positively correlated with fetal growth [52]. Dietary sources of riboflavin include liver, almonds, soy nuts, shellfish, eggs, and dairy products.

Vitamin B_3 (niacin)

Vitamin B_3 is a water-soluble vitamin. It is metabolized to niacinamide, an essential component of nicotinamide adenine dinucleotide (NAD) and nicotinamide adenine dinucleotide phosphate (NADP) coenzymes for glycogenesis, tissue respiration, and lipid metabolism. One study suggested that periconceptional intake of vitamin B_3 decreased the risk of orofacial clefts [53]. Dietary sources of vitamin B_3 include meat, nuts, and cereals.

Vitamin B_5 (pantothenic acid)

Pantothenic acid is a water-soluble vitamin that is an important component of the coenzyme A in the transfer of acyl groups in the oxidation and synthesis of fatty acids and in the metabolism of carbohydrates, fats, and proteins [54]. Elevated circulating levels of pantothenic acid are detected in the fetus [55]. Maternal pantothenic acid deficiency can result in teratogenic effects [55]. Animal studies have also suggested protection against NTDs [56]. Dietary sources of pantothenic acid include liver, beef, and sunflower seeds.

Vitamin B_6 (pyridoxine)

Vitamin B_6 is a water-soluble vitamin that is essential for the metabolism of amino acids and fatty acids for normal nerve function and formation of antibodies and red blood cells. Vitamin B_6 has been help-ful in the management of nausea and vomiting during pregnancy [57]. Dietary sources of vitamin B_6 include bananas, carrots, nuts, fish, liver, and whole grains.

Vitamin B_9 (folic acid)

Vitamin B_9 is a water-soluble vitamin that is essential in the formation of red blood cells and genetic material. Folic acid is required for the synthesis of methionine from homocysteine [58]. Methionine is a cofactor for many methylation reactions including the methylation of deoxyribonucleic acid (DNA), ribonucleic acid (RNA), proteins, and neurotransmitters [59–62]. Therefore, all new-cell formation is dependent on an adequate supply of folic acid. Folate deficiency in rapidly dividing cells may lead to alterations in DNA synthesis and chromosomal aberrations, resulting in impaired cell formation and tissue growth; consequently maternal folate requirements increase during pregnancy [60, 63, 64].

Folic acid has long been known to decrease the risk of NTDs. One small double-blinded trial randomized women who had previously delivered a child with NTD to receive 4 mg folic acid supplementation or placebo [65]. In none of the 44 children were NTDs observed in the supplemented group, whereas 6 of 61 NTDs were observed in the unsupplemented group [65]. Similarly, an observational study reported a 0 in 227 recurrence of NTDs in a folic acid–supplemented group, whereas 2 in 213 NTDs were observed in the unsupplemented group [66]. A cohort study of women supplementing with 5 mg of folic acid also observed no recurrence of NTDs in supplemented women, whereas a 3% recurrence was observed in unsupplemented women [67]. Many other trials have examined the effect of folic acid during pregnancy and have also observed a reduction in risk for NTDs [68, 69].

To investigate whether the dosage of folic acid affects the rate of reduction of NTDs, the California Birth Defects Monitoring Program conducted a case-control study comparing 538 children with NTDs and 540 controls [70]. Women who reported any use of folic acid from 3 months before or 3 months after conception had an overall lower risk of having a child with NTDs (OR = 0.60, 95% CI 0.46–0.79) [70]. Women taking folic acid 0.4 to 0.9 mg had a further reduced risk. Women who supplemented with less than 0.4 mg did not have important reductions in risk (OR = 0.99) [70]. The only available study investigating serum folate concentrations found an inverse relation between maternal cell folate and the risk of NTD [71]. Daly et al. showed in a case-control study that women receiving less than 150 μg or more than 400 μg of folic acid had a 6.6 in 1 000 and 0.8 in 1 000 chance of delivering a child with NTD, respectively [72]. Supplementation at different doses of 100 μg, 200 μg, and 400 μg resulted in a 22%, 41%, and 47% decreased risk in NTD, respectively [72]. Another study investigating dosing variations of folic acid corroborated this result, noting that 100 μg, 200 μg, and 400 μg folic acid decreased NTD by 18%, 35%, and 53%, respectively [73].

An interventional time series analysis observed a 0.157 in 1 000 to 0.062 in 1 000 decrease in the incidence of neuroblastoma after the introduction of folic acid fortification of flour with an adjusted incidence (RR = 0.38, 95% CI 0.23–0.62) [74]. Not only is folic acid beneficial in decreasing the risk for birth defects, it can also treat anemia during pregnancy [75] and decrease the risk of premature births [76].

Folic acid is especially important for women who are using folate antagonists (e.g. valproic acid, methotrexate) or have medical conditions (e.g. celiac disease) in which folate is poorly absorbed. Women using folate antagonists are generally recommended to use 5 mg of folate. Some people have questioned whether folic acid is associated with an increased rate of cancers. Studies have suggested that it is protective against some cancers [77–85]. Because folic acid plays an important role in the cell cycle, theoretically, if all cells were healthy, then there would not be an issue. It is only if there are cancerous cells that folate would assist in their replication. However, the majority of existing literature supports a relationship of cancer protection.

The minimum recommendation by health authorities is 0.4 mg folic acid supplementation for pregnancy [86–88]. Studies of folic acid dosing have ranged up to 10 mg during pregnancy without any reported adverse events. Recently the U.S. Centers for Disease Control and Prevention and a Canadian study reported that women of childbearing age did not have protective levels of folate in their blood [89, 90]. Daly et al. showed that protective levels should be 900 nM folate [72]. In light of this information, it has been suggested that the current requirements of folic acid should be increased to 5 mg in prenatal multivitamins [91]. Previous studies of women receiving 5 mg of folic acid reported no adverse effects toward the fetus [67]. Because half of pregnancies are unplanned, women discovering that

they are pregnant who have not begun supplementing may benefit from supplementing with 5 mg of folic acid in their multivitamin to increase the available folate in their bloodstream quickly. One manufacturer has already begun manufacturing a prenatal multivitamin contain 5 mg folic acid, which can be purchased by prescription. Dietary sources of folate include fortified grains and green leafy vegetables.

Vitamin B$_{12}$ (cobalamin)

Vitamin B$_{12}$ is a water-soluble vitamin required for growth, cell production, DNA synthesis, and erythropoiesis. Cobalamin is a cofactor in folate-dependent homocysteine metabolism. It is involved in the methylation of homocysteine to form methionine and tetrahydrofolate as well as the conversion of methylmalonyl-coenzyme A to succinyl-coenzyme A [92]. Humans are unable to synthesize cobalamin [93]. Vitamin B$_{12}$ deficiency can result in defective DNA synthesis, reduced rate of cell multiplication, and metabolism disorders, which may lead to a megaloblastic anemia or neurological abnormalities [94, 95].

Vitamin B$_{12}$ deficiency is uncommon because dietary requirements are usually met with the omnivorous diet, and the vitamin is conserved efficiently by enterohepatic circulation [96]. Cobalamin deficiency may occur because of low dietary intake (strict vegetarian diets) but also because of disturbance of the absorption, transport, or cellular uptake or genetic variations in transcobalamin II [97, 98]. Vitamin B$_{12}$ deficiency has been associated with folate deficiency (methyl-folate trap) [99–101].

A steady fall in serum cobalamin level has been shown throughout pregnancy [102]. This fall is rationalized by increase plasma volume, changes in hormonal status, and increased vitamin requirements [103]. During pregnancy, blood homocysteine levels decrease during the first and second trimesters and slightly increase during the third trimester [104]. Deficiency may result in hyperhomocysteinemia [92, 105].

Hyperhomocysteinemia has been associated with several pregnancy complications including repeated miscarriages [106, 107], preeclampsia [108, 109], abruptio placentae [110, 111], NTDs [112–115], intrauterine growth retardation [111, 116], and fetal death [111]. It is also hypothesized that hyperhomocysteinemia may increase the risk for megaloblastic anemia and neuropsychiatric symptoms, which may occur even before the onset of megaloblastic anemia [117–120] and thrombosis in pregnancy and postpartum [121, 122]. Dietary sources of vitamin B_{12} include liver, dairy products, and fortified cereals.

Vitamin C (ascorbic acid)

Vitamin C is a water-soluble vitamin required for collagen formation for bone and connective tissue and various other metabolic processes, including the conversion of folic acid to folinic acid and iron metabolism. In addition, this antioxidant maintains the mechanical strength of amniotic membranes and assists in the absorption of iron.

Pregnant women exposed to less than 2 000 mg vitamin C reported no adverse effects [123]. A meta-analysis of vitamin C in pregnancy revealed similar results [124]. One study suggested an association between low maternal ascorbic acid levels and increased frequency of premature rupture of amniotic membranes [125]. This prompted investigations of vitamin C in preventing preeclampsia. High doses of vitamin C and vitamin E in combination to treat preeclampsia initially suggested a protective effect [126]. However, this combination has recently been associated with low birth weight [127, 128]. One study suggested that this effect may be due to vitamin E [129]. Further studies need to be undertaken to determine the effects of vitamin C during pregnancy. Dietary sources of vitamin C include oranges, fruits, and vegetables.

Vitamin D

Vitamin D is a fat-soluble vitamin required for the absorption of calcium and phosphorus. A study of 15 mothers supplementing with vitamin D to treat hypoparathyroidism observed that 107 000 IU daily did not increase the risk for malformations, and follow-up at 16 years of age also observed no differ-ences [130]. Another study of mothers treated with 0.25 to 3.25 μg/day calcitriol (1,25(OH)2D3, a vitamin D analogue) for hypoparathyroidism observed no adverse effects in the babies [131]. Daily vitamin D requirements can be met with adequate sun/ultraviolet light exposure.

Vitamin E (tocopherol)

Vitamin E is a fat-soluble vitamin that is important in maintaining the integrity of the cell membrane, and it protects cells against oxidative damage by free radicals. Four double-blinded trials in women at high risk of preeclampsia randomized participants to receive high doses of vitamin E (400–800 IU) in the second and third trimesters of pregnancy [126, 132, 133]. No difference was observed between supplemented and unsupplemented women for the risk of stillbirth, perinatal death, preterm birth, intrauterine growth restriction, or mean birth weight [134]. One study reported that concentrations of vitamin E were positively related to increased fetal growth [135].

Vitamin C and vitamin E have a synergistic effect as antioxidants. High doses of vitamin C and vitamin E were used in combination to treat preeclampsia. Recently it was shown that this combination may result in low birth weight [128]. A cohort study of women exposed to 400 to 1 200 IU of vitamin E during the first trimester of pregnancy observed no significant differences in rates of live births, preterm deliveries, miscarriages, stillbirths, or malformations. There was, however, an apparent decrease in mean birth weight in the supplemented group compared with controls ($p = 0.001$) [129]. Dietary sources of vitamin E include wheat germ oil, sunflower oil, green leafy vegetables, and peanuts.

Conclusion

Prenatal multivitamin supplementation is beneficial to the development of the fetus, and therefore, women actively planning pregnancy should supplement daily.

References

1. Wilson CW, Letter: vitamin C and fertility. *Lancet* (1973), **7833**:859–60.

2. Arey LB, *Developmental Anatomy: A Textbook and Laboratory Manual of Embryology* (Philadelphia: Saunders, 1974).

3. Smithells RW, Incidence of congenital abnormalities in Liverpool, 1960–64. *Br J Prev Soc Med* (1968), **1**:36–7.

4. Milunsky A, Jick H, Jick SS, Bruell CL, MacLaughlin DS, Rothman KJ, and Willett W, Multivitamin/folic acid supplementation in early pregnancy reduces the prevalence of neural tube defects. *JAMA* (1989), **20**:2847–52.

5. Czeizel AE and Dudas I, Prevention of the first occurrence of neural-tube defects by periconceptional vitamin supplementation. *N Engl J Med* (1992), **26**:1832–5.

6. Czeizel AE, Dobó M, and Vargha P, Hungarian cohort-controlled trial of periconceptional multivitamin supplementation shows a reduction in certain congenital abnormalities. *Birth Defects Res A Clin Mol Teratol* (2004), **11**:853–61.

7. MRC Vitamin Study Research Group, Prevention of neural tube defects: results of the Medical Research Council Vitamin Study. *Lancet* (1991), **8760**:131–7.

8. Goh YI, Bollano E, Einarson TR, and Koren G, Prenatal multivitamin supplementation and rates of congenital anomalies: a meta-analysis. *J Obstet Gynaecol Can* (2006), **8**:680–9.

9. Briggs RM, Vitamin supplementation as a possible factor in the incidence of cleft lip/palate deformities in humans. *Clin Plast Surg* (1976), **4**:647–52.

10. Tolarova M and Harris J, Reduced recurrence of orofacial clefts after periconceptional supplementation with high-dose folic acid and multivitamins. *Teratology* (1995), **2**:71–8.

11. Shaw GM, O'Malley CD, Wasserman CR, Tolarova MM, and Lammer EJ, Maternal periconceptional use of multivitamins and reduced risk for conotruncal heart defects and limb deficiencies among offspring. *Am J Med Genet* (1995), **4**:536–45.

12. Shaw GM, Lammer EJ, Wasserman CR, O'Malley CD, and Tolarova MM, Risks of orofacial clefts in children born to women using multivitamins containing folic acid periconceptionally. *Lancet* (1995), **8972**:393–6.

13. Badovinac RL, Werler MM, Williams PL, Kelsey KT, and Hayes C, Folic acid-containing supplement consumption during pregnancy and risk for oral clefts: A meta-analysis. *Birth Defects Res A Clin Mol Teratol* (2007), **1**:8–15.

14. Czeizel AE and Susanszky E, Diet intake and vitamin supplement use of Hungarian women during the preconceptional period. *Int J Vitam Nutr Res* (1994), **4**:300–5.

15. Botto LD, Khoury MJ, and Mulinare J, *Periconceptional Use of Vitamins and the Prevention of Conotruncal Heart Defects: Evidence From a Population-Based Case-Control Study*. Presented at the 4th Annual Epidemic Intelligence Service Conference, 1995.

16. Botto LD, Mulinare J, and Erickson JD, Occurrence of congenital heart defects in relation to maternal mulitivitamin use. *Am J Epidemiol* (2000), **9**:878–84.

17. Czeizel AE, Dudas I, and Metneki J, Pregnancy outcomes in a randomised controlled trial of periconceptional multivitamin supplementation. Final report. *Arch Gynecol Obstet* (1994), **3**:131–9.

18. Li DK, Daling JR, Mueller BA, Hickok DE, Fantel AG, and Weiss NS, Periconceptional multivitamin use in relation to the risk of congenital urinary tract anomalies. *Epidemiology* (1995), **3**:212–18.

19. Botto LD, Mulinare J, and Erickson JD, Occurrence of omphalocele in relation to maternal multivitamin use: a population-based study. *Pediatrics* (2002), **5**:904–8.

20. Correa-Villaseñor A, Cragan J, Kucik J, O'Leary L, Siffel C, and Williams L, The Metropolitan Atlanta Congenital Defects Program: 35 years of birth defects surveillance at the Centers for Disease Control and Prevention. *Birth Defects Res A Clin Mol Teratol* (2003), **9**:617–24.

21. Myers MF, Li S, Correa-Villasenor A, Li Z, Moore CA, Hong SX, and Berry RJ, Folic acid supplementation and risk for imperforate anus in China. *Am J Epidemiol* (2001), **11**:1051–6.

22. Preston-Martin S, Yu MC, Benton B, and Henderson BE, N-Nitroso compounds and childhood brain tumors: a case-control study. *Cancer Res* (1982), **12**:5240–5.

23. Preston-Martin S, Pogoda JM, Mueller BA, Holly EA, Lijinsky W, and Davis RL, Maternal consumption of cured meats and vitamins in relation to pediatric brain tumors. *Cancer Epidemiol Biomarkers Prev* (1996), **8**:599–605.

24. Preston-Martin S, Pogoda JM, Mueller BA, Lubin F, Modan B, Holly EA, et al., Prenatal vitamin supplementation and pediatric brain tumors: huge international variation in use and possible reduction in risk. *Childs Nerv Syst* (1998), **10**:551–7.

25. Bunin GR, Kuijten RR, Buckley JD, Rorke LB, and Meadows AT, Relation between maternal diet and subsequent primitive neuroectodermal brain tumors in

young children. *N Engl J Med* (1993), **8**:536–41.

26. Bunin GR, Buckley JD, Boesel CP, Rorke LB, and Meadows AT, Risk factors for astrocytic glioma and primitive neuroectodermal tumor of the brain in young children: a report from the Children's Cancer Group. *Cancer Epidemiol Biomarkers Prev* (1994), **3**:197–204.

27. Thorne RN, Pearson AD, Nicoll JA, Coakham HB, Oakhill A, Mott MG, and Foreman NK, Decline in incidence of medulloblastoma in children. *Cancer* (1994), **12**:3240–4.

28. Goh YI, Bollano E, Einarson TR, and Koren G, Prenatal multivitamin supplementation and rates of pediatric cancers: a meta-analysis. *Clin Pharmacol Ther* (2007), **5**:685–91.

29. Sarasua S and Savitz DA, Cured and broiled meat consumption in relation to childhood cancer: Denver, Colorado (United States). *Cancer Causes Control* (1994), **2**:141–8.

30. Wen W, Shu XO, Potter JD, Severson RK, Buckley JD, Reaman GH, and Robison LL, Parental medication use and risk of childhood acute lymphoblastic leukemia. *Cancer* (2002), **8**:1786–94.

31. Michalek AM, Buck GM, Nasca PC, Freedman AN, Baptiste MS, and Mahoney MC, Gravid health status, medication use, and risk of neuroblastoma. *Am J Epidemiol* (1996), **10**:996–1001.

32. Olshan AF, Smith JC, Bondy ML, Neglia JP, and Pollock BH, Maternal vitamin use and reduced risk of neuroblastoma. *Epidemiology* (2002), **5**:575–80.

33. Fawzi WW, Msamanga GI, Kupka R, Spiegelman D, Villamor E, Mugusi F, et al., Multivitamin supplementation improves hematologic status in HIV-infected women and their

children in Tanzania. *Am J Clin Nutr* (2007), **5**:1335–43.

34. Irlam JH, Visser ME, Rollins N, and Siegfried N, Micronutrient supplementation in children and adults with HIV infection. *Cochrane Database Syst Rev* (2005), **4**:CD003650.

35. Merchant AT, Msamanga G, Villamor E, Saathoff E, O'Brien M, Hertzmark E, et al., Multivitamin supplementation of HIV-positive women during pregnancy reduces hypertension. *J Nutr* (2005), **7**:1776–81.

36. McGrath N, Bellinger D, Robins J, Msamanga GI, Tronick E, and Fawzi WW, Effect of maternal multivitamin supplementation on the mental and psychomotor development of children who are born to HIV-1-infected mothers in Tanzania. *Pediatrics* (2006), **2**:e216–25.

37. Fawzi WW, Msamanga GI, Urassa W, Hertzmark E, Petraro P, Willett WC, and Spiegelman D, Vitamins and perinatal outcomes among HIV-negative women in Tanzania. *N Engl J Med* **14** (2007), 1423–31.

38. Postma MJ, Londeman J, Veenstra M, de Walle HE, and deJong-vandenBerg LT, Cost-effectiveness of periconceptional supplementation of folic acid. *Pharm World Sci* (2002), **1**:8–11.

39. Jentink J, vandeVrie-Hoekstra NW, deJong-vandenBerg LT, and Postma MJ, Economic evaluation of folic acid food fortification in The Netherlands. *Eur J Public Health* (2008), **3**:270–274.

40. Grosse SD, Ouyang L, Collins JS, Green D, Dean JH, and Stevenson RE, Economic evaluation of a neural tube defect recurrence-prevention program. *Am J Prev Med* (2008), **6**:572–7.

41. Llanos A, Hertrampf E, Cortes F, Pardo A, Grosse SD, and Uauy R, Cost-effectiveness of a folic acid fortification program in Chile.

Health Policy (2007), 2–3:295–303.

42. Forrest JD, Epidemiology of unintended pregnancy and contraceptive use. *Am J Obstet Gynecol* (1994), **5**:1485–9.

43. Thylefors B, Negrel AD, and Pararajasegaram R, Epidemiologic aspects of global blindness prevention. *Curr Opin Ophthalmol* (1992), **6**:824–34.

44. Hartong DT, Berson EL, and Dryja TP, Retinitis pigmentosa. *Lancet* (2006), **9549**:1795–1809.

45. Rosa FW, Wilk AL, and Kelsey FO, Teratogen update: vitamin A congeners. *Teratology* (1986), **3**:355–64.

46. Mills JL, Simpson, JL, Cunningham GC, Conley MR, and Rhoads GG, Vitamin A and birth defects. *Am J Obstet Gynecol* (1997), **1**:31–6.

47. Rothman KJ, Moore LL, Singer MR, Nguyen US, Mannino S, and Milunsky A, Teratogenicity of high vitamin A intake. *N Engl J Med* (1995), **21**:1369–73.

48. Rassin DK, Nutritional requirements for the fetus and the neonate. In: Ogra PL ed., Neonatal Infections-Nutritional and Immunological Interactions (Orlando, FL: Grune and Stratton, 1984), p. 227.

49. Butterworth RF, Gaudreau C, Vincelette J, Bourgault AM, Lamothe F, and Nutini AM, Thiamine deficiency and Wernicke's encephalopathy in AIDS. *Metab Brain Dis* (1991), **4**:207–12.

50. Heinze T and Weber W, Determination of thiamine (vitamin B1) in maternal blood during normal pregnancies and pregnancies with intrauterine growth retardation. *Z Ernahrungswiss* (1990), **1**:39–46.

51. Butterworth RF, Maternal thiamine deficiency. A factor in intrauterine growth retardation.

Ann N Y Acad Sci (1993), **678**:325–9.

52. Badart-Smook A, vanHouwelingen AC, Al MD, Kester AD, and Hornstra G, Fetal growth is associated positively with maternal intake of riboflavin and negatively with maternal intake of linoleic acid. *J Am Diet Assoc* (1997), **8**:867–70.

53. Krapels IP, van Rooij I, Ocke MC, West CE, VanDerHorst CM, and Steegers-Theunissen RP, Maternal nutritional status and the risk for orofacial cleft offspring in humans. *J Nutr* (2004), **11**:3106–13.

54. Fox HM, Pantothenic acid. In: Machlin LJ, ed., Handbook of Vitamins (New York: Marcel Dekker, 1984), p. 437.

55. Baker H, Frank O, Thomson AD, Langer A, Munves ED, De Angelis B, and Kaminetzky HA, Vitamin profile of 174 mothers and newborns at parturition. *Am J Clin Nutr* (1975), **1**:59–65.

56. Sato M, Shirota M, and Nagao T, Pantothenic acid decreases valproic acid-induced neural tube defects in mice (I). *Teratology* (1995), **3**:143–8.

57. Jewell D and Young G, Interventions for nausea and vomiting in early pregnancy. *Cochrane Database Syst Rev* (2003), **4**:CD000145.

58. Stover PJ, Physiology of folate and vitamin B12 in health and disease. *Nutr Rev* (2004), **6**:S3–12.

59. Kruschwitz HL, McDonald D, Cossins EA, and Schirch V, 5-Formyltetrahydropteroylpolyglutamates are the major folate derivatives in *Neurospora crassa* conidiospores. *J Biol Chem* (1994), **46**:28757–63.

60. Locksmith GJ and Duff P, Preventing neural tube defects: the importance of periconceptional folic acid supplements. *Obstet Gynecol* (1998), **6**:1027–34.

61. Hall J and Solehdin F, Folic acid for the prevention of congenital anomalies. *Eur J Pediatr* (1998), **6**:445–50.

62. Clarke S and Banfield K, S-adenosylmethionine-dependent methyltransferases. In: ed. Carmel R and Jacobsen DW, Homocysteine in Health and Disease (Cambridge: Cambridge University Press, 2001), pp. 63–78.

63. Heath CW Jr., Cytogenetic observations in vitamin B12 and folate deficiency. *Blood* (1966), **6**:800–15.

64. Sutherland GR and Ledbetter DH, Report of the committee on cytogenetic markers. *Cytogenet Cell Genet* (1989), **1–4**:452–8.

65. Laurence KM, James N, Miller MH, Tennant GB, and Campbell H, Double-blind randomised controlled trial of folate treatment before conception to prevent recurrence of neural-tube defects. *Br Med J (Clin Res Ed)* (1981), **6275**:1509–11.

66. Sheppard S, Nevin NC, Seller MJ, Wild J, Smithells RW, Read AP, et al., Neural tube defect recurrence after 'partial' vitamin supplementation. *J Med Genet* (1989), **5**:326–9.

67. Vergel RG, Sanchez LR, Heredero BL, Rodriguez PL, and Martinez AJ, Primary prevention of neural tube defects with folic acid supplementation: Cuban experience. *Prenat Diagn* (1990), **3**:149–2.

68. Werler MM, Hayes C, Louik C, Shapiro S, and Mitchell AA, Multivitamin supplementation and risk of birth defects. *Am J Epidemiol* (1999), **7**:675–82.

69. Berry RJ, Li Z, Erickson JD, Li S, Moore CA, Wang H, et al., Prevention of neural-tube defects with folic acid in China. China-U.S. Collaborative Project for Neural Tube Defect Prevention. *N Engl J Med* (1999), **20**:1485–90.

70. Shaw GM, Schaffer D, Velie EM, Morland K, and Harris JA, Periconceptional vitamin use, dietary folate, and the occurrence of neural tube defects. *Epidemiology* (1995), **3**:219–26.

71. Daly LE, Kirke PN, Molloy A, Weir DG, and Scott JM, Folate levels and neural tube defects. Implications for prevention. *JAMA* (1995), **21**:1698–702.

72. Daly S, Mills JL, Molloy AM, Conley M, Lee YJ, Kirke PN, et al., Minimum effective dose of folic acid for food fortification to prevent neural-tube defects. *Lancet* (1997), **9092**:1666–9.

73. Wald NJ, Law M, and Jordan R, Folic acid food fortification to prevent neural tube defects. *Lancet* (1998), **9105**:834–5.

74. French AE, Grant R, Weitzman S, Ray JG, Vermeulen MJ, Sung L, et al., Folic acid food fortification is associated with a decline in neuroblastoma. *Clin Pharmacol Ther* (2003), **3**:288–94.

75. Studies in "pernicious anaemia" of pregnancy. I. Preliminary report. *Indian J Med Res*, (1930), **17**:777–92.

76. Metz J, Stevens K, Krawitz S, and Brandt V, The plasma clearance of injected doses of folic acid as an index of folic acid deficiency. *J Clin Pathol* (1961), **14**:622–5.

77. Graham S, Hellmann R, Marshall J, Freudenheim J, Vena J, Swanson M, et al., Nutritional epidemiology of postmenopausal breast cancer in western New York. *Am J Epidemiol* (1991), **6**:552–66.

78. Zhang S, Hunter DJ, Hankinson SE, Giovannucci EL, Rosner BA, Colditz GA, et al., A prospective study of folate intake and the risk of breast cancer. *JAMA* (1999), **17**:1632–7.

79. Negri E, La Vecchia C, and Franceschi S, Re: dietary folate consumption and breast cancer risk. *J Natl Cancer Inst* (2000), **15**:1270–1.

80. Rohan TE, Jain MG, Howe GR, and Miller AB, Dietary folate consumption and breast cancer risk. *J Natl Cancer Inst* (2000), **3**:266–9.

81. Shrubsole MJ, Jin F, Dai Q, Shu XO, Potter JD, Hebert JR, et al., Dietary folate intake and breast cancer risk: results from the Shanghai Breast Cancer Study. *Cancer Res* (2001), **19**:7136–41.

82. Schabath MB, Spitz MR, Lerner SP, Pillow PC, Hernandez LM, Delclos GL, et al., Case-control analysis of dietary folate and risk of bladder cancer. *Nutr Cancer* (2005), **2**:144–51.

83. Kune G and Watson L, Colorectal cancer protective effects and the dietary micronutrients folate, methionine, vitamins B6, B12, C, E, selenium, and lycopene. *Nutr Cancer* (2006), **1**:11–21.

84. Larsson SC, Giovannucci E, and Wolk A, Folate intake, MTHFR polymorphisms, and risk of esophageal, gastric, and pancreatic cancer: a meta-analysis. *Gastroenterology* (2006), **4**:1271–83.

85. Navarro Silvera SA, Jain M, Howe GR, Miller AB, and Rohan TE, Dietary folate consumption and risk of ovarian cancer: a prospective cohort study. *Eur J Cancer Prev* (2006), **6**:511–15.

86. Department of Health (U.K.), Thinking of having a baby: folic acid-an essential ingredient in making babies (2004). Available at: http://www.dh.gov.uk/en/Publicationsandstatistics/Publications/Publications-PolicyAndGuidance/DH_4081396. Accessed 2009.

87. Health Canada, Folic acid and birth defects (2005). Available at: http://www.hc-sc.gc.ca/hl-vs/iyh-vsv/med/folic-folique-eng.php. Accessed 2009.

88. National Academy of Sciences, Dietary Reference Intakes (DRIs): Recommended intakes for individuals, vitamins (2004).

89. Available at: http://www.iom.edu/object.file-master/21/372/0.pdf.

90. Kapur BM, Bar-Oz B, Koren G, and Nguyen P, Folate fortification and supplementation – are we there yet? *Can J Clin Pharmacol* (2007), **2**:104–204.

90. Pfeiffer CM, Johnson CL, Jain RB, Yetley EA, Picciano MF, Rader JI, et al., Trends in blood folate and vitamin B-12 concentrations in the United States, 1988–2004. *Am J Clin Nutr* (2007), **3**:718–27.

91. Wald NJ, Law MR, Morris JK, and Wald DS, Quantifying the effect of folic acid. *Lancet* (2001), **9298**:2069–73.

92. Chanarin I, The Megaloblastic Anemias, 3rd edn (Oxford: Blackwell, 1990).

93. Briddon A, Homocysteine in the context of cobalamin metabolism and deficiency states. *Amino Acids* (2003), **1–2**:1–12.

94. Chanarin I, Folate and cobalamin. *Clin Haematol* (1985), **3**:629–41.

95. Thompson WG and Freedman ML, Vitamin B_{12} and geriatrics: unanswered questions. *Acta Haematol* (1989), **4**:169–74.

96. Herbert V, Vitamin B_{12}. *Am J Clin Nutr* (1981), **5**:971–2.

97. Scott JM, Folate and vitamin B_{12}. *Proc Nutr Soc* (1999), **2**:441–8.

98. Afman LA, Lievers KJ, VanDerPut NM, Trijbels FJ, and Blom HJ, Single nucleotide polymorphisms in the transcobalamin gene: relationship with transcobalamin concentrations and risk for neural tube defects. *Eur J Hum Genet* (2002), **7**:433–8.

99. Tisman G and Herbert V, B 12 dependence of cell uptake of serum folate: an explanation for high serum folate and cell folate depletion in B 12 deficiency. *Blood* (1973), **3**:465–9.

100. Chanarin I, Deacon R, Perry J, and Lumb M, How vitamin B12 acts. *Br J Haematol* (1981), **4**:487–91.

101. Scott JM and Weir DG, The methyl folate trap. A physiological response in man to prevent methyl group deficiency in kwashiorkor (methionine deficiency) and an explanation for folic-acid induced exacerbation of subacute combined degeneration in pernicious anaemia. *Lancet* (1981), **8242**:337–40.

102. Hytten FE, Nutrition in pregnancy. *Postgrad Med J* (1979), **643**:295–302.

103. VanDenBerg H, Vitamin and mineral status in healthy pregnant women. *Symposium Nestle-Hoffmann-La Roche Workshop Series* (1988), **16**:93–108.

104. Walker MC, Smith GN, Perkins SL, Keely EJ, and Garner PR, Changes in homocysteine levels during normal pregnancy. *Am J Obstet Gynecol* (1999), **3**:660–4.

105. Carmel R, Green R, Rosenblatt DS, and Watkins D, Update on cobalamin, folate, and homocysteine. *Hematol Am Soc Hematol Educ Program* (2003), 62–81.

106. Wouters MG, Boers GH, Blom HJ, Trijbels FJ, Thomas CM, Borm GF, et al., Hyperhomocysteinemia: a risk factor in women with unexplained recurrent early pregnancy loss. *Fertil Steril* (1993), **5**:820–5.

107. Aubard Y, Darodes N, and Cantaloube M, Hyperhomocysteinemia and pregnancy – review of our present understanding and therapeutic implications. *Eur J Obstet Gynecol Reprod Biol* (2000), **2**:157–65.

108. Roberts JM, Taylor RN, Musci TJ, Rodgers GM, Hubel CA, and McLaughlin, MK, Preeclampsia: an endothelial cell disorder. *Am J Obstet Gynecol* (1989), **5**:1200–4.

109. Roberts JM and Hubel CA, Is oxidative stress the link in the two-stage model of pre-eclampsia? *Lancet* (1999), **9181**:788–9.

110. Goddijn-Wessel TA, Wouters MG, vandeMolen EF, Spuijbroek MD, Steegers-Theunissen RP, Blom HJ, et al., Hyperhomocysteinemia: a risk factor for placental abruption or infarction. *Eur J Obstet Gynecol Reprod Biol* (1996), **1**:23–9.

111. deVries JI, Dekker GA, Huijgens PC, Jakobs C, Blomberg BM, and vanGeijn HP, Hyperhomocysteinaemia and protein S deficiency in complicated pregnancies. *Br J Obstet Gynaecol* (1997), **11**:1248–54.

112. Smithells RW, Sheppard S, and Schorah CJ, Vitamin deficiencies and neural tube defects. *Arch Dis Child* (1976), **12**:944–50.

113. Schorah CJ, Smithells RW, and Scott J, Vitamin B$_{12}$ and anencephaly. *Lancet* (1980), **8173**:880.

114. Steegers-Theunissen RP, Boers GH, Trijbels FJ, Finkelstein JD, Blom HJ, Thomas CM, et al., Maternal hyperhomocysteinemia: a risk factor for neural-tube defects? *Metabolism* (1994), **12**:1475–80.

115. Eskes TK, Open or closed? A world of difference: a history of homocysteine research. *Nutr Rev* (1998), **8**:236–44.

116. Burke G, Robinson K, Refsum H, Stuart B, Drumm J, and Graham I, Intrauterine growth retardation, perinatal death, and maternal homocysteine levels. *N Engl J Med* (1992), **1**:69–70.

117. Lindenbaum J, Healton EB, Savage DG, Brust JC, Garrett TJ, Podell ER, et al., Neuropsychiatric disorders caused by cobalamin deficiency in the absence of anemia or macrocytosis. *N Engl J Med* (1988), **26**:1720–8.

118. Savage DG and Lindenbaum J, Neurological complications of acquired cobalamin deficiency: clinical aspects. *Baillieres Clin Haematol* (1995), **3**:657–78.

119. Lovblad K, Ramelli G, Remonda L, Nirkko AC, Ozdoba C, and Schroth G. Retardation of myelination due to dietary vitamin B12 deficiency: cranial MRI findings. *Pediatr Radiol* (1997), **2**:155–8.

120. Monagle PT and Tauro GP, Infantile megaloblastosis secondary to maternal vitamin B12 deficiency. *Clin Lab Haematol* (1997), **1**:23–5.

121. Quere I, Bellet H, Hoffet M, Janbon C, Mares P, and Gris JC, A woman with five consecutive fetal deaths: case report and retrospective analysis of hyperhomocysteinemia prevalence in 100 consecutive women with recurrent miscarriages. *Fertil Steril* (1998), **1**:152–4.

122. Bonnar J, Green R, and Norris L, Inherited thrombophilia and pregnancy: the obstetric perspective. *Semin Thromb Hemost* (1998), **24**(Suppl 1):49–53.

123. Korner WF and Weber F, [Tolerance for high dosages of ascorbic acid]. *Int J Vitam Nutr Res* (1972), **4**:528–44.

124. Rumbold A and Crowther CA, Vitamin C supplementation in pregnancy. *Cochrane Database Syst Rev* (2005), **2**:CD004072.

125. Barrett B, Gunter E, Jenkins J, and Wang M, Ascorbic acid concentration in amniotic fluid in late pregnancy. *Biol Neonate* (1991), **5**:333–5.

126. Chappell LC, Seed PT, Kelly FJ, Briley A, Hunt BJ, Charnock-Jones DS, et al., Vitamin C and E supplementation in women at risk of preeclampsia is associated with changes in indices of oxidative stress and placental function. *Am J Obstet Gynecol* (2002), **3**:777–84.

127. Rumbold AR, Crowther CA, Haslam RR, Dekker GA, and Robinson JS, Vitamins C and E and the risks of preeclampsia and perinatal complications. *N Engl J Med* (2006), **17**:1796–1806.

128. Poston L, Briley AL, Seed PT, Kelly FJ, and Shennan AH, Vitamin C and vitamin E in pregnant women at risk for pre-eclampsia (VIP trial): randomised placebo-controlled trial. *Lancet* (2006), **9517**:1145–54.

129. Boskovic R, Gargaun L, Oren D, Djulus J, and Koren G, Pregnancy outcome following high doses of vitamin E supplementation. *Reprod Toxicol* (2005), **1**:85–8.

130. Goodenday LS, and Gordon GS, No risk from vitamin D in pregnancy. *Ann Intern Med* (1971), **5**:807–8.

131. Callies F, Arlt W, Scholz HJ, Reincke M, and Allolio B, Management of hypoparathyroidism during pregnancy – report of twelve cases. *Eur J Endocrinol* (1998), **3**:284–9.

132. Gulmezoglu AM, Hofmeyr GJ, and Oosthuisen MM, Antioxidants in the treatment of severe pre-eclampsia: an explanatory randomised controlled trial. *Br J Obstet Gynaecol* (1997), **6**:689–96.

133. Beazley D, Ahokas R, Livingston J, Griggs M, and Sibai BM, Vitamin C and E supplementation in women at high risk for preeclampsia: a double-blind, placebo-controlled trial. *Am J Obstet Gynecol* (2005), **2**:520–1.

134. Rumbold A and Crowther CA, Vitamin E supplementation in pregnancy. *Cochrane Database Syst Rev* (2005), **2**:CD004069.

135. Scholl TO, Chen X, Sims M, and Stein TP, Vitamin E: maternal concentrations are associated with fetal growth. *Am J Clin Nutr* (2006), **6**:1442–8.

17

Determinants of egg and embryo quality: long-term effects of maternal diet and assisted reproduction

Kevin D. Sinclair and Wing Yee Kwong

Introduction

Reproductive rate in humans is in decline, while the incidence of obesity and metabolic-related diseases are increasing. Recent World Bank statistics reveal that, although the pace of decline in reproductive rate over the past 50 years differs between regions, this phenomenon is global, occurring in both developed and developing countries. Statistics based on the U.S. government's Centers for Disease Control and Prevention's National Center for Health Statistics, for the period 1960 to 2002, confirm these trends in the United States [1]. Similarly, although the proportion of clinically obese individuals is greatest in developed countries, the problem of obesity and obesity-related diseases is increasing most rapidly in developing countries [2]. These trends in human health can largely be attributed to changing lifestyles but may also be due to environmental exposure to endocrine-disrupting chemicals and, of particular relevance to this chapter, diet at key stages during early development [3–5].

At this juncture, the discussion could develop in one of two ways. There is compelling evidence that exposure in utero to environmentally prevalent endocrine-disrupting chemicals can lead to impaired reproductive development and the programming of obesity and related metabolic disorders in animals and humans. These topics have been extensively reviewed elsewhere [6–8]. Similarly, there is compelling evidence, from both epidemiological studies in humans and direct interventionist studies with animals, that many late-onset adult diseases arise as a consequence of malnutrition during in utero life [9], although direct effects on fecundity are less clear [10]. Although most studies to date have investigated these effects during the greater part of pregnancy and infancy, much less attention has been directed toward understanding the effects of environment and diet on the mammalian egg and preimplantation embryo, although it is now widely recognized that these early stages of development may be the most environmentally sensitive [11, 12].

Consequently, set in the context of pregnancy establishment and long-term developmental programming, this chapter provides a contemporary overview of the key developmental processes that take place during the earliest stages of mammalian development, highlighting their sensitivity to environmental influences in a manner that can determine fertility, pregnancy outcome, and offspring health.

Ovarian folliculogenesis and oocyte maturation

In sexually mature adults, the process of ovarian folliculogenesis, from when primordial follicles leave their resting state to when they reach the preovulatory stage, typically takes between 6 and 7 months, although the active period of growth is estimated to be around 12 weeks [14] and witnesses a 400-fold increase in follicle volume [14] (Figure 17.1). Although the corresponding increase in oocyte volume (40-fold) may appear more modest, it nevertheless represents a significant increase in mass and highlights the extent of cellular biosynthesis that takes place in the germ cell during this period of development. It further emphasizes the protracted period of time during which environmental determinants of egg quality can exert their effects.

Transcriptional activity and DNA methylation

Transcript profiling during mouse oocyte development has revealed the primordial-to-primary follicle transition to be a major transitional stage; changes in transcriptional activity, observed for approximately 33% oocyte genes, were greater at this than at any other stage of folliculogenesis [15] (Figure 17.1).

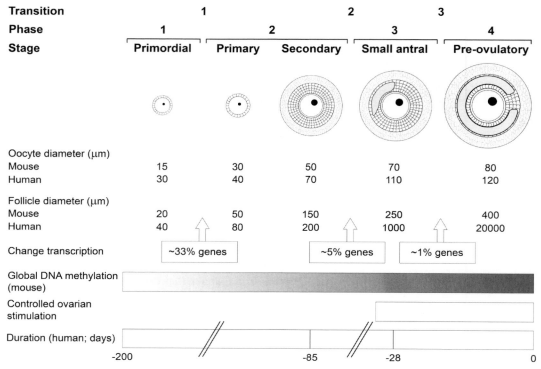

Transition		1		2	3	
Phase	**1**		**2**	**3**	**4**	
Stage	**Primordial**	**Primary**	**Secondary**	**Small antral**	**Pre-ovulatory**	

Oocyte diameter (μm)					
Mouse	15	30	50	70	80
Human	30	40	70	110	120

Follicle diameter (μm)					
Mouse	20	50	150	250	400
Human	40	80	200	1000	20000

Change transcription	~33% genes	~5% genes	~1% genes

Global DNA methylation (mouse)

Controlled ovarian stimulation

Duration (human; days)			
-200	-85	-28	0

Figure 17.1 Schematic representation of ovarian folliculogenesis and oocyte growth in the postnatal mouse and sexually mature human, highlighting molecular events that occur during each of three key transitionary periods.

A second major change in transcriptional activity occurs between the secondary and tertiary (small antral) stages of follicular development. Here transcriptional activity is altered in fewer (~5%) genes, but many are associated with DNA synthesis and cell cycle regulation. Oocytes from preantral follicles are incapable of resuming meiosis, whereas oocytes from small antral follicles have acquired this capacity [16]. A third key transitional event occurs during antral follicle development (coincident with follicular selection and dominance in mono-ovular species). Although transcriptional activity was altered in only approximately 1% of mouse genes [15], once again they were mostly genes involved in cell cycle progression and chromatin remodeling. The proportion of oocytes that successfully reach metaphase II, and develop following fertilization, progressively increases with antral follicle size [17], indicating that significant "maturational" events occur during the latter stages of antral follicle development.

The temporal patterns of transcript expression described here are integrally linked to ongoing epigenetic modifications to DNA and associated proteins,

although at present these are poorly characterized in the germline [18]. The available evidence points to a genomewide loss of DNA methylation before meiotic arrest, although this is thought to vary among single copy genes and repetitive sequences. Remethylation of the female germline occurs during oocyte growth (Figure 17.1), but much of our knowledge on the timing of this process is limited to the remethylation of a group of imprinted genes and repeat sequences in the mouse [19]. Although the precise timing of methylation acquisition varied between genes in that study, the most active period of DNA methylation was around 15 days post conception, coincident with the formation of antral follicles. More recent studies in the mouse and sheep, using an immunofluorescence staining approach to measure global DNA methylation, have since identified the most rapid phase of DNA methylation to occur in growing oocytes around the time of antrum formation in the follicle [20, 21].

Ovarian stimulation and oocyte maturation

The foregoing discussion highlights how key molecular events change in the days and weeks leading up to conception. Given that a typical in vitro fertilization (IVF) cycle, involving the use of gonadotropin-releasing hormone (GnRH) agonists and gonadotrophins, can last 3 to 4 weeks, it follows that some of these molecular events may be disturbed in a manner that could jeopardize pregnancy outcome. A number of animal studies (albeit mostly with mice) support this premise. For example, using an immunostaining approach with an antibody against 5-methyl cytosine, Shi and Haaf [22] showed that the DNA methylation pattern of two-cell mouse embryos differed between superovulated and nonstimulated females. Abnormal patterns of DNA methylation were associated with reduced preimplantation development in vitro. More recently, superovulation followed by in vivo development (i.e. embryo transfer to pseudopregnant females) led to aberrant patterns of methylation and a loss of imprinting at specific loci in mid-gestation mouse placenta [23]. There is an emerging consensus that trophectoderm-derived tissues may be more susceptible to loss of imprinting than the embryo proper. Importantly, the results of that study indicated that it is not the establishment of imprinting that is affected but rather its maintenance. However, this may merely reflect the timing of intervention. The methylation status of several imprinted genes has also been reported in oocytes from stimulated and non-stimulated cycles in both the human and mouse [24]. Modest gains in methylation at the *H19* differentially methylated region were observed in some oocytes from both species, although in the case of human oocytes, the effects of superovulation could not be distinguished from those of donor age and fertility. The biological significance of these latter observations is therefore uncertain, and there is generally a lack of compelling evidence of a significant clinical problem in human pregnancies following ovarian stimulation [25]. Poor perinatal outcomes in ovarian stimulated IVF cycles can often be explained by the confounding factors of advanced maternal age and subfertility.

Similar reservations relate to statistics on pregnancy and perinatal outcomes following in vitro maturation (IVM). In many instances the retrieval of germinal vesicle-stage oocytes for IVM is performed in women for whom polycystic ovarian syndrome (PCOS) has been diagnosed, so that the effects of IVM cannot be separated from the underlying causes of subfertility [25]. Long-term developmental consequences of IVM have been largely unexplored in animal studies, but postfertilization development is usu-

ally impaired and pregnancy rates following transfer reduced [26]. However, it has seldom been possible to separate the effects of IVM from those of in vitro fertilization or culture (discussed later).

Maternal diet and egg quality

Because of the dramatic increase in obesity levels referred to earlier, a considerable amount of research effort has been devoted to understanding the effects of obesity on fertility. Overweight women are more likely to encounter menstrual dysfunction and anovulation [27]. Furthermore, women with a body mass index 25 kg/m^{-2} or greater have a lower chance of pregnancy following IVF and have an increased miscarriage rate [28]. A contributing factor in these cases is impaired egg quality associated with insulin resistance. Much of the human data in this area is derived from patients with PCOS [29]. We have shown that antral follicle development and egg quality are both impaired in clinically obese and hyperinsulinemic young female cattle [30]. In that study, oocytes were retrieved from donors using ultrasound-guided follicular aspiration and matured, fertilized, and cultured in vitro. Detailed analysis revealed that the negative relationship between insulin and egg quality (defined as the proportion of inseminated oocytes that developed to the blastocyst stage) increased over time (Figure 17.2). This effect could be due to the duration of exposure of oocytes to elevated levels of insulin but also suggests that oocytes exposed to high levels of insulin during the preantral stages of follicular development may be most sensitive. Recently, the ability of insulin-sensitizing agents 5-aminoimidazole 4-carboxamide-riboside (AICAR), sodium salicylate, and rosiglitazone to enhance the postfertilization developmental potential of oocytes was determined in obese C57BL/6 mice offered a high-fat diet [31]. Rosiglitazone, a potent agonist for the nuclear receptor peroxisome proliferator-activated receptor gamma (PPAR gamma), was most effective in lowering blood insulin and triglyceride concentrations and restoring postfertilization development of in vivo–derived zygotes cultured in vitro. Within the mouse ovary, PPAR gamma is most highly expressed in granulosa cells [32], where it can interact with target genes such as *Cd36* and *Scarb1* involved in lipid uptake and metabolism [31].

PCOS is a heterogeneous syndrome affecting 5% to 10% of women of reproductive age and is generally characterized by oligo-anovulation, clinical

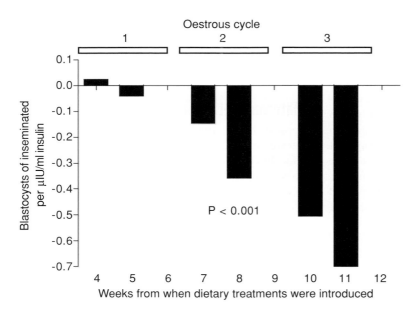

Figure 17.2 Regression coefficients for blastocysts of cleaved against plasma insulin concentrations determined at each of two oocyte recovery sessions within each of three successive estrous cycles from the study of Adamiak et al. [30]. Heifers were moderately fat at the beginning of the experimental period and were offered a high-calorie diet at a level equivalent to twice their metabolizable energy requirements for maintenance. Oocytes were matured, fertilized, and cultured to the blastocyst stage in vitro. Mean plasma insulin concentration for these animals was 48 μIU/ml.

or biochemical hyperandrogenism, and/or polycystic ovaries [33]. It is also frequently associated with insulin resistance and hyperinsulinemia. Oocytes from obese and hyperinsulinemic PCOS patients frequently fail to fertilize, and those that do often fail to implant, even following surrogate embryo transfer [34]. Microarray analysis of metaphase II oocytes from normal ovulatory women and women with PCOS identified a subset of differentially expressed genes associated with chromosome alignment and segregation during meiosis, and genes containing putative androgen receptor and PPAR gamma binding sites [35]. These observations may help explain impaired oocyte quality and pregnancy establishment in PCOS subjects, but longer term developmental consequences are not known.

In fact, few studies have specifically assessed the long-term developmental consequences of maternal diet on oocyte quality. Most, including studies at the author's laboratory, have had protracted treatment periods that extended into early pregnancy [36]. One study, however, assessed the effects of maternal low-protein diet (LPD; 9% casein) restricted to one ovulatory cycle before natural conception in mice [37]. The authors observed no effects on pregnancy establishment or outcome but reported increased anxiety-related behavior in offspring. Furthermore, male mice exhibited elevated systolic blood pressure at 9 and 15

weeks, and systolic blood pressure was elevated in both sexes at 21 weeks. A feature of this study and that of Minge et al. [31], however, was that fertilization occurred in vivo while dams were still on their experimental treatments, so that dietary effects on fertilization and related-related events (discussed later) cannot be ruled out.

Summary 17.1

- Although a number of animal studies indicate that ovarian stimulation can impair egg quality, postfertilization development, and pregnancy outcome, there is a lack of compelling evidence to indicate that this is the case in human assisted reproduction, where factors such as subfertility, maternal age, and embryo culture confound interpretation.

- Overweight women, excluding those with PCOS, face a lower likelihood of pregnancy establishment and an increased risk of miscarriage following IVF.

- Although recent animal studies have demonstrated significant improvements in oocyte quality following the treatment of obese egg donors with insulin-sensitizing agents, their efficacy in assisting with ovulation induction and pregnancy establishment in PCOS women is variable, and so routine use is currently not recommended.

> - The metabolite composition of follicular fluid and granulosa cells, normally discarded at the time of egg recovery in IVF cycles, can be used to predict postfertilization development.

Fertilization

There is sparse information concerning the effects of maternal diet on the processes involved in fertilization, although it is now apparent that events during this period can have a profound effect on long-term development. The sperm in mammals does not appear to provide the egg activation signal by the conventional interaction with a receptor linked to the production of the Ca^{2+} releasing messenger inositol triphosphate (IP_3); rather, it uses a more direct route by introducing a soluble signaling molecule that triggers endogenous Ca^{2+} release. Upon membrane fusion, a novel sperm-specific form of phospholipase C, referred to as PLCζ (zeta), is released into the ooplasm, and this triggers endogenous Ca^{2+} oscillations by increasing intracellular concentrations of IP_3 [38]. This mechanism appears to be highly conserved across species. Indeed, the injection of primate PLCζ into mouse eggs has been shown to induce Ca^{2+} oscillations and to activate development [39].

Developmental legacy of calcium signaling

Of particular interest to the current thesis are the recent observations in mice that perturbations to Ca^{2+} oscillatory signaling during the first few hours following insemination can have long-term effects on development. It has been known for some time that the pattern of Ca^{2+} transients during parthenogenetic activation of rabbit eggs can influence the proportion of embryos that reach the compacted morula or blastocyst stage [40]. A recent study in mice, however, used a number of recognized agents, including the protein synthesis inhibitor cycloheximide, which does not rely on the actions of Ca^{2+}, to parthenogenetically activate eggs [41]. These authors also conducted a microarray analysis of gene expression in eight-cell embryos. A greater proportion of embryos that underwent Ca^{2+} oscillations or a single Ca^{2+} increase developed to the blastocyst stage than those from the cycloheximide-activated group, which experienced no Ca^{2+} oscillations. Furthermore, those cycloheximide-

activated embryos that developed to the blastocyst stage had a reduced inner-cell mass and a higher number of TUNEL-positive cells. Microarray analysis identified in excess of 800 genes that were differentially expressed between the treatments. Significantly, cell cycle–related and growth arrest genes, together with apoptosis-related genes, appeared to be overexpressed in the activated-activated embryos.

Calcium oscillations around fertilization are known to have longer-term consequences on development, influencing implantation in rabbit parthenogenotes [42] and, more recently, term development following fertilization in the mouse [43]. In the latter study, Ca^{2+} oscillations were either inhibited or overridden and experimentally increased following the first few endogenous oscillations induced by the fertilizing sperm. In either case, development to the blastocyst stage was unaffected, but development to term was compromised. When the natural pattern of signaling was prematurely interrupted, implantation rate was reduced. In contrast, when Ca^{2+} oscillations around fertilization were experimentally increased, implantation rates were not affected, but resorption rates increased. Furthermore, there appeared to be long-term effects on weight variation in offspring derived from this latter treatment group. Microarray analysis of gene expression in blastocysts revealed that approximately 20% of transcripts were misregulated when too few oscillations occurred. In contrast, only approximately 3% of transcripts were misregulated when Ca^{2+} oscillations were increased. In the former case, genes involved in transcription regulation, mRNA processing, and cell adhesion were preferentially misexpressed, whereas in the latter case, genes involved in metabolism were dysregulated. The mechanisms of action of Ca^{2+} oscillations on gene expression, however, are not understood, so that it is currently not possible to gain further insights into these differential effects. It is also not known what effects maternal nutrition or media metabolite composition may have on these processes. However, Ca^{2+} oscillations are influenced by oxidative stress through the generation of reactive oxygen species (ROS) from the mitochondria in aged oocytes [44]. The culture of mouse embryos in the presence of both n-3 and n-6 polyunsaturated fatty acids (PUFAs) increased lipid peroxidation and intracellular ROS, and decreased embryo development, an effect attenuated by the addition of antioxidants [45].

More recently, ROS production was increased and intracellular Ca^{2+} homeostasis perturbed in mature oocytes from mice offered n-3 PUFA-enriched diets, resulting in a reduced proportion of cleaved zygotes [46]. Once again, the precise mechanisms of action of these dietary effects are not understood, and long-term developmental consequences remain to be established.

These observations, however, may have profound implications for the safety of assisted reproductive techniques such as intracytoplasmic sperm injection (ICSI) and the formulation of culture media for IVF. The current consensus, based on ICSI outcome studies in humans, is that there is a significant, albeit low, increased risk of preterm delivery, low birth weights, and perinatal mortality in both single and multiple births, although it is difficult to isolate completely the effects of ICSI from the recognized risk factors of maternal age and infertility [25]. ICSI not only bypasses membrane fusion of gametes but leads to the delivery of a membrane-intact sperm head, which could impair the release of sperm factor. Indeed, ICSI-generated zygotes in the mouse cleaved at a slower rate, had lower cell numbers, and had lower hatching rates [47]. This was associated with shorter duration Ca^{2+} oscillations. Curiously, ICSI is much less successful in the bovine. The problem here appears to lie in the initiation of Ca^{2+} oscillations following injection. For reasons that remain unclear, the majority of bovine oocytes appear unable to mount such oscillations and subsequently fail to cleave [48].

Intercourse and seminal plasma

Studies across a broad range of mammalian species indicate that semen introduced to the female reproductive tract elicits a cascade of molecular and cellular changes that can promote conception and improve pregnancy outcome [49, 50]. Seminal plasma induces the synthesis and release of embryotrophic cytokines and chemokines from estrogen-primed oviductal and uterine epithelial cells, which can interact with the cleavage-stage embryo before implantation. Transforming growth factor beta (in particular, TGFβ1) is a cytokine present in abundance in seminal plasma and is one of the principal factors responsible for initiating this inflammatory response [51]. One of the key pro-inflammatory cytokines for which expression is upregulated by TGFβ1 is granulocyte-macrophage colony-stimulating factor (GM-CSF), which has been shown to promote preimplantation development of 8-cell mouse embryos in vitro by increasing the number of viable blastomeres and by enhancing glucose uptake [52]. Embryotrophic effects of GM-CSF in vitro have been reported in other species, including the cow [53] and human [54]. Significantly, this latter group found that GM-CSF added to mouse embryo culture media alleviated at least some of the effects of in vitro culture on fetal and postnatal development [55]. The inclusion of GM-CSF in media used to culture two-cell mouse embryos to the blastocyst stage before transfer led to increased litter sizes, improvements in near-term fetal weights, and a normalization of postweaning growth relative to offspring from nontreated in vitro cultured embryos. GM-CSF was unable, however, to overcome the increased levels of obesity, particularly central obesity, observed in adult offspring from cultured embryos, indicating that more than one mechanistic pathway is involved in this pathology.

Summary 17.2

- Intercourse, specifically exposure to semen, around the time of embryo transfer can increase the likelihood of pregnancy establishment in humans.
- Be wary of natural conception, which can arise if oocytes not collected during follicular aspiration become fertilized, because this can lead to multiple pregnancies.
- Prolonged exposure to semen and/or seminal plasma from a single source, a feature of monogamous relationships, can further induce functional tolerance to male antigens, enhancing placental-fetal development during late gestation and minimizing the risk of preeclampsia.
- Although the underlying mechanisms of these effects are not fully understood, current models in the mouse are investigating the effects of TGFβ1, which can induce a state of systemic functional tolerance to paternal major histocompatibility complex class I antigens.

Preimplantation development

Preimplantation development can also be characterized by three major transitions. The first transition concerns activation of the embryonic genome, the timing of which varies between species [56]. The second is compaction, where adhesive junctions form between individual blastomeres to create the first transporting epithelium [57]. The third transition is blastocyst formation, where the outermost cells of the embryo differentiate to form the trophectoderm, which gives rise to extraembryonic tissue. These events occur during a comparatively short period of time (< 7 days in most mammalian species) where, curiously, embryo metabolism operates at a relatively low level [58]. However, although nutrient demands of the embryo during this period are quantitatively small, they are, nevertheless, qualitatively specific and reflect the changing needs of the embryo in response to nutrient supply during its migration from the oviduct to the uterine lumen [59].

Transcriptional activity and DNA methylation

Transcript profiling during mouse embryo development has characterized the three transitional periods referred to earlier [60]. The first of these spans the period from oocyte maturation to the onset of embryonic transcription, during which time more than 90% of maternal RNA is destroyed. A large subset of these genes is involved in cell-to-cell communication, signal transduction, and cell adhesion required to maintain bidirectional communication between the oocyte and surrounding cumulus. The rapid demise of these pathways is hypothesized to "insulate" the embryo during this transitional period from extracellular signals to maintain its totipotent state. Interestingly, metabolic activity during these early cleavage stages (i.e. to approximately the eight-cell stage) is comparatively low in terms of adenosine triphosphate (ATP) production and de novo protein synthesis [59], and subsequent embryo viability is inversely related to the level of metabolic activity during this period [61]. Indeed, the early embryo would appear to exert a high degree of autonomy and relies heavily on utilizing endogenous reserves of protein and energy, mostly in the form of triglycerides [62]. These observations, however, belie the incredible turmoil that occurs upon sperm-egg union and egg activation (discussed earlier), pro-nuclear formation, DNA replication, and chromatin modifications.

Epigenetic programming during this early period of embryo development has been best studied in the mouse, where the paternally derived genome, which is packaged densely with protamines, is actively (in the absence of DNA replication) demethylated during the first cell cycle [63, 64]. The maternal genome, in contrast, is passively demethylated during the first few cell cycles. Approximately equivalent levels of hypomethylation are attained by each genome around the 16-cell stage, after which the combined genomes undergo de novo methylation in a cell lineage specific manner. Although similar patterns of global DNA demethylation of the paternal genome have been observed in the rat, cow, and human zygote, this has not been observed in either the rabbit or sheep zygote [65]. Although the functional significance of these species-related differences in DNA methylation is unclear, they may partly reflect preexisting levels of methylation in the male pronucleus at the time of syngamy, which are comparatively low in the sheep [66], or differential expression patterns of DNA methyltransferases in the oocyte and preimplantation embryo [67, 68].

A dramatic increase in biosynthesis follows compaction (typically around 8 to 16 cells [59]). In the mouse, this is immediately preceded by the activation of a series of related genes involved in ribosome biogenesis, and protein and phospholipid synthesis [60]. In contrast, a smaller set of genes, mostly involved in metabolism, are turned on in the blastocyst. On an embryo basis, the generation of ATP increases exponentially following compaction and blastocele formation although, at a cellular level, oxidative and glycolytic activities alter little [59]. The β-oxidation of fatty acids by apposing mitochondria is believed to generate much of the water and at least some of the energy necessary for blastocele formation.

Embryo culture

Early embryo culture media formulations were adapted from those used for cell culture, and subsequent modifications were largely empirical. These media were often complex with many components included at nonphysiological levels [69]. Serum was commonly included, often with somatic support cells to promote embryo development beyond the cleavage stage. Indeed, interest in the use of co-culture systems for human embryo culture persists [70]. Most laboratories, however, have abandoned such systems in favor of more chemically defined and "sequential" media formulations that have contributed to the significant improvement in postfertilization development and clinical pregnancies observed over the past decade following assisted reproduction (ART) [71].

The incentive to remove both serum and somatic support cells from culture arose from reports that emerged during the 1990s of aberrant in utero development, leading to large offspring, in both cattle and sheep following the transfer of embryos that had been cultured in the presence of these components [11]. Referred to as the "large offspring syndrome" (LOS), characteristic features of this phenomenon, other than its sporadic occurrence, include in utero overgrowth and perturbed growth allometry, congenital anomalies involving the central nervous system, gastrointestinal tract, and cardiovascular system, polyhydramnios, and allantoic aplasia [72, 73]. Often newborns from in vitro–produced ruminant embryos experience greater difficulties in adjusting to extrauterine life. Many exhibit aberrant metabolic activity including hypothyroidism, hypoxemia, hypoglycemia, hyperinsulinemia, and metabolic acidosis. Importantly, a number of features of this syndrome are strikingly similar to several naturally occurring overgrowth syndromes in humans, most notably Beckwith-Wiedemann syndrome (BWS), which is associated with abnormalities in an imprinted cluster of genes on chromosome 11 (11p15.5) [11]. In our studies with sheep, exposure to serum throughout the 5-day period of embryo culture or during the first 3 days of culture had the most dramatic effect on ovine fetal development [74]. We had earlier demonstrated that these effects were associated with a loss of imprinting (loss of methylation on the second intron differentially methylated region) of the normally active maternal allele of the type 2 insulin-like growth factor receptor gene ($Igf2R$), which resulted in a significant reduction in its expression in all affected tissues within LOS fetuses [75]. Similar imprinting anomalies have since been reported in mice [76], and, of most concern, in humans following ART [77].

The absolute risk of inducing imprinting disorders in human ART pregnancies, however, would appear to be small. For example, analysis of data from several studies indicates that the incidence of BWS following ART may increase to 1 in 4500 relative to the natural incidence of imprinting anomalies associated with BWS of 1 in 28 000. To date it has not been possible to attribute this phenomenon to any specific component of culture media, to manipulative procedures such as ICSI or, indeed, to the type of infertility in humans [77]. It is noteworthy, however, that extended periods of culture to the blastocyst stage are routinely practiced in ruminant embryo production, so that the relatively high incidence of imprinting anomalies in these species may be a feature of extended culture following IVM and/or ovarian stimulation.

Maternal diet and embryo quality

Evidence that subtle alterations to the in vivo environment of the early cleavage-stage embryo can lead to long-term effects on fetal development came from some of our earlier studies into LOS where we temporarily (for 3 days) exposed Day 3 sheep embryos to an advanced uterine environment. Although there was no effect on pregnancy establishment and no gross effect fetal mass [78], myogenic regulatory pathways were altered. These included a temporal shift in the expression of Myf5 protein (a member of the *MyoD* gene family responsible for myoblast proliferation), leading to an increase in muscle fiber number and the ratio of secondary to primary muscle fibers [79].

One of the first studies to show that maternal diet during the preimplantation period can have a long-term effect on development and offspring health was conducted in the rat. A maternal LPD (described earlier) given to dams from Day 0 to 4.25 altered postnatal growth and hypertension in male pups at 12 weeks of age [80]. Subsequent follow-up studies by this group also pointed to sex-specific programming of imprinted gene expression as a possible contributory factor in this phenomenon [81]. Curiously, the expression of both *H19* and *Igf2* was reduced in only male embryos and fetal tissues. It would appear that in a nutrient-restricted (i.e. LPD) environment, the early embryo is capable of activating a series of as yet poorly defined mechanisms that attempt to normalize conceptus growth and postnatal fitness but may predispose offspring to certain adult diseases [82].

Effect of B vitamins in the periconceptional diet

Given that sweeping epigenetic modifications to DNA and related proteins take place during the periconceptional period (discussed earlier), we recently tested the hypothesis that a restricted supply of specific B vitamins (i.e. vitamin B_{12} and folate) and sulphur amino acids (in particular, methionine) from the diet of adult female sheep, from 8 weeks preceding until 6 days following conception, would lead to epigenetic modifications to DNA methylation and affect adult health in offspring [83]. The duration of exposure to "methyl-deficient" diets ensured that the critical periods of DNA methylation programming that occur in both the oocyte (Figure 17.1) and embryo were incorporated. The transfer of Day 6 embryos to normally fed surrogates further ensured that the timing of dietary treatments was limited specifically to the periods of oocyte growth and early postfertilization development. We observed no effects on pregnancy establishment or birth weight, but adult offspring were heavier and fatter, elicited altered immune responses to antigenic challenge, were insulin resistant, and had elevated blood pressure. Curiously, these effects were most obvious in male offspring. Furthermore, the altered methylation status of 4% of 1400 CpG islands examined by restriction landmark genome scanning in the fetal liver revealed compelling evidence of a widespread epigenetic mechanism associated with this nutritionally programmed effect. These findings in a large outbred species, in which pre- and postnatal development and physiological approximates that of humans, have profound implications for nutritional advice offered to intending mothers, where the message to date has focused on the protective effects of folic acid around the time of conception against the development of neural tube defects.

Conclusions

The major changes in transcriptional activity and the extent of epigenetic reprogramming that take place around the time of conception make it a particularly sensitive period to environmental influences, including maternal diet. The success of ART has, to a large extent, relied on the remarkable tolerance of mammalian gametes and cleavage-stage embryos to physical manipulations and alterations to their chemical environment. There is emerging evidence from studies in both animals and humans, however, that the ability of these "germ cells" to recapitulate the normal pro-

cess of development accurately under such conditions may be compromised. Thus far, the consequences for human development and health either have been too subtle or have occurred too infrequently to be adequately determined. They are also confounded by factors such as underlying infertility and maternal age. The longer-term effects of maternal diet around the time of conception have, until comparatively recently, been poorly investigated. Animal studies once again, however, point to very subtle programming effects that may not affect fertility and pregnancy outcome but that may manifest as disease in adult life.

Summary 17.3

- Given the relatively high incidence of genomic imprinting-related anomalies in animal studies following ovarian stimulation and/or following extended periods of gamete/embryo culture, the widespread uptake of procedures such as oocyte in vitro maturation and blastocyst culture should proceed with caution.

- Noninvasive assessments of preimplantation embryo development to the blastocyst stage in vitro have developed to usefully combine morphological, kinetic, and metabolic criteria. Such developments have the potential to further improve predictions of pregnancy outcome, in which more simple measures of embryo metabolism have already been found to correlate with clinical pregnancy rates following embryo transfer in humans.

- In addition to the well-documented protective effects of folic acid against the development of neural tube defects, maternal B vitamin status during the periconceptional period can have a major impact on fertility, pregnancy establishment, and term delivery and can determine pregnancy outcome in clinical IVF cycles. New data now indicate that there may also be more subtle, long-term developmental consequences of deficiencies in these vitamins around the time of conception that determine offspring adult health.

References

1. Hamilton BE and Ventura SJ, Fertility and abortion rates in the United States, 1960–2002. *Int J Androl* (2006), **29**:34–45.

2. Popkin BM, Understanding global nutrition dynamics as a step towards controlling cancer incidence. *Nat Rev Cancer* (2007), 7:61–7.

3. Heindel JJ, Endocrine disruptors and the obesity epidemic. *Toxicol Sci* (2003) 76:247–9.

4. Skakkebaek NE, Jorgensen N, Main KM, Rajpert-De Meyts E, Leffers H, Andersson AM, et al., Is human fecundity declining? *Int J Androl* (2006), 29:2–11.

5. Batsis JA, Nieto-Martinez RE, and Lopez-Jimenez F, Metabolic syndrome: from global epidemiology to individualized medicine. *Clin Pharmacol Ther* (2007), **82**:509–524.

6. Toppari J, Larsen JC, Christiansen P, Giwercman A, Grandjean P, Guillette LJ, Jr., et al., Male reproductive health and environmental xenoestrogens. *Environ Health Perspect* (1996), **104**(Suppl 4):741–803.

7. Henley DV and Korach KS, Endocrine-disrupting chemicals use distinct mechanisms of action to modulate endocrine system function. *Endocrinology* (2006), 147:S25–S32.

8. Newbold RR, Padilla-Banks E, Snyder RJ, and Jefferson WN, Perinatal exposure to environmental estrogens and the development of obesity. *Mol Nutr Food Res* (2007), 51:912–917.

9. McMillen IC and Robinson JS Developmental origins of the metabolic syndrome: prediction, plasticity, and programming. *Physiol Rev* (2005), 85:571–633.

10. Gardner DS, Lea RG, and Sinclair KD, Developmental programming of reproduction and fertility: what is the evidence? *Animal* (in press).

11. Sinclair KD, Young LE, Wilmut I, and McEvoy TG, In-utero overgrowth in ruminants following embryo culture: lessons from mice and a warning to men. *Hum Reprod* (2000), **15**(Suppl 5):68–86.

12. Fleming TP, Kwong WY, Porter R, Ursell E, Fesenko I, Wilkins A, et al., The embryo and its future. *Biol Reprod* (2004), **71**:1046–54.

13. Gougeon A, Regulation of ovarian follicular development in primates: facts and hypotheses. *Endocr Rev* (1996), **17**:121–55.

14. Griffin J, Emery BR, Huang I, Peterson CM, and Carrell DT, Comparative analysis of follicle morphology and oocyte diameter in four mammalian species (mouse, hamster, pig, and human). *J Exp Clin Assist Reprod* (2006), 3:2.

15. Pan H, O'Brien MJ, Wigglesworth K, Eppig JJ, and Schultz RM, Transcript profiling during mouse oocyte development and the effect of gonadotropin priming and development in vitro. *Dev Biol* (2005), **286**:493–506.

16. Miyano T and Manabe N, Oocyte growth and acquisition of meiotic competence. *Soc Reprod Fertil Suppl* (2007), **63**:531–8.

17. Sirard MA, Richard F, Blondin P, and Robert C, Contribution of the oocyte to embryo quality. *Theriogenology* (2006), **65**:126–36.

18. Allegrucci C, Thurston A, Lucas E, and Young L. Epigenetics and the germline. *Reproduction* (2005), **129**:137–49.

19. Lucifero D, Mann MR, Bartolomei MS, and Trasler JM, Gene-specific timing and epigenetic memory in oocyte imprinting. *Hum Mol Genet* (2004), 13:839–49.

20. Kageyama S, Liu H, Kaneko N, Ooga M, Nagata M, and Aoki F, Alterations in epigenetic modifications during oocyte growth in mice. *Reproduction* (2007), **133**:85–94.

21. Russo V, Martelli A, Berardinelli P, Di Giacinto O, Bernabo N, Fantasia D, et al., Modifications in chromatin morphology and organization during sheep oogenesis. *Microsc Res Tech* (2007), **70**:733–44.

22. Shi W and Haaf T, Aberrant methylation patterns at the two-cell stage as an indicator of early developmental failure. *Mol Reprod Dev* (2002), **63**:329–334.

23. Fortier AL, Lopes FL, Darricarrere N, Martel J, and Trasler JM, Superovulation alters the expression of imprinted genes in the midgestation mouse placenta. *Hum Mol Genet* (2008), 17:1653–65.

24. Sato A, Otsu E, Negishi H, Utsunomiya T, and Arima T, Aberrant DNA methylation of imprinted loci in superovulated oocytes. *Hum Reprod* (2007), **22**:26–35.

25. Sinclair KD, Assisted reproductive technologies and pregnancy outcomes: mechanistic insights from animal studies. *Semin Reprod Med* (2008), 26:153–61.

26. Banwell KM and Thompson JG, In vitro maturation of Mammalian oocytes: outcomes and consequences. *Semin Reprod Med* (2008), 26:162–74.

27. Clark AM, Ledger W, Galletly C, Tomlinson L, Blaney F, Wang X, and Norman RJ, Weight loss results in significant improvement in pregnancy and ovulation rates in anovulatory obese women. *Hum Reprod* (1995), **10**:2705–12.

28. Maheshwari A, Stofberg L, and Bhattacharya S, Effect of overweight and obesity on assisted reproductive technology – a systematic review. *Hum Reprod Update* (2007), 13:433–44.

29. Jungheim ES and Moley KH, The impact of type 1 and type 2 diabetes mellitus on the oocyte and the preimplantation embryo. *Semin Reprod Med* (2008), 26:186–95.

30. Adamiak SJ, Mackie K, Watt RG, Webb R, and Sinclair KD, Impact of nutrition on oocyte quality: cumulative effects of body composition and diet leading to hyperinsulinemia in cattle. *Biol Reprod* (2005), **73**:918–26.

31. Minge CE, Bennett BD, Norman RJ, and Robker RL, Peroxisome proliferator-activated receptor-gamma agonist rosiglitazone reverses the adverse effects of diet-induced obesity on oocyte quality. *Endocrinology* (2008), **149**:2646–56.

32. Minge CE, Ryan NK, Van Der Hoek KH, Robker RL, and Norman RJ, Troglitazone regulates peroxisome proliferator-activated receptors and inducible nitric oxide synthase in murine ovarian macrophages. *Biol Reprod* (2006), **74**:153–60.

33. Thessaloniki ESHRE/ASRM-Sponsored PCOS Consensus Workshop Group, Consensus on infertility treatment related to polycystic ovary syndrome. *Hum Reprod* (2008), **23**:462–77.

34. Dumesic DA, Padmanabhan V, and Abbott DH Polycystic ovary syndrome and oocyte developmental competence. *Obstet Gynecol Surv* (2008), **63**:39–48.

35. Wood JR, Dumesic DA, Abbott DH, and Strauss JF III, Molecular abnormalities in oocytes from women with polycystic ovary syndrome revealed by microarray analysis. *J Clin Endocrinol Metab* (2007), **92**:705–13.

36. Sinclair KD and Singh R, Modelling the developmental origins of health and disease in the early embryo. *Theriogenology* (2007), **67**:43–53.

37. Watkins AJ, Ursell E, Panton R, Papenbrock T, Hollis L, Cunningham C, et al., Adaptive responses by mouse early embryos to maternal diet protect fetal growth but predispose to adult onset disease. *Biol Reprod* (2008), **78**:299–306.

38. Swann K, Saunders CM, Rogers NT, and Lai FA, PLCzeta(zeta): a sperm protein that triggers Ca2+ oscillations and egg activation in mammals. *Semin Cell Dev Biol* (2006), **17**:264–73.

39. Cox LJ, Larman MG, Saunders CM, Hashimoto K, Swann K, and Lai FA. Sperm phospholipase Czeta from humans and cynomolgus monkeys triggers Ca2 +oscillations, activation and development of mouse oocytes. *Reproduction* (2002), **124**: 611–23.

40. Ozil JP, The parthenogenetic development of rabbit oocytes after repetitive pulsatile electrical stimulation. *Development* (1990), **109**:117–27.

41. Rogers NT, Halet G, Piao Y, Carroll J, Ko MS, and Swann K, The absence of a Ca(2+) signal during mouse egg activation can affect parthenogenetic preimplantation development, gene expression patterns, and blastocyst quality. *Reproduction* (2006), **132**:45–57.

42. Ozil JP and Huneau D, Activation of rabbit oocytes: the impact of the Ca2+ signal regime on development. *Development* (2001), **128**:917–28.

43. Ozil JP, Banrezes B, Toth S, Pan H, and Schultz RM, Ca2+ oscillatory pattern in fertilized mouse eggs affects gene expression and development to term. *Dev Biol* (2006), **300**:534–44.

44. Takahashi T, Takahashi E, Igarashi H, Tezuka N, and Kurachi H, Impact of oxidative stress in aged mouse oocytes on calcium oscillations at fertilization. *Mol Reprod Dev* (2003), **66**:143–52.

45. Nonogaki T, Noda Y, Goto Y, Kishi J, and Mori T, Developmental blockage of mouse embryos caused by fatty acids.

J Assist Reprod Genet (1994), **11**:482–8.

46. Wakefield SL, Lane M, Schulz SJ, Hebart ML, Thompson JG, and Mitchell M, Maternal supply of omega-3 polyunsaturated fatty acids alter mechanisms involved in oocyte and early embryo development in the mouse. *Am J Physiol Endocrinol Metab* (2008), **294**:E425–34.

47. Kurokawa M and Fissore RA, ICSI-generated mouse zygotes exhibit altered calcium oscillations, inositol 1,4,5-trisphosphate receptor-1 down-regulation, and embryo development. *Mol Hum Reprod* (2003), **9**:523–33.

48. Malcuit C, Maserati M, Takahashi Y, Page R, and Fissore RA, Intracytoplasmic sperm injection in the bovine induces abnormal [Ca2+]i responses and oocyte activation. *Reprod Fertil Dev* (2006), **18**:39–51.

49. Tremellen KP, Valbuena D, Landeras J, Ballesteros A, Martinez J, Mendoza S, et al., The effect of intercourse on pregnancy rates during assisted human reproduction. *Hum Reprod* (2000), **15**:2653–8.

50. Robertson SA, Seminal fluid signaling in the female reproductive tract: lessons from rodents and pigs. *J Anim Sci* (2007), **85**:E36–44.

51. Robertson SA, Bromfield JJ, and Tremellen KP, Seminal "priming" for protection from pre-eclampsia – a unifying hypothesis. *J Reprod Immunol* (2003), **59**:253–65.

52. Robertson SA, Sjoblom C, Jasper MJ, Norman RJ, and Seamark RF, Granulocyte-macrophage colony-stimulating factor promotes glucose transport and blastomere viability in murine preimplantation embryos. *Biol Reprod* (2001), **64**:1206–15.

53. de Moraes AA and Hansen PJ, Granulocyte-macrophage

colony-stimulating factor promotes development of in vitro produced bovine embryos. *Biol Reprod* (1997), **57**:1060–5.

54. Sjöblom C, Wikland M, and Robertson SA, Granulocyte-macrophage colony-stimulating factor promotes human blastocyst development in vitro. *Hum Reprod* (1999), **14**:3069–76.

55. Sjöblom C, Roberts CT, Wikland M, and Robertson SA, Granulocyte-macrophage colony-stimulating factor alleviates adverse consequences of embryo culture on fetal growth trajectory and placental morphogenesis. *Endocrinology* (2005), **146**:2142–53.

56. Betteridge KJ, Phylogeny, Ontogeny and embryo transfer. *Theriogenology* (1995), **44**:1061–98.

57. Eckert JJ and Fleming TP, Tight junction biogenesis during early development. *Biochim Biophys Acta* (2008), **1778**:717–28.

58. Leese HJ, Quiet please, do not disturb: a hypothesis of embryo metabolism and viability. *Bioessays* (2002), **24**:845–9.

59. Sinclair KD, Rooke JA, and McEvoy TG, Regulation of nutrient uptake and metabolism in pre-elongation ruminant embryos. *Reprod Suppl* (2003), **61**:371–85.

60. Zeng F, Baldwin DA, and Schultz RM, Transcript profiling during preimplantation mouse development. *Dev Biol* (2004), **272**:483–96.

61. Baumann CG, Morris DG, Sreenan JM, and Leese HJ, The quiet embryo hypothesis: molecular characteristics favoring viability. *Mol Reprod Dev* (2007), **74**:1345–53.

62. Ferguson EM and Leese HJ, A potential role for triglyceride as an energy source during bovine oocyte maturation and early embryo development. *Mol Reprod Dev* (2006), **73**:1195–201.

63. Schultz RM, The molecular foundations of the maternal to zygotic transition in the preimplantation embryo. *Hum Reprod Update* (2002), **8**:323–31.

64. Morgan HD, Santos F, Green K, Dean W, and Reik W, Epigenetic reprogramming in mammals. *Hum Mol Genet* (2005), **14**(Spec No 1):R47–58.

65. Beaujean N, Taylor J, Gardner J, Wilmut I, Meehan R, and Young L, Effect of limited DNA methylation reprogramming in the normal sheep embryo on somatic cell nuclear transfer. *Biol Reprod* (2004), **71**:185–93.

66. Young LE and Beaujean N, DNA methylation in the preimplantation embryo: the differing stories of the mouse and sheep. *Anim Reprod Sci* (2004), **82–83**:61–78.

67. Golding MC and Westhusin ME, Analysis of DNA (cytosine 5) methyltransferase mRNA sequence and expression in bovine preimplantation embryos, fetal and adult tissues. *Gene Expr Patterns* (2003), **3**:551–8.

68. Vassena R, Dee SR, and Latham KE, Species-dependent expression patterns of DNA methyltransferase genes in mammalian oocytes and preimplantation embryos. *Mol Reprod Dev* (2005), **72**:430–6.

69. Steele W, Allegrucci C, Singh R, Lucas E, Priddle H, Denning C, Sinclair K, and Young L, Human embryonic stem cell methyl cycle enzyme expression: modelling epigenetic programming in assisted reproduction? *Reprod Biomed Online* (2005), **10**:755–66.

70. Urman B and Balaban B, Is there still a place for co-cultures in the era of sequential media? *Reprod Biomed Online* (2005), **10**:492–6.

71. Quinn P, The development and impact of culture media for assisted reproductive technologies. *Fertil Steril* (2004), **81**:27–9.

72. Maxfield EK, Sinclair KD, Dunne LD, Broadbent PJ, Robinson JJ, Stewart E, et al., Temporary exposure of ovine embryos to an advanced uterine environment does not affect fetal weight but alters fetal muscle development. *Biol Reprod* (1998), **59**:321–5.

73. Sinclair KD, McEvoy TG, Maxfield EK, Maltin CA, Young LE, Wilmut I, et al., Aberrant fetal growth and development after in vitro culture of sheep zygotes. *J Reprod Fertil* (1999), **116**:177–86.

74. Rooke JA, McEvoy TG, Ashworth CJ, Robinson JJ, Wilmut I, Young LE, and Sinclair KD, Ovine fetal development is more sensitive to perturbation by the presence of serum in embryo culture before rather than after compaction. *Theriogenology* (2007), **67**:639–47.

75. Young LE, Fernandes K, McEvoy TG, Butterwith SC, Gutierrez CG, Carolan C, et al., Epigenetic change in IGF2R is associated with fetal overgrowth after sheep embryo culture. *Nat Genet* (2001), **27**:153–4.

76. Fernandez-Gonzalez R, Moreira P, Bilbao A, Jimenez A, Perez-Crespo M, Ramirez MA, et al., Long-term effect of in vitro culture of mouse embryos with serum on mRNA expression of imprinting genes, development, and behavior. *Proc Natl Acad Sci USA* (2004), **101**:5880–5.

77. Lawrence LT and Moley KH, Epigenetics and assisted reproductive technologies: human imprinting syndromes. *Semin Reprod Med* (2008), **26**:143–52.

78. Sinclair KD, Dunne LD, Maxfield EK, Maltin CA, Young LE, Wilmut I, et al., Fetal growth and development following temporary exposure of day 3 ovine embryos to an advanced uterine environment. *Reprod Fertil Dev* (1998), **10**:263–9.

79. Maxfield EK, Sinclair KD, Broadbent PJ, McEvoy TG, Robinson JJ, and Maltin CA, Short-term culture of ovine embryos modifies fetal myogenesis. *Am J Physiol* (1998), **274**:E1121–3.

80. Kwong WY, Wild AE, Roberts P, Willis AC, and Fleming TP, Maternal undernutrition during the preimplantation period of rat development causes blastocyst abnormalities and programming of postnatal hypertension.

Development (2000), **127**:4195–202.

81. Kwong WY, Miller DJ, Ursell E, Wild AE, Wilkins AP, Osmond C, et al., Imprinted gene expression in the rat embryo-fetal axis is altered in response to periconceptional maternal low protein diet. *Reproduction* (2006), **132**:265–77.

82. Watkins AJ, Wilkins A, Cunningham C, Perry VH, Seet MJ, Osmond C, et al., Low protein diet fed exclusively during mouse oocyte maturation leads to behavioural and cardiovascular abnormalities in offspring. *J Physiol* (2008), **586**:2231–44.

83. Sinclair KD, Allegrucci C, Singh R, Gardner DS, Sebastian S, Bispham J, et al., DNA methylation, insulin resistance, and blood pressure in offspring determined by maternal periconceptional B vitamin and methionine status. *Proc Natl Acad Sci USA* (2007), **104**:19351–6.

Specialized requirements

Nutrition, environment, and epigenetics

Ian M. Morison and Wolf Reik

Key messages

Epigenetics. In this chapter, we refer to epigenetic modifications of the genome, which include deoxyribonucleic acid (DNA) methylation and histone modifications. These modifications result in structural changes to chromosomal regions, resulting in altered activity states [1]. In other words, epigenetic modifications have the potential to cause mitotically and/or meiotically heritable changes in gene function that are not attributable to changes in DNA sequence.

Maternal dietary manipulation. Changes in DNA methylation and phenotype that occur after maternal dietary manipulations in mutant Agouti and Axin1 mouse models provide convincing evidence for the role of epigenetics in shaping adult phenotypes. It is plausible that similar changes in human maternal diet will affect the epigenotype of children, thereby affecting their phenotype including their lifelong susceptibility to disease.

Environmental manipulation. The use of assisted reproductive technologies in humans and animals is associated with altered epigenetic states in a small minority of children and in a substantial proportion of animals. The identification of factors that contribute to these epigenetic changes has important implications for reproductive technologies and also for the role of the environment in epigenetic plasticity.

Introduction

The growth and physiological function of cells and organs within a fetus, child, and adult rely on appropriate switching and regulation of approximately 20 000 genes that make up the human genome. During development, pluripotent embryonic and trophoblastic cells differentiate into cells and organs with specific functions and heritable memories of their identities. A cell's identity is controlled by many factors. Endocrine signalling, physiological cues, and signals from neighboring cells contribute to the gene activity (expression) of a cell, but gene expression is also regulated by long-term modifications to the DNA and chromatin itself, referred to as epigenetic modifications. Through the effects of DNA methylation, together with other epigenetic modifications, genes can be permanently silenced. As development and differentiation proceed, differentiated cells accumulate epigenetic marks that differ from those of pluripotent cells and distinguish cells of different lineages.

Epigenetic regulation has a well-defined role in the normal physiological events of X chromosome inactivation, genomic imprinting (discussed later), the maintenance of genomic integrity, and the silencing of retrotransposon elements. Its role in defining cell fate and lineage determination during organ development is being documented in increasing detail. An important recent development is the recognition of plasticity within the epigenetic modifications of the genome, and with it, the potential for the epigenome to be modified by environmental factors, including the nutritional state of the fetus.

Environmental factors can modify epigenetic programming at many stages of development, and in so doing epigenetics provides an organism with a mechanism by which it might "remember" its past exposures. For example, it is now clear that the environment of a cultured preimplantation embryo can affect its epigenetic modifications. In utero, maternal dietary manipulation is clearly associated with changes in epigenetically controlled phenotypes in mouse models such as the agouti[vy] mouse. During the postnatal period, maternal behavior can permanently modify the behavior of offspring through mechanisms that might include epigenetic modifications.

The focus of this chapter is to highlight developmental opportunities for nutritionally induced variation within the epigenotype (Figure 18.1). In addition, normal programmed, epigenetic modifications

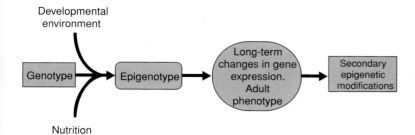

Figure 18.1 Epigenetic modification, influenced by nutritional and environmental exposures, is superimposed on the genome and contributes to long-term regulation of gene expression. Secondary epigenetic modifications, resulting from changes in gene expression, can be difficult to distinguish from primary epigenetic changes.

are critical for nutrient supply to the fetus. This aspect is discussed with reference in particular to the role of imprinted genes in placental function.

Epigenetic modifications

DNA methylation

DNA methylation and histone protein modifications interact to provide a stable epigenetic mechanism by which genes are made accessible for activation or rendered inactive. DNA methylation changes the chemical structure of the base within the double helix itself, whereas histones affect the structure of the nucleosome, and thereby the openness of the chromatin. Interactions between DNA methylation and histone modifications are being progressively elucidated. In vertebrates, DNA methylation almost exclusively affects cytosine nucleotides in the context of cytosine guanine dinucleotides (CpGs) (the "p" denotes the intervening phosphate group). Throughout the genome, the majority of CpG-associated cytosines are methylated, gene promoter regions being the exception in that they usually remain unmethylated [2]. Because every CpG dinucleotide is inevitably associated with a reciprocal CpG on the opposite strand, the cytosines on both strands can be, and are, reciprocally methylated. This reciprocal methylation provides the basis for the heritability of the epigenetic modification to daughter cells, in that, following DNA replication, the hemimethylated CpG provides the template for the maintenance DNA methyltransferase, DNMT1, which restores the original pattern of DNA methylation to the newly replicated strand of DNA.

Roles of DNA methylation

DNA methylation has multiple roles in regulating and maintaining the integrity of the genome. Its role may have originated as a mechanism to silence newly retro-transposed retroelements, given the need to maintain genomic integrity by preventing the transcription of mutagenic retrotransposons [3]. Methylation is also required for preservation of genome stability through its effects on pericentromeric and other repetitive DNA [4].

Methylation that is associated with gene promoters is likely to be of physiological relevance because it has the potential to alter gene expression and thus a cell's phenotype. The promoters and first exon of approximately 70% of genes contain regions that have a high density of CpGs often referred to as CpG islands [5]. These CpG-rich promoter regions remain unmethylated in most genes, but in a minority, they acquire methylation, often in a tissue-specific manner [6]. The consequence is gene silencing, which is often irreversible. The best-studied examples of gene promoter methylation involve genes on the inactivated X chromosome and imprinted genes. Imprinted genes comprise a group of approximately 100 genes for which gene expression is dependent on the parent from which the allele was inherited [7]. The silencing or activation of one parental copy of imprinted genes is mediated by methylation marks that are applied to imprint control regions during gametogenesis. Of the imprinted genes, approximately 20 are directly controlled by a differentially methylated region overlapping with their promoter. The parental allele that is methylated is silent, whereas the unmethylated allele is expressed. The remaining imprinted genes are controlled through secondary modifications that do not usually involve methylation.

Although anticipated for many years [8], a role for methylation in cell differentiation has only recently been confirmed. For some genes, early steps of differentiation involve tissue-specific methylation to maintain silencing permanently. For example, *Oct4* and *Nanog*, genes critically important for maintaining pluripotency in embryonic stem cells, become

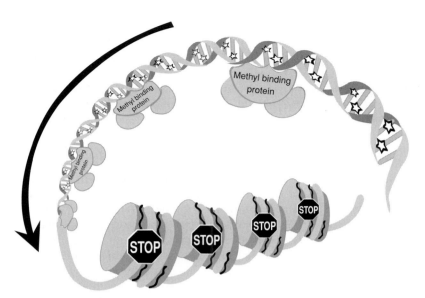

Figure 18.2 DNA methylation and histone modifications together make up the best-studied epigenetic modifications. The presence of DNA methylation (stars) attracts DNA binding proteins, which in turn recruit proteins that induce repressive histone modifications (stop signs) and lead to compact chromatin with repressed gene transcription.

methylated in differentiated tissues to prevent inappropriate pluripotency [9, 10]. Increasing numbers of developmental epigenetic switches are being identified [11], but key questions remain. How many developmental epigenetic switches are plastic, that is, how many genes can be influenced by extrinsic factors? During which phases of development can stable long-lasting epigenetic modifications be made? Are these switches binary (on or off), or variable as in a rheostat?

Histone modifications

DNA is wrapped around histones to form nucleosomes. Each nucleosome comprises two of each of the core histones H2A, H2B, H3, and H4 together with approximately 146 bp of DNA wrapped around the histone octamer.

The histones are modified by a plethora of post-translational protein modifications, predominantly within the amino terminal tails that project externally from the nucleosome [12]. These modifications determine the structure and compaction of the chromatin and are associated with the level of transcriptional activity. For example, methylation of specific lysines (H3 lysine 4 and H3 lysine 36) is often associated with active genes, whereas methylation of other lysines is associated with gene repression (H3 lysine 9, H3 lysine 27, and H4 lysine 20). The heritability and stability of the histone modifications remain poorly understood [13]. Histone acetylation is a transient modification, observed in genes that are being actively transcribed.

In contrast, lysine methylation states may be associated with long-term heritable states of gene activity [14]. Specific histone modifications can be recognized by specific "reader" proteins (such as HP1 for H3K9 methylation), which in turn can be associated with transcriptional repressors or activators [14].

Interaction between DNA methylation and histone modification is bidirectional [15] (Figure 18.2). For example, DNA methyltransferase enzymes are recruited to complexes associated with the repressive histone 3 lysine 9 methylation. Conversely, methylated DNA can be bound by DNA methyl-binding proteins, which in turn recruit chromatin remodelling co-repressor complexes. MBD1, for example, associates with the histone methyltransferase SetDB1, thereby coupling DNA methylation to repressive histone methylation. Although most of the examples provided here relate to observations of DNA methylation, it should be noted that commensurate alterations of the neighboring histones might also be occurring.

Cycles of epigenetic modification

The cycle of mammalian life entails a progression from the totipotency of an early embryo, through to the loss of multipotency associated with differentiation of somatic and extraembryonic tissues, but then reprogramming of the germ cells to provide a return to totipotency in the next generation. This cycle is accompanied by series of epigenetic events, each of which provides a potential opportunity for natural or pathological variation.

To summarize these epigenetic steps, we choose an arbitrary beginning point of the epigenetic cycle, that is, the fusion of the gametes at fertilization. The oocytes and sperm carry epigenetic marks that reflect their tissue type and their parental origin, but within hours of fertilization, a wave of epigenetic reprogramming occurs. This reprogramming includes genomewide DNA demethylation in the zygote, together with changes in histone modifications [16]. The wave of DNA demethylation presumably exists to erase epigenetic modifications that were specifically required for germ cell and gamete development. Within a few cell divisions, however, repressive epigenetic modifications begin to be applied to the early embryo. These epigenetic changes include consolidation of the parental imprints, X chromosome inactivation in females, inactivation of retrotransposons, and the early stages of lineage commitment and differentiation. As development proceeds in the embryo and newborn, there are ongoing modifications to the epigenome, some of which may be influenced by the environment of the developing animal. The germ cells of the developing fetus begin a distinct branch of the cycle, wherein the epigenetic marks of the embryo are erased, wiping the slate clean for the new generation. The developing germ cells and gametes then acquire new epigenetic marks including the imprinting marks that signal the parent-of-origin-specific gene expression and the repressive modifications required to silence (retro)transposons [3].

Each of these steps has the potential to be affected during normal and aberrant development. For some of these modification steps, there is evidence of developmental plasticity that might allow for environmentally or nutritionally induced modification of the epigenetic program, and consequently the phenotype.

Epigenetics of the early embryo

Epigenetic programming in the zygote

The process of fertilization sets in motion a massive reprogramming of the epigenome. In the early mouse embryo, the parental genomes undergo extensive demethylation, the paternal genome being actively demethylated within a few hours, whereas the maternal genome is progressively demethylated up to the morula stage. From the time of the late morula–early

blastocyst transition, the methylation of the genome is restored, progressively to adult levels. It is interesting to note that average methylation of the trophectoderm DNA is lower than that in the inner cell mass, indicating that different tissues can modulate their genomic methylation. Of note, the kinetics of demethylation and remethylation vary between different mammalian species [17].

The dynamic and massive changes in methylation during the first few cell divisions and days of life have multiple implications for human development. First, the opportunities for generalized perturbation or manipulation of epigenetic programming may be at their greatest at this stage. More specifically, if the efficiency of either, or both, demethylation and remethylation is affected by the environment, through the availability of methyl donors or by other features of maternal nutritional state, then there is the opportunity for epigenetic variation in the offspring. Second, in the assisted reproductive technologies (ART), it is this stage of development that occurs in vitro in artificial media. Third, if epigenetic modifications applied to the gametes (discussed later) are to have an effect on a child, those modifications must survive the epigenetic erasure in the zygote.

Diet-associated hypomethylation in sheep

The methylation of cytosine requires donation of a methyl group by S-adenosyl methionine (SAM). If the dynamics of demethylation and remethylation in the zygote are affected by the availability of methyl donors, it follows that SAM levels might influence the overall methylation state of an organism. SAM provides methyl groups not only for DNA but also for protein and lipid methylation, and its levels are affected by changes in the B_{12} and folate pathways (Figure 18.3). It must be remembered, however, that the functions of folate and other constituents of the pathway extend well beyond the supply of methyl donors.

To address the role of vitamin B_{12}, folate, and methionine in periconceptual sheep development, Sinclair and colleagues [18] induced "methyl-deficiency" in maternal sheep and, following transfer of the embryos to recipient ewes, demonstrated long-term epigenetic and phenotypic changes in adult offspring. Methyl deficiency was achieved by reducing the dietary cobalt and sulphur levels, thus diminishing the capacity of the rumen organisms to synthesize sulphur amino acids (including methionine) and vitamin B_{12}.

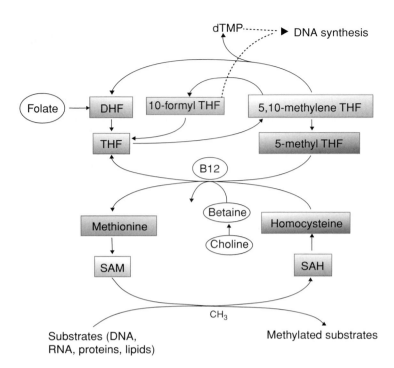

Figure 18.3 Simplified overview of folate metabolism. Dietary factors (folate, vitamin B₁₂, choline, and betaine) that might affect methylation are shown. DHF, dihydrofolate; THF, tetrahydrofolate; SAM, S-adenosylmethionine; SAH, S-adenosylhomocysteine.

Although the levels of plasma vitamin B_{12}, folate, and methionine in the donor ewes remained within normal physiological ranges, they were significantly reduced compared with control animals. "Deficient" and control Day 6 blastocyst embryos were then transferred to normally fed surrogate ewes. As adults, male offspring of treated ewes showed increased weight and were fatter, had impaired insulin sensitivity, and had higher blood pressure. Putative epigenetic modifications, most of which involved reduced DNA methylation, appeared to affect 4% of the genes studied.

This study indicates that nutritional modification of early embryos can have lasting phenotypic effects, notably affecting physiological functions that are relevant to the detrimental effects of famine and low birth weight in humans (discussed later). Questions of cause and effect remain. What is the role of altered DNA methylation? Does it constitute the heritable memory that brings about adverse phenotypic changes in adulthood, or is it simply a consequence of altered cell metabolism?

Diet-induced hypermethylation in the agouti^{vy} mouse

The agouti viable yellow (A^{vy}) mouse model provides another useful example of the potential for dietary manipulation of the epigenotype. The A^{vy} mutation resulted from insertion of an intracisternal A-particle (IAP) retrotransposon in the promoter of the agouti gene. When the IAP is active, the coat color is abnormal (yellow), and the mice become obese and develop tumors, but when the IAP element is silenced by methylation, the phenotype is normal. In any one litter, the mice can show the full range of coat colors that vary from yellow (unmethylated), through mottled, to normal (so called pseudo-agouti; fully methylated). This intra- and intermouse variation in coat color indicates the occurrence of epigenetic variability, the level of which is set early in embryogenesis before lineage-specific tissue differentiation has occurred [19].

The key point about the A^{vy} mouse model is that a supplemented maternal diet (enriched with methyl donors: folate [3-fold enrichment compared with NIH-31 diet], vitamin B [12] [20-fold], betaine, and choline [3-fold]) shifts the average coat color of the offspring toward normal [20] and that this normalization is associated with an increase in methylation of the IAP retrotransposon [21]. It has been proposed that the altered maternal diet increases the availability of methyl donors, which then modulate the epigenetic modifications of the IAP promoter at the mutant *agouti* gene.

The observations on the methyl-deficient sheep and the A^{vy} mice raise profound questions for the role of diet in human epigenetic programming. How many genes might be affected by the changes in the apparent abundance of methyl donors? Given that pseudoagouti A^{vy} mice are leaner and longer lived than agouti A^{vy} mice [20, 22], it might be predicted that a methyl-supplemented diet would have beneficial effects, such as reducing the obesity and tumor predisposition of these mice. In contrast, human birth weight is positively correlated with maternal folate status [23]. Obviously the long-term effects and mechanisms of action of methyl-donor supplementation need to be determined.

Can the lessons from nutritional manipulation be generalized, or are changes restricted to genes that contain IAP and related elements? Would it be expected that a mother who has a diet rich in folate and other methyl donors would have hypermethylated offspring compared with the hypomethylated offspring of folate-deficient mothers? What is the mechanism by which maternal diet modifies the epigenome of the offspring?

Notably the administration of genistein, a soy-derived phyto-estrogen, to mice similarly increases the average level of methylation of the A^{vy} IAP, altering coat color and protecting against later obesity [24]. Conversely, the estrogenic xenobiotic chemical bisphenol A (BPA) that is used in the manufacture of polycarbonate plastic and epoxy resins was shown to reduce methylation of this IAP element. These last observations increase the range of maternal ingestible compounds that might affect methylation in offspring but also broaden the range of mechanisms through which they might directly or indirectly induce epigenetic change.

Are diet-induced epigenetic changes restricted to a subset of genes?

The A^{vy} model is unusual in that the mutation is caused by the insertion of a retrotransposon upstream of the gene promoter. Invading retrotransposons appear to be a specific target for the methylation machinery, and thus the effects of diet might be observed in similarly affected genes. Indeed, the $Axin1^{Fu}$ mouse provides another example of an IAP insertion in which methylation can be manipulated by diet. The kinky-tailed phenotype of the $Axin1^{Fu}$ mouse results from insertion of an IAP into the $Axin1$ gene, and the penetrance of the mutation is inversely correlated with the degree of methylation of the IAP [25]. As for the A^{vy} mouse, methylation levels are concordant across multiple tissues (liver, kidney, brain), reflecting similar modifications in each of the different germ layers of the early embryo. Furthermore, modification of mothers' diet, by addition of folate, vitamin B_{12}, choline, and betaine, resulted in a substantial reduction in the severity of the kinked-tail phenotype, which was associated with increased methylation of the IAP element [26].

Epigenetic variation in human *AXIN1* methylation

A fascinating human parallel with the $Axin1^{Fu}$ mouse might be provided by the human congenital disorder caudal duplication anomaly in which there is duplication of the distal spine and pelvic organs. In a pair of monozygotic twins discordant for the caudal duplication anomaly, the affected twin was found to have significantly more *AXIN1* promoter methylation than the unaffected twin and controls [27], suggesting that silencing of the *AXIN1* gene played a causative role and that nongenetic factors can influence the level of methylation. Furthermore, in the control population, there was variation in the degree of *AXIN1* methylation, thus establishing *AXIN1* as a candidate gene for environmentally induced epigenetic variation.

Neural tube defects

In view of the success of maternal folate supplementation in reducing the incidence of neural tube defects, it has been speculated that epigenetic mechanisms may be involved in the disease etiology and its prevention [28]. This hypothesis is especially attractive given the epigenetic variability reported for the human *AXIN1* gene. There are several mouse models of neural tube defects, many of which are folate responsive, but despite the obvious efficacy of folate therapy, the mechanism of its action remains unknown [29]. As noted earlier, the effect of folate supplementation might not be limited to the availability of methyl donors because this vitamin has pleiotropic effects including effects on purine and pyrimidine synthesis, amino acid metabolism, and DNA, protein, and lipid methylation (Figure 18.3).

Human IVF demonstrates an environmental effect

Data from human in vitro fertilization (IVF) suggest that epigenetic perturbation is possible during the first few days of development. A petri dish of synthetic media provides a markedly abnormal environment for the developing embryo and there is evidence that this abnormal environment is associated with epigenetic aberrations in children conceived by IVF. For example, the incidence of Beckwith-Wiedemann syndrome (BWS) appears to be increased, as is that of Angelman syndrome (AS) [30]. In a population-wide study in Australia, the incidence of BWS was approximately 9 times greater in children conceived by IVF than in the general population (i.e. 1 in ~4000 after IVF, compared with 1 in ~36 000 in the general population). That children conceived by IVF who have BWS almost all share a single epigenetic defect – hypomethylation of the *KCNQ1OT1* gene promoter – provides additional evidence that the procedure itself is responsible for the aberrant epigenetic modification. Although epidemiological evidence for an increase in the incidence of AS is less strong, the molecular studies of many IVF-associated AS cases reveal a rare mechanism for AS (hypomethylation at the imprint control region), suggesting a causal association.

If the abnormal in vitro environment of IVF can induce major epigenetic aberration at low frequency, then does IVF induce minor epigenetic change at higher frequencies? The observation that children conceived by IVF are, on average, taller with higher insulin-like growth factor 1 (IGF-1) and IGF-2 levels and have more favorable lipid profiles than control children, points to common changes with IVF [31]. Furthermore, if perturbed environment within a petri dish can alter epigenetic programming, can an imbalanced in vivo environment do likewise? That is, can the periconceptual nutritional state of the mother affect the epigenome in naturally conceived children?

Epigenetic aberrations after animal embryo culture

Animal studies certainly confirm the increase in epigenetic abnormalities that can be associated with in vitro embryo culture. However, the lessons from animals might not be directly applicable to early human embryo development.

Mouse embryos show frequent epigenetic aberrations when exposed to an abnormal environment and media. One of the earliest examples of this is altered methylation and expression of specific genes in adult mice following nuclear transplantation [32]. More recently, aberrant loss of imprinting (biallelic expression) of one or more genes occurred in 80% to 90% of placentas and 17% of fetuses following embryo transfer and culture [33]. IVF shows an increased rate of epigenetic aberrations compared with culture alone [34]. Mouse embryo culture has been associated with higher blood pressure in adult mice and changes in the activity of physiological regulators, suggesting that culture-induced epigenetic changes can have a phenotypic impact [35]. In contrast, the phenotypic consequences of abnormal imprinting in mouse or human placentas are not yet clear.

A feature that clearly distinguishes some published animal culture results from human IVF is the use of serum within the culture media. The addition of serum reduces viability of mouse embryos and was associated with a decrease in expression from both *H19* and *Igf2* (a pair of reciprocally imprinted genes) and a small increase in *H19* methylation [36].

Additional manipulation of the mouse culture environment may provide candidate procedures for improvement of human and animal artificial reproductive techniques. If the nutrient balance of the culture media alters epigenetic programming in embryos, then not only is early nutrition important for children conceived by IVF, it also suggests that the environment provided by mothers in normal in vivo conceptions may influence offspring. However, the rate of imprinting abnormalities detected by molecular techniques (17%) in mice after embryo transfer and culture is approximately 700-fold higher than the rate of phenotypically detected imprinting abnormalities in humans. Furthermore, the potential to modify the nutrient composition of the human oviduct and uterine fluids may be insignificant compared to that occurring in vitro, and the lessons from IVF may not be easily generalizable to in vivo conception.

Mouse studies suggest that the composition of the media is important in causing epigenetic aberrations, but other in vitro factors such as temperature fluctuations, absence of a hypoxia, or altered growth kinetics may play a role. Furthermore, although animals clearly show epigenetic abnormalities from artificial reproductive techniques, it remains controversial whether humans do. Given that infertility itself appears to be associated with epigenetic abnormalities of the sperm, and an increase in BWS and AS, it is not clear how many of the human IVF-associated imprinting abnormalities reflect the procedure versus infertility itself [37].

Cow and sheep IVF

The occurrence of aberrant phenotypes following in vitro culture in cows and sheep has reinforced concerns about the potential for human IVF to affect phenotype. Large offspring syndrome, associated with cloning and embryo culture, is characterized by placental and fetal overgrowth with abnormal organ and skeletal development. In cultured sheep embryos, the syndrome is associated with a reduction in methylation of the DMR that controls *Igf2R* imprinting, with consequent reduction in levels of IGF2R, explaining the enhanced fetal growth [38]. It occurs after both cloning (nuclear transfer) and culture, but the mechanisms are not necessarily the same, because cloning requires the additional step of erasure of somatic epigenetic modifications. Importantly, however, this extreme example of embryo culture–associated epigenetic aberration is predominantly associated with the use of serum in the culture media [39]. Not only does this suggest a growth factor–related etiology, but the lessons are probably not applicable to human IVF, in which the use of serum is no longer recommended. At this stage, results from animal and human IVF do not allow general conclusions to be drawn about the optimal nutrient environment for the developing zygote.

Environmental effects during embryogenesis

After early postimplantation development, the global DNA methylation status of an embryo and its extra-embryonic tissues remains relatively stable. However, continuing epigenetic modification does occur during the process of tissue differentiation. For example, as neural progenitor cells differentiate from mouse embryonic stem cells, numerous genes undergo epigenetic modification, reflected by changes in histone modification [40], whereas differentiating embryonic or extraembryonic cells, or differentiating fat cells show modifications of DNA methylation [11, 41]. In utero development, essentially an accumulating sequence of differentiation events, will obviously

include numerous epigenetic modifications that alter the physiology of the developing organs.

The ability to manipulate the maternal environment to optimize the health of offspring is a key focus of this chapter. This section considers the possibility that offsprings' epigenotypes can be altered by changes in maternal factors.

Metabolic syndrome, diabetes, and insulin resistance

There is considerable evidence that poor fetal growth can influence the phenotype of adults. To explain the adult "memory" of fetal exposures, it has been speculated that these effects are mediated by epigenetic mechanisms, although the evidence so far remains scant.

A role for epigenetic modification has been proposed, for example, in Type II diabetes on the basis of observations that various maternal interventions in rats result in diabetes or insulin resistance in adult offspring. Specific evidence for the involvement of epigenetic factors comes from observed changes in DNA methylation and histone modifications in offspring of rats with intrauterine growth restriction (IUGR). In a commonly used model, a hypoxic, vascular insult from bilateral uterine artery ligation 3 days before birth rapidly induces IUGR, which is associated with reduced pancreatic beta-cell mass, reduced insulin secretion, insulin resistance, and, consequently, Type II diabetes in adults. Within 24 hours of the onset of growth retardation, the level of expression from the *Pdx1* (pancreatic and duodenal homeobox 1) gene was halved. Subsequently, histone modifications that are associated with gene silencing were observed in the *Pdx1* promoter, that is, histone deacetylation, reduced histone 3 lysine 4 methylation, and increased histone 3 lysine 9 methylation, along with increasing promoter DNA methylation as the animals age [42, 43].

A change in epigenetic modification, however, does not necessarily reflect a causal effect. For example, DNA methylation can occur as a consequence, rather than a cause, of gene silencing [44], whereas histone acetylation is a short-term labile modification that merely reflects the activity state of that gene rather than its long-term epigenetic state [45]. Many of the histone modifications are more stable than acetylation, but the extent to which they contribute to long-term heritable gene activity states remains controversial [13, 14]. Epigenetic changes that have been reported to date might constitute part of the permanent metabolic memory that causes persistence of the diabetic phenotype into adulthood, but they might also reflect physiological changes mediated by other mechanisms. For example, the memory of the fetal environment may reside predominantly within anatomical changes induced in the developing organs such as the pancreas.

Feeding pregnant rats with a low-protein (high-carbohydrate) diet from conception to delivery provides another model that has been used to study epigenetic modification. The glucocorticoid receptor and PPARα genes (GR and PPARA) have been the specific targets of study, because upregulation of their expression occurs with disturbed metabolic control in rats. PPARα, one of the peroxisome proliferator-activated nuclear receptors, has roles in fatty acid oxidation, lipid metabolism, and inflammation, and its expression is increased under conditions of fasting to manage energy substrates for survival. Glucocorticoid receptor, ubiquitously expressed in all tissues, mediates the multiple roles of glucocorticoids, effectors of the stress system. PPARA promoter methylation has been quantified by using pyrosequencing of liver DNA from offspring of pregnant rats fed a low-protein (high-carbohydrate) diet [46]. The average methylation of PPARA was reduced from 6.1% to 4.5%, raising the possibility that profound dietary changes might induce subtle, graded changes in the epigenotype. Previous studies have also suggested reduction in methylation of the GR gene, but quantitative data are not yet available.

Nutritional studies in India point to associations between vitamin B_{12} and folate status, intrauterine growth retardation, and childhood insulin resistance. In particular, high red cell folate levels were positively associated with insulin resistance [47]. These findings are interesting, particularly in view of the evidence implicating altered B_{12} and folate with epigenetic change in mice and sheep.

Hypertension

Human epidemiological studies and animal models both implicate a role for fetal undernutrition in adult hypertension [48]. The in utero effects of altered maternal diet include reduction in nephron number, modification of the renin-angiotensin system, endothelial dysfunction, and increased birth weight, confounded by postnatal catch-up growth and obesity. Epigenetic

mechanisms have been considered as mediators of these developmental changes.

Using the maternal low-protein (high-carbohydrate) rat model, methylation of, and expression from, the angiotensin II receptor, type 1b gene (Agtr1b) has been studied [49]. The low-protein diet was associated with a reduction in Agtr1b methylation from 22% in controls to 7% in the whole adrenal of treated animals. Concurrently, threefold greater expression of Agtr1b was detected in treated animals. Because Agtr1b expression is predominantly from the adrenal cortex, which constitutes only a small minority of adrenal cells, the apparent correlation between cortical expression and whole adrenal methylation requires further investigation.

Animal models, and some human epidemiological data, point toward an association between maternal diet and birth weight and the number of nephrons in adult kidney [50]. Retarded renal growth is possibly associated with adult hypertension [51]. Although epigenetic changes may be associated with the changes in gene expression that accompany fetal kidney growth retardation [52], it is also possible that altered anatomical structures themselves could provide a legacy of the uterine environment.

Postnatal programming

The potential for maternal effects on epigenetic modification might not be restricted to pregnancy. Behavioral changes in nursing rat mothers, which induce long-term physiological changes in offspring, might affect DNA methylation. Mothers that exhibit high levels of licking and grooming of their pups caused increased expression of the estrogen receptor alpha in the hypothalamus, and of the glucocorticoid receptor in the hippocampus in offspring. These changes in receptor expression were paralleled by changes in methylation of the 1b and exon 1_7 promoters, respectively; pups from high licking and grooming mothers showing lower methylation for these genes than pups from low licking and grooming mothers [53, 54].

It remains plausible, yet currently unproven, that epigenetic change can be induced after birth, by changes in nutrition. Indeed, excessive catch-up growth in low birth weight infants is associated with long-term obesity [55], which might be mediated by anatomical or physiological changes supported by epigenetic modification.

Suggestions that DNA methylation within the brain shows plasticity and that nutritional status may be important in its maintenance herald the possibility that lifelong nutritional status may play a role in epigenetic programming [56]. However, evidence for this is provided only by a small group of preliminary reports of altered epigenetic DNA methylation.

Altered epigenetics during germ cell development

Modification of the germ cells constitutes completion of the epigenetic cycle, albeit in a specialized branch of development distinct from the other somatic tissues of the embryo. Epigenetic marks required for successful imprinting and differentiation of the embryo are erased in the early germ cells in preparation for totipotency. During this erasure or reprogramming, there is substantial loss of repressive epigenetic modifications such as DNA methylation and repressive histone methylation (e.g. histone 3-lysine 9 dimethylation) [57].

Subsequently, during germ cell maturation and gametogenesis, a new round of epigenetic modifications is applied to this "clean slate." Presumably within germ cells, oocytes, and sperm, epigenetic modifications are applied to restrict gene expression to a relevant subset of developmental genes. In addition, during gametogenesis, it is critically important to minimize activity and mobility of retrotransposons within the genome. These repetitive retroelements are held in check by DNA methylation [3], preventing increased mutational load in the species.

Impact of imprinted genes on resources and placental growth

The focus of the previous sections has been on potential effects of maternal nutrients on epigenetic modifications. In addition, the epigenetically controlled imprinted genes appear to play a major role in controlling nutrient transfer at the maternal-fetal interface [58, 59]. Because genomic imprinting arose at the time of evolution of lactation and placentation, we have proposed that imprinting has a key role in the allocation of maternal resources across the placenta to the developing embryo. The conflict, or kinship, theory of imprinting evolution postulates a conflict between maternal and paternal genomes, in that the fitness of the paternal genes is enhanced by extracting the maximum quantity of resources at the expense of offspring from other fathers. Conversely, the fitness of the maternal genome is enhanced if maternal resources are conserved and distributed to as many offspring as possible during the mother's reproductive life.

In accordance with the predictions of the conflict hypothesis, the effect of parental imprinting on placental growth and efficiency differs between maternally and paternally expressed genes. That is, in general, paternally expressed (maternally suppressed) imprinted genes enhance placental growth, surface area, and nutrient transport, whereas the maternally expressed genes suppress placental growth [60].

By using knockout mouse models to reduce the number of functional copies of the imprinted genes even further (i.e. to zero), the role of imprinting in placental growth can be inferred. These mouse models suggest that a role of maternal suppression of $Igf2$, $Peg1$, and $Peg3$ is to decrease placental size. Similarly, knockout of paternally suppressed genes, $Igf2r$, $Cdkn1c$, $H19$, $Phlda2$, and $Grb10$, results in enhanced placental growth. Therefore, by controlling the size of the placenta during normal development, epigenetic control of these imprinted genes has the potential to control global nutrient transfer to the fetus.

More detailed assessment has confirmed key functional roles for some of these genes. $Igf2$, for example, has a placenta-specific transcript (P0), deletion of which results in marked placental growth retardation [58]. The constraint on fetal growth imposed by the small placenta is demonstrated by postnatal catch-up growth. Although the efficiency of the small placenta was shown to be enhanced, it was clearly insufficient to meet the nutritional requirements of the developing fetus. The placentomegaly that results from loss of $Igf2$ imprinting (which causes a double dose of $Igf2$) confirms the role of maternal suppression of this gene in restricting resource allocation to her offspring. In addition, these models demonstrate the requirement for coordinated supply (placental) and demand (fetal) and point to the possibility that uncoordinated growth may have maladaptive consequences such as excess postnatal catch-up growth, with its negative consequences in adult life [55].

The coordination between placental nutrient supply and fetal demand is further demonstrated by the crosstalk between paternally expressed $Igf2$ and another imprinted gene $Slc38a4$. When $Igf2$-controlled fetal demand exceeded supply, Slc38a4, a System A amino acid transporter, was upregulated, thereby increasing placental efficiency [61]. The interaction between paternally expressed *Igf2* and paternally expressed *Slc38a4* shows the importance of epigenetic gene regulation (i.e. genomic imprinting) in controlling nutrient demand and supply. In addition, the roles of both proteins are consistent with the hypothesis that paternally expressed imprinted genes contribute to the extraction of maternal resources. Reciprocally, suppression of the maternally inherited allele is an important mechanism by which a mother controls the allocation of her resources, thus enhancing her lifelong reproductive fitness.

A key question is whether physiological or pathological alterations within the cells that give rise to the trophoblast and placenta during the first 3 to 4 days of life can additionally influence placental function. In mice, as noted earlier, embryo culture and IVF are associated with a high rate of aberrant methylation of imprinted genes in the placenta. In cattle, placentomegaly is a prominent feature of the large offspring syndrome, which is associated with embryo culture [38]. It is interesting to note that in vitro–produced pregnancies were associated with increased glucose and fructose accumulation in fetal plasma and associated fluids, suggesting that placentomegaly and enhanced transport capacity are closely related [62]. In addition, in humans, placental overgrowth is a characteristic feature of the somatic overgrowth imprinting disorder Beckwith-Wiedemann syndrome [63].

A more subtle response to an altered nutritional environment at conception might lead to modulation of placental imprinting. This would result in a direct relationship between maternal nutritional state and feto-placental growth at the earliest stages of development.

Transgenerational epigenetic modification

The earlier sections have considered the potential for a mother to modify her offspring epigenetically, but to what extent can the effects of the maternal or paternal environment induce any transgenerational epigenetic effects? Epidemiological evidence highlights the potential for grandparental nutrition to impact on the phenotype of the grandchildren. The food supply of paternal grandfathers during their prepubertal slow growth period (age 9–12 years) has been linked to the mortality of the grandsons, and that of the paternal grandmothers to the granddaughters. In both situations, good food supply was associated with an increased risk of premature death in the grandchildren [64].

The ability to inherit the consequences of grandparental food supply suggests the occurrence of transgenerational nongenetic inheritance. Although the mechanism has yet to be determined, these observations raise the possibility that germline epigenetic marks can survive germ cell reprogramming and zygotic demethylation. Importantly, transmission through the paternal line appears to exclude maternal lineage effects (discussed later). Confirmation of these results and determination of the mechanism of transmission might have implications for future nutritional manipulation.

When considering maternal transgenerational transmission, it is important to consider that a change in the maternal environment could potentially exert direct epigenetic and genetic effects on the offspring itself but also, through modification of the offspring's germ cells, the subsequent generation (i.e. grandchildren). The following generation is, therefore, the first to be not directly exposed to the environmental exposure of interest, and thus, it is not until this third generation that one can conclude the occurrence of transgenerational inheritance of an epigenetic modification [65].

For intergenerational epigenetic inheritance to occur, a modification within a gamete must survive the epigenetic programming that occurs in the zygote. As imprinted genes attest, not all DNA methylation is erased in the zygote, given that approximately 20 imprint control regions must maintain differential methylation throughout this stage. In addition to imprint gene control regions, it is known that the methylation of IAP retroelements is relatively resistant to erasure in the zygote [66]. The extent to which these and other gametic modifications survive the postconception erasure essentially defines the potential for intergenerational epigenetic inheritance. Germline epigenetic marks that survive zygotic reprograming to manifest themselves in the second generation are indeed of considerable interest, in that it would provide a mechanism by which the environment of the grandmother could affect the grandchild's phenotype. Epigenetic inheritance for an additional generation (i.e. true transgenerational inheritance) has the additional requirement of surviving the reprogramming that occurs in primordial germ cells.

Table 18.1 Examples of putative epigenetic modifications associated with environmental factors or ancestral phenotypes

Timing	Factor	Model	Putative epigenetic modification	References
Grandparental	Food supply	Human	Unknown	
Transgenerational	Endocrine disruptors	Rat	DNA meth	
Maternal soma and germ cells	Maternal coat color	A^{vy} mouse	DNA meth	
Parental soma and germ cells	Parental tail shape	$Axin1^{Fu}$ mouse	DNA meth	
Paternal germ cells	Nuclear transfer	Mouse	DNA meth	
Periconception	Methyl donor "deficiency"	Sheep	DNA hypometh	
Periconception	Methyl donor supplements	A^{vy} and $Axin1^{Fu}$ mice	DNA hypermeth	[21], [26]
Periconception	In vitro fertilization	Human	DNA hypometh at KCNQTOT1, SNRPN	
Periconception	Embryo culture, in vitro fertilization	Mouse	Altered DNA meth	[33], [34]
Periconception	Embryo culture (with serum)	Cow, sheep	DNA hypometh at IGF-2R	
Embryogenesis	Placental ischemia with intrauterine growth restriction	Rat	Altered histones; DNA meth at Pdx1	[42], [43]
Embryogenesis	Maternal low-protein/high-carbohydrate diet	Rat	Reduced DNA meth at Ppara	
Embryogenesis	Maternal low-protein/high-carbohydrate diet	Rat	Reduced DNA meth Agtr1b	
Postnatal	Maternal behavior	Rat	Altered DNA meth gene name ERA, GR?	[53], [54]

It is further important to distinguish maternal epigenetic inheritance from maternal lineage effects: a phenotype could be inherited through the maternal lineage simply because of altered phenotype of the mother, causing altered phenotype of the daughter and so on. There is, for example, a consistent positive correlation between the birth weights of mothers and their offspring, the consequence of which is to perpetuate, over multiple generations, the phenotypic response to food deprivation [67]. Fortunately, maternal lineage effects can be experimentally dissociated from maternal epigenetic inheritance by embryo transfers.

Lessons from animal models

Manipulation of early embryos, by culture or nuclear transfer, is associated with perturbed epigenetic modifications, some of which may be capable of transgenerational transmission. For example, manipulation of zygotes by transfer of the pronuclei into recipient eggs of a different genetic background resulted in increased gene methylation and repressed expression of major urinary protein (MUP), as well as reduced adult body weight [32]. Importantly, probable transgeneration epigenetic inheritance occurred after transmission to the next generation through the male germline [68]. More than half of the offspring of manipulated males showed similar reduction of MUP expression, along with increased Mup methylation. Furthermore, adult body weight was also reduced in these offspring.

As noted earlier, the phenotype of A^{vy} mice depends on the degree of methylation of an IAP retrotransposon within the agouti gene promoter. Compared with those with agouti (yellow) coat color, agouti mothers with a normal coat color (i.e. heavily methylated IAP) have a higher proportion of offspring with normal coat color, suggesting the persistence of an epigenetic signal through erasure in the germ cells and post fertilization [22]. Thus, the mothers' gametes carry an epigenetic record that parallels her somatic phenotype, and this record is not completely erased in the zygote. Similar observations with respect to parental transmission of the kinky-tail phenotype of the $Axin1^{Fu}$ mouse support the case that transgenerational epigenetic inheritance can occur [25]. Curiously, the A^{vy} IAP is completely demethylated in the early embryo, showing that the intergenerational epigenetic mark may not be DNA methylation [69].

The next question is whether nutritional manipulation of an F0 mother can alter the long-term epigenotype of the "unexposed" grand (F2)-offspring. Indeed Cropley et al. showed that a high-methyl-donor supplemented maternal (F0) diet (vitamin B_{12}, folate, betaine, choline, zinc, and methionine) normalized not only the coat color of the F1 offspring (maternal effect) but also that of the F2 generation [70]. Because the germ cells of the F1 females were exposed to, and presumably modified by, the supplemented diet during their embryogenesis, this experiment indicates that the oocyte-associated epigenetic modifications are not completely erased in the F2 zygote. Thus, this dietary intervention experiment is consistent with previous observations that a mother's somatic epigenotype can influence the epigenotype of her offspring.

Can these modifications be transmitted yet another generation and influence the epigenotype of F3 offspring, the true test of transgenerational inheritance? [65] When A^{vy} mice were fed with methyl-supplemented diets for successive generations, there was no cumulative effect across generations, suggesting that diet-induced epigenetic change is not inherited in a transgenerational manner [19].

Although a role for diet in mediating transgenerational epigenetic inheritance has not been demonstrated, such inheritance has been observed after exposure of rats to estrogenic and antiandrogenic endocrine disruptors (methoxychlor and vinclozolin, respectively) that induce decreased spermatogenic capacity and increased infertility [71]. The effects of these drugs were transferred through the male germline to the fourth generation of offspring, with a penetrance inconsistent with genetic inheritance. Epigenetic differences were observed in affected F2 to F4 mice, suggesting that the phenotype may be attributable to nongenetic mechanisms. Thus, the potential for transgenerational inheritance has been demonstrated, suggesting that the epigenetic reprograming that occurs during germ cell development and after fertilization can potentially be circumvented by undefined mechanisms.

Summary

Epigenetic modification provides an important mechanism through which the totipotent resources of the genome are managed to create tissue-specific differences in gene expression and cellular function. In addition to its role in specifying tissue differentiation within an individual, studies in genetically identical animals indicate the potential for epigenetic modification to create interindividual phenotypic variation. A wide range of environmental changes (Table 18.1), including in vitro embryo culture, dietary methyl donor content or protein-carbohydrate balance, tissue ischemia, and possibly maternal behavior, have the capacity to modify an organism's epigenome. The extent to which such factors contribute to adult phenotypes and common diseases is an area of intense research activity. Furthermore, the extent to which acquired epigenetic modifications can be transmitted to future generations is of great interest for biomedicine. It is likely that future recommendations for maternal nutrition and postpartum behavior will be, in part, based on their epigenetic consequences.

References

1. Bird A, Perceptions of epigenetics. *Nature* (2007), **447**:396–8.

2. Bird A, DNA methylation patterns and epigenetic memory. *Genes Dev* (2002), **16**:6–21.

3. Bourc'his D and Bestor TH, Meiotic catastrophe and retrotransposon reactivation in male germ cells lacking Dnmt3L. *Nature* (2004), **431**:96–9.

4. Ehrlich M, DNA methylation in cancer: too much, but also too little. *Oncogene* (2002), 12; 21:5400–13.

5. Saxonov S, Berg P, and Brutlag DL, A genome-wide analysis of CpG dinucleotides in the human genome distinguishes two distinct classes of promoters. *Proc Natl Acad Sci U S A* (2006), **103**:1412–7.

6. Weber M, Hellmann I, Stadler MB, Ramos L, Paabo S, Rebhan M, et al., Distribution, silencing potential and evolutionary impact of promoter DNA methylation in the human genome. *Nat Genet* (2007), **39**:457–66.

7. Morison IM, Ramsay JP, and Spencer HG, A census of mammalian imprinting. *Trends Genet* (2005), **21**:457–65.

8. Razin A and Riggs AD, DNA methylation and gene function. *Science* (1980), **210**:604–10.

9. Hattori N, Nishino K, Ko YG, Hattori N, Ohgane J, and Tanaka S, et al., Epigenetic control of mouse Oct-4 gene expression in embryonic stem cells and trophoblast stem cells. *J Biol Chem* (2004), **279**:17063–9.

10. Deb-Rinker P, Ly D, Jezierski A, Sikorska M, and Walker PR, Sequential DNA methylation of the Nanog and Oct-4 upstream regions in human NT2 cells during neuronal differentiation. *J Biol Chem* (2005), **280**:6257–60.

11. Farthing CR, Ficz G, Ng RK, Chan C-F, Andrews S, Dean W, et al., Global mapping of DNA methylation in mouse promoters reveals epigenetic reprogramming of pluripotency genes. *PLoS Genet* (2008), 4:e1000116.

12. Bernstein BE, Meissner A, and Lander ES, The mammalian epigenome. *Cell* (2007), **128**:669–81.

13. Ptashne M, On the use of the word "epigenetic." *Curr Biol* (2007), **17**:R233–6.

14. Turner BM, Defining an epigenetic code. *Nat Cell Biol* (2007), **9**:2–6.

15. Stancheva I, Caught in conspiracy: cooperation between DNA methylation and histone H3K9 methylation in the establishment and maintenance of heterochromatin. *Biochem Cell Biol* (2005), **83**:385–95.

16. Morgan HD, Santos F, Green K, Dean W, and Reik W, Epigenetic reprogramming in mammals. *Hum Mol Genet* (2005), **14**(Spec No 1):R47–58.

17. Young LE and Beaujean N, DNA methylation in the preimplantation embryo: the differing stories of the mouse and sheep. *Anim Reprod Sci* (2004), **82–83**:61–78.

18. Sinclair KD, Allegrucci C, Singh R, Gardner DS, Sebastian S, Bispham J, et al., DNA methylation, insulin resistance, and blood pressure in offspring determined by maternal periconceptional B vitamin and methionine status. *Proc Natl Acad Sci U S A* (2007), **104**:19351–6.

19. Waterland RA and Michels KB, Epigenetic epidemiology of the developmental origins hypothesis. *Annu Rev Nutr* (2007), **27**:363–88.

20. Wolff GL, Kodell RL, Moore SR, and Cooney CA, Maternal epigenetics and methyl supplements affect agouti gene expression in Avy/a mice. *FASEB J* (1998), **12**:949–57.

21. Waterland RA and Jirtle RL, Transposable elements: targets for early nutritional effects on epigenetic gene regulation. *Mol Cell Biol* (2003), **23**:5293–300.

22. Morgan HD, Sutherland HG, Martin DI, and Whitelaw E, Epigenetic inheritance at the agouti locus in the mouse. *Nat Genet* (1999), **23**:314–18.

23. Takimoto H, Mito N, Umegaki K, Ishiwaki A, Kusama K, Abe S, et al., Relationship between dietary folate intakes, maternal plasma total homocysteine and B-vitamins during pregnancy and fetal growth in Japan. *Eur J Nutr* (2007), **46**:300–6.

24. Dolinoy DC, Weidman JR, Waterland RA, and Jirtle RL, Maternal genistein alters coat color and protects Avy mouse offspring from obesity by modifying the fetal epigenome. *Environ Health Perspect* (2006), **114**:567–72.

25. Rakyan VK, Chong S, Champ ME, Cuthbert PC, Morgan HD, Luu KV, et al., Transgenerational inheritance of epigenetic states at the murine Axin(Fu) allele occurs after maternal and paternal transmission. *Proc Natl Acad Sci U S A* (2003), **100**: 2538–43.

26. Waterland RA, Dolinoy DC, Lin JR, Smith CA, Shi X, and Tahiliani KG, Maternal methyl supplements increase offspring DNA methylation at Axin Fused. *Genesis* (2006), **44**:401–6.

27. Oates NA, van Vliet J, Duffy DL, Kroes HY, Martin NG, Boomsma DI, et al., Increased DNA methylation at the *AXIN1* gene in a monozygotic twin from a pair discordant for a caudal duplication anomaly. *Am J Hum Genet* (2006), **79**:155–62.

28. Dunlevy LP, Burren KA, Chitty LS, Copp AJ, and Greene ND, Excess methionine suppresses the methylation cycle and inhibits neural tube closure in mouse embryos. *FEBS Lett* (2006), **580**:2803–7.

29. Ernest S, Carter M, Shao H, Hosack A, Lerner N, Colmenares C, et al., Parallel changes in metabolite and expression profiles in crooked-tail mutant and folate-reduced wild-type mice. *Hum Mol Genet* (2006), **15**:3387–93.

30. Paoloni-Giacobino A, Epigenetics in reproductive medicine. *Pediatr Res* (2007), **61**(5 Pt 2):51R–7R.

31. Miles HL, Hofman PL, Peek J, Harris M, Wilson D, Robinson EM, et al., In vitro fertilization improves childhood growth and metabolism. *J Clin Endocrinol Metab* (2007), **92**:3441–5.

32. Reik W, Romer I, Barton SC, Surani MA, Howlett SK, and Klose J, Adult phenotype in the mouse can be affected by epigenetic events in the early embryo. *Development* (1993), **119**:933–42.

33. Rivera RM, Stein P, Weaver JR, Mager J, Schultz RM, Bartolomei MS, Manipulations of mouse embryos prior to implantation result in aberrant expression of imprinted genes on day 9.5 of development. *Hum Mol Genet* (2008), **17**:1–14.

34. Fauque P, Jouannet P, Lesaffre C, Ripoche MA, Dandolo L, Vaiman D, et al., Assisted reproductive technology affects developmental kinetics, H19 imprinting control region methylation and H19 gene expression in individual mouse embryos. *BMC Dev Biol* (2007), **7**:116.

35. Watkins AJ, Platt D, Papenbrock T, Wilkins A, Eckert JJ, Kwong WY, et al., Mouse embryo culture induces changes in postnatal phenotype including raised systolic blood pressure. *Proc Natl Acad Sci U S A* (2007), **104**:5449–54.

36. Khosla S, Dean W, Brown D, Reik W, Feil R, Culture of preimplantation mouse embryos affects fetal development and the expression of imprinted genes.

37. Doornbos ME, Maas SM, McDonnell J, Vermeiden JP, Hennekam RC, Infertility, assisted reproduction technologies and imprinting disturbances: a Dutch study. *Hum Reprod* (2007), **22**:2476–80.

38. Young LE, Fernandes K, McEvoy TG, Butterwith SC, Gutierrez CG, and Carolan C, et al., Epigenetic change in IGF2R is associated with fetal overgrowth after sheep embryo culture. *Nat Genet* (2001), **27**:153–4.

39. Young LE, Sinclair KD, and Wilmut I, Large offspring syndrome in cattle and sheep. *Rev Reprod* (1998), **3**:155–63.

40. Mikkelsen TS, Ku M, Jaffe DB, Issac B, Lieberman E, Giannoukos G, et al., Genome-wide maps of chromatin state in pluripotent and lineage-committed cells. *Nature* (2007), **448**:553–60.

41. Sakamoto H, Kogo Y, Ohgane J, Hattori N, Yagi S, Tanaka S, et al., Sequential changes in genome-wide DNA methylation status during adipocyte differentiation. *Biochem Biophys Res Commun* (2008), **366**:360–6.

42. Simmons RA, Role of metabolic programming in the pathogenesis of beta-cell failure in postnatal life. *Rev Endocr Metab Disord* (2007), **8**:95–104.

43. Simmons RA, Developmental origins of beta-cell failure in type 2 diabetes: the role of epigenetic mechanisms. *Pediatr Res* (2007), **61**(5 Pt 2):64R–7R.

44. Stirzaker C, Song JZ, Davidson B, and Clark SJ, Transcriptional gene silencing promotes DNA hypermethylation through a sequential change in chromatin modifications in cancer cells. *Cancer Res* (2004) **64**:3871–7.

45. Li B, Carey M, and Workman JL, The role of chromatin during transcription. *Cell* (2007), **128**:707–19.

Biol Reprod (2001), **64**:918–26.

46. Lillycrop KA, Phillips ES, Torrens C, Hanson MA, Jackson AA, Burdge GC, Feeding pregnant rats a protein-restricted diet persistently alters the methylation of specific cytosines in the hepatic PPARalpha promoter of the offspring. *Br J Nutr* (2008), **11**:1–5.

47. Yajnik CS, Deshpande SS, Jackson AA, Refsum H, Rao S, Fisher DJ, et al., Vitamin B and folate concentrations during pregnancy and insulin resistance in the offspring: the Pune Maternal Nutrition Study. *Diabetologia* (2008), **51**:29–38.

48. McMillen IC and Robinson JS, Developmental origins of the metabolic syndrome: prediction, plasticity, and programming. *Physiol Rev* (2005), **85**:571–633.

49. Bogdarina I, Welham S, King PJ, Burns SP, and Clark AJ, Epigenetic modification of the renin-angiotensin system in the fetal programming of hypertension. *Circ Res* (2007), **100**:520–6.

50. Welham SJ, Wade A, and Woolf AS, Protein restriction in pregnancy is associated with increased apoptosis of mesenchymal cells at the start of rat metanephrogenesis. *Kidney Int* (2002), **61**:1231–42.

51. Keller G, Zimmer G, Mall G, Ritz E, and Amann K, Nephron number in patients with primary hypertension. *N Engl J Med* (2003), **348**:101–8.

52. Welham SJ, Riley PR, Wade A, Hubank M, Woolf AS, Maternal diet programs embryonic kidney gene expression. *Physiol Genomics* (2005), **22**:48–56.

53. Weaver IC, Cervoni N, Champagne FA, D'Alessio AC, Sharma S, Seckl JR, et al., Epigenetic programming by maternal behavior. *Nat Neurosci* (2004), **7**:847–54.

54. Champagne FA, Weaver IC, Diorio J, Dymov S, Szyf M, Meaney MJ, Maternal care

associated with methylation of the estrogen receptor-alpha1b promoter and estrogen receptor-alpha expression in the medial preoptic area of female offspring. *Endocrinology* (2006), **147**:2909–15.

55. Ong KK, Ahmed ML, Emmett PM, Preece MA, Dunger DB, Association between postnatal catch-up growth and obesity in childhood: prospective cohort study. *BMJ* (2000), **320**:967–71.

56. Liu L, van Groen T, Kadish I, Tollefsbol TO, DNA methylation impacts on learning and memory in aging. *Neurobiol Aging* (2007), 10.

57. Seki Y, Hayashi K, Itoh K, Mizugaki M, Saitou M, and Matsui Y, Extensive and orderly reprogramming of genome-wide chromatin modifications associated with specification and early development of germ cells in mice. *Dev Biol* (2005), **278**:440–58.

58. Constância M, Hemberger M, Hughes J, Dean W, Ferguson-Smith A, Fundele R, et al., Placental-specific IGF-II is a major modulator of placental and fetal growth. *Nature* (2002), **417**:945–8.

59. Reik W, Constancia M, Fowden A, Anderson N, Dean W, Ferguson-Smith A, et al., Regulation of supply and demand for maternal nutrients in mammals by imprinted genes. *J Physiol* (2003), **547**(Pt 1):35–44.

60. Angiolini E, Fowden A, Coan P, Sandovici I, Smith P, Dean W, et al. Regulation of placental efficiency for nutrient transport by imprinted genes. *Placenta* (2006), **27**(Suppl A):S98–102.

61. Constancia M, Angiolini E, Sandovici I, Smith P, Smith R, Kelsey G, et al., Adaptation of nutrient supply to fetal demand in the mouse involves interaction between the *Igf2* gene and placental transporter systems. *Proc Natl Acad Sci U S A* (2005) **102**:19219–24.

62. Bertolini M, Moyer AL, Mason JB, Batchelder CA, Hoffert KA, Bertolini LR, et al., Evidence of increased substrate availability to in vitro-derived bovine foetuses and association with accelerated conceptus growth. *Reproduction* (2004), **128**:341–54.

63. Martinez Y and Martinez R, Clinical features in the Wiedemann-Beckwith syndrome. *Clin Genet* (1996), **50**:272–4.

64. Kaati G, Bygren LO, Pembrey M, and Sjöström M, Transgenerational response to nutrition, early life circumstances and longevity. *Eur J Hum Genet* (2007), **15**:784–90.

65. Skinner MK, What is an epigenetic transgenerational phenotype? F3 or F2. *Reprod Toxicol* (2008), **25**:2–6.

66. Lane N, Dean W, Erhardt S, Hajkova P, Surani A, Walter J, et al., Resistance of IAPs to methylation reprogramming may provide a mechanism for epigenetic inheritance in the mouse. *Genesis* (2003 Feb), **35**:88–93.

67. Stein AD and Lumey LH, The relationship between maternal and offspring birth weights after maternal prenatal famine exposure: the Dutch Famine Birth Cohort Study. *Hum Biol* (2000), **72**:641–54.

68. Roemer I, Reik W, Dean W, and Klose J, Epigenetic inheritance in the mouse. *Curr Biol* (1997), **7**:277–80.

69. Blewitt ME, Vickaryous NK, Paldi A, Koseki H, and Whitelaw E, Dynamic reprogramming of DNA methylation at an epigenetically sensitive allele in mice. *PLoS Genet* (2006), **2**:e49.

70. Cropley JE, Suter CM, Beckman KB, and Martin DI, Germ-line epigenetic modification of the murine A vy allele by nutritional supplementation. *Proc Natl Acad Sci U S A* (2006), **103**:17308–12.

71. Anway MD, Cupp AS, Uzumcu M, and Skinner MK, Epigenetic transgenerational actions of endocrine disruptors and male fertility. *Science* (2005), **308**:1466–9.

Index